Register
Access

MW00843611

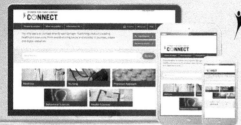

Titles in *The Physician Assistant Student's Guide to the Clinical Year* Series

Family Medicine

Gerald Kayingo
Deborah Opacic
Mary Carcella Allias

Internal Medicine

David Knechtel
Deborah Opacic

Emergency Medicine

Dipali Yeh
Erin Marthedal

Surgery

Brennan Bowker

OB-GYN

Elyse Watkins

Pediatrics

Tanya L. Fernandez
Amy Akerman

Behavioral Health

Jill Cavalet

THE PHYSICIAN ASSISTANT STUDENT'S GUIDE

to the Clinical Year

Gerald Kayingo, PhD, PA-C, is the director of the Master of Health Services, Physician Assistant Studies Program, and an associate clinical professor at the University of California (UC), Davis. Prior to his UC Davis appointment in 2014, he was a faculty member at the Yale School of Medicine Physician Associate Program and practiced at the Yale New Haven Hospital Primary Care Center in Connecticut. Dr. Kayingo has extensive experience in scholarship, education, clinical practice, and global health. He is a graduate of the Management Development Program at the Harvard Institutes for Higher Education, following a master of medical science–physician assistant degree at Yale University School of Medicine, and a PhD in microbiology from Orange Free State University in South Africa. He completed his postdoctoral education in infectious diseases at Yale, where he studied microbial pathogenesis, membrane transport, and signal transduction. He is a recent graduate of the UC Davis Interprofessional Teaching Scholars Program. Nationally, Dr. Kayingo serves as a trustee of the Physician Assistant Foundation, serves on the editorial board for the *Journal of BMC Health Services Research*, and is a member of the PAEA board of directors. He is a coeditor of the *Health Professions Educator: A Practical Guide for New and Established Faculty*. He was recently inducted into the prestigious Uganda National Academy of Sciences and has been widely published in several peer-reviewed journals.

Deborah Opacic, MMS, EdD, PA-C, DFAAP, received a bachelor of science–physician assistant degree at St. Francis University in Loretto, Pennsylvania, in 1982. She completed her graduate studies and received a master of medical science degree at St. Francis in 1994, and a doctoral degree in educational leadership from Duquesne University in 2001. Dr. Opacic has held clinical and academic appointments at the Western Psychiatric Institute and Clinic, the University of Pittsburgh, Duquesne University, and Allegheny General Hospital. Her clinical experience is in adult psychiatry; hematology/oncology; cardiothoracic surgery; heart, lung, and liver transplantation; and gastroenterology. During her 12-year tenure at Duquesne University, Dr. Opacic served as academic coordinator, clinical coordinator, and vice chair of the Department of Physician Assistant Studies. Dr. Opacic is the founding director of the physician assistant studies program at the University of Pittsburgh. She recently returned to clinical practice in the Division of Gastroenterology at the Allegheny Health Care Network. Dr. Opacic received both the Pennsylvania Society of Physician Assistants Award as PA Educator of the Year 2010 and the Pennsylvania Society of Physician Assistants Award as Humanitarian of the Year 2018 for her work as a primary care volunteer provider and grant writer for Sheep Inc. Free Health Care Center located in East Pittsburgh, Pennsylvania. She is a distinguished fellow of the American Academy of Physician Assistants (AAPA), member of the AAPA's Research and Strategic Initiatives Commission, and a fellow of the Society of Gastroenterology Physician Assistants and the Pennsylvania Society of Physician Assistants.

Mary Carcella Allias, MPAS, PA-C, is the director of Didactic Education and an assistant professor in the Physician Assistant Studies Program at the University of Pittsburgh. Her instructional themes include health policy, clinical reasoning, therapeutic communication, and medical care across the life span. She is a graduate of Saint Francis University, earning bachelor of science and master of physician assistant science degrees there. She is currently a doctoral student in the School of Education at the University of Pittsburgh. Ms. Allias has received awards for distinguished teaching and for her use of standardized patients in the curriculum, and has also been awarded a University of Pittsburgh Office of Diversity and Inclusion grant. She has practiced clinically in Emergency Medicine and currently practices in Family Medicine. She has presented her work at state and national forums. Her memberships in professional organizations have been highlighted by committee service and leadership roles including serving as a committee chairperson, proposal reviewer, and coordinator of scholarly poster presentations.

Maureen Knechtel, MPAS, PA-C (Series Editor), received a bachelor's degree in health science and a master's degree in physician assistant (PA) studies from Duquesne University in Pittsburgh, Pennsylvania. She is the author of the textbook *EKGs for the Nurse Practitioner and Physician Assistant*, first and second editions. Ms. Knechtel is a fellow member of the Physician Assistant Education Association, the American Academy of Physician Assistants, and the Tennessee Academy of Physician Assistants. She is the academic coordinator and an assistant professor with the Milligan College Physician Assistant Program in Johnson City, Tennessee, and practices as a cardiology PA with the Ballad Health Cardiovascular Associates Heart Institute. Ms. Knechtel has been a guest lecturer nationally and locally on topics including EKG interpretation, chronic angina, ischemic and hemorrhagic stroke, hypertension, and mixed hyperlipidemia.

THE PHYSICIAN ASSISTANT STUDENT'S GUIDE

to the Clinical Year

Gerald Kayingo, PhD, PA-C
Deborah Opacic, MMS, EdD, PA-C, DFAAP
Mary Carcella Allias, MPAS, PA-C

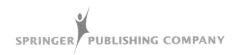

SPRINGER PUBLISHING COMPANY

Copyright © 2020 Springer Publishing Company, LLC

Springer Publishing Company, LLC
11 West 42nd Street
New York, NY 10036
www.springerpub.com
http://connect.springerpub.com/home

Acquisitions Editor: Suzanne Toppy
Compositor: diacriTech

ISBN: 978-0-8261-9522-7
ebook ISBN: 978-0-8261-9532-6
DOI: 10.1891/9780826195326

19 20 21 22 / 5 4 3 2 1

The author and the publisher of this Work have made every effort to use sources believed to be reliable to provide information that is accurate and compatible with the standards generally accepted at the time of publication. Because medical science is continually advancing, our knowledge base continues to expand. Therefore, as new information becomes available, changes in procedures become necessary. We recommend that the reader always consult current research and specific institutional policies before performing any clinical procedure or delivering any medication. The author and publisher shall not be liable for any special, consequential, or exemplary damages resulting, in whole or in part, from the readers' use of, or reliance on, the information contained in this book. The publisher has no responsibility for the persistence or accuracy of URLs for external or third-party Internet websites referred to in this publication and does not guarantee that any content on such websites is, or will remain, accurate or appropriate.

CIP data is on file at the Library of Congress.
Library of Congress Control Number: 2019910966

Contact us to receive discount rates on bulk purchases.
We can also customize our books to meet your needs.
For more information please contact: sales@springerpub.com

Publisher's Note: New and used products purchased from third-party sellers are not guaranteed for quality, authenticity, or access to any included digital components.

Printed in the United States of America.

To Jane, Geri, Grace, and Ethan. Your love is the kerosene that keeps the candle burning day and night.

—GERALD KAYINGO

For my family, especially Ethan and Abigail, who always encourage me to dare greatly.

—MARY CARCELLA ALLIAS

CONTENTS

Contributors

David C. Beck, MPAS, PA-C, DFAAPA   Program Director, Assistant Professor, Physician Assistant Studies Program, University of Pittsburgh, Pittsburgh, Pennsylvania

Felix D. Emond, Jr., MS, PA-C, DFAAPA   Assistant Clinical Professor, PA Program, University of California–Davis

Rosa Fannie, MPA, PA-C   Assistant Professor, Clinical Coordinator, School of Health and Rehabilitation Sciences, Physician Assistant Studies Program, University of Pittsburgh, Pittsburgh, Pennsylvania

Jennifer Feirstein, MSPAS, PA-C, DFAAPA   Academic Coordinator and Assistant Clinical Professor, Physician Assistant Studies Program, Northern Arizona University, Flagstaff, Arizona

Jamie Hammond, MS, MPAS, PA-C   Assistant Professor, Physician Assistant Studies Program, University of Pittsburgh, Pittsburgh, Pennsylvania

Jason W. Hare, MPAS, PA-C   Assistant Professor, Physician Assistant Studies Program, University of Pittsburgh, Pittsburgh, Pennsylvania

Christopher Holland, MPAS, PA-C   Adjunct Assistant Professor, Physician Assistant Studies Program, University of Pittsburgh, Pittsburgh, Pennsylvania

Lucy Kibe, DrPH, PA-C   Chief Quality Officer, Community Access Clinic, Lynchburg, Virginia

Vasco Deon Kidd, DHSc, MPH, MS, PA-C   Orthopaedic Surgery PA Fellowship Director/Chief Administrative PA, Assistant Professor in the Doctor of Medical Science Program at Lynchburg College, Arrowhead Regional Medical Center, Lynchburg, Virginia

Brent Luu, PharmD   Assistant Clinical Professor, UC Davis, Sacramento, California

Stephen Noe, DMS, MPAS, PA-C   Assistant Professor and Director of Didactic Education, Lincoln Memorial University, DeBusk College of Osteopathic Medicine PA Program, Harrogate, Tennessee

Peer Reviewers

Jennifer Feirstein, MSPAS, PA-C, DFAAPA   Academic Coordinator and Assistant Clinical Professor, Physician Assistant Studies Program, Northern Arizona University, Flagstaff, Arizona. *Jennifer Feirstein is an item writer for the PAEA PACKRAT Exam Development Board and did not write or review any practice questions for this book.*

Leslie Milteer, MPAS, PA-C, DFAAPA   Assistant Professor, Saint Catherine University, MPAS Program, St. Paul, Minnesota

Elyse Watkins, DHSc, PA-C, DFAAPA   Associate Professor, University of Lynchburg School of PA Medicine, Lynchburg, Virginia; Lecturer, Florida State University, School of Physician Assistant Practice, Tallahassee, Florida

Foreword

The alignment between the specialty of family medicine and the physician assistant (PA) profession is hard to ignore. Founded in 1969, the family medicine specialty sought to fix the decline of general medicine while providing outstanding care to people from all socioeconomic backgrounds throughout the United States. Family medicine has since grown to represent over 131,400 physicians while continuing to focus on its historical roots.[1] Dr. G. Gayle Stephens, the founding father of the family medicine specialty, wrote that "medicine is always the child of its time and cannot escape being influenced and shaped by contemporary ideas and social trends."[2] The PA profession, created over 50 years ago, was also a child of its time. Founded in the 1960s, the PA profession initially sought to impact the rural communities of North Carolina, and general medicine was at the core of its roots.[3] Although the PA profession has evolved, family medicine is still the largest specialty choice for graduates today.[4]

The Physician Assistant Student's Guide to the Clinical Year: Family Medicine by Kayingo, Opacic, and Allias is a critical step to increasing the competence and comfort of students who are engaging in a family medicine experience during their PA education. This book includes the holistic aspects of patient care that are indelibly marked in the family medicine specialty, including common presentations, diseases, diagnostics, management, procedures, and patient education and counseling, which is a hallmark of the specialty. Additional case studies and review questions are available through the e-Chapters. The guide should provide every student seeking additional insights into family medicine key learning objectives needed for success. The authors have a combined 50+ years of experience in primary care and PA education that contribute to a rich guide to this important chapter in PA education.

In closing, the heart of family medicine includes a commitment to social justice and focus on three important components of health: (a) primary prevention; (b) a holistic approach to patients; and (c) a commitment to caring for all patients, regardless of socioeconomic background. The tools in this book will provide a strong foundation in learning the core principles in family medicine.

KEVIN LOHENRY, PHD, PA-C

References

1. American Academy of Family Physicians. Family medicine specialty. https://www.aafp.org/about/the-aafp/family-medicine-specialty.html
2. Stephens G. *The Intellectual Basis of Family Practice*. Greensburg, IN: Winter Publishing Company; 1982.
3. Cawley JF. Physician assistant education: an abbreviated history. *J Physician Assist Educ*. 2007;18(3):6–15.
4. American Academy of Physician Assistants. 2018 AAPA salary report. https://www.aapa.org/download/36360

Preface

For a physician assistant student, the clinical year marks a time of great excitement and anticipation. It is a time to hone the skills you have learned in your didactic training and work toward becoming a competent and confident healthcare provider. After many intense semesters in the classroom, you will have the privilege of participating in the practice of medicine. Each rotation will reinforce, refine, and enhance your knowledge and skills through exposure and repetition. When you look back on this time, you will likely relish the opportunities, experiences, and people involved along the way. You may find an affinity for a medical specialty you did not realize you enjoyed. You will meet lifelong professional mentors and friends. You may even be hired for your first job.

While excitement is the overlying theme, some amount of uncertainty is bound to be present as you progress from rotation to rotation, moving through the various medical specialties. You have gained a vast knowledge base during your didactic training, but may be unsure of how to utilize it in a fast-paced clinical environment. As a clinical year physician assistant student, you are not expected to know everything, but you are expected to seek out resources that can complement what you will learn through hands-on experience. Through an organized and predictable approach, this book series should serve as a guide and companion to help you feel prepared for what you will encounter during the clinical year.

Each book was written by physician assistant educators, clinicians, and preceptors who are experts in their respective fields. Their knowledge from years of experience is laid out in the pages before you. Each book will answer questions such as "What does my preceptor want me to know?" "What should I be familiar with prior to this rotation?" "What can I expect to encounter during this rotation?" This is followed by a guided approach to the clinical decision-making process for common presenting complaints, detailed explanations of common disease entities, and specialty-specific patient education.

Chapters are organized in a way that will allow you to quickly access vital information that can help you recognize, diagnose, and treat commonly seen conditions. You can easily review suggested labs and diagnostic imaging for a suspected diagnosis, find a step-by-step guide to frequently performed procedures, and review urgent management of conditions specific to each rotation. Electronic resources are available for each book. These include case studies with explanations to evaluate your clinical reasoning process, and review questions to assist in self-evaluation and preparation for your end of rotation examinations as well as the Physician Assistant National Certifying Exam.

As a future physician assistant, you have already committed to being a lifelong learner of medicine. It is my hope that this book series will outline expectations, enhance your medical knowledge base, and provide you with the confidence you need to be successful in your clinical year.

MAUREEN KNECHTEL, **MPAS, PA-C**
Series Editor
The Physician Assistant Student's Guide to the Clinical Year

Introduction

The Approach to the Patient in Family Medicine

WHAT TO EXPECT

Every clinical rotation has a defined set of guidelines that must be met. It is critical that each student observe these instructions in order to have a successful learning experience. The variability between clinical sites is why flexibility as a physician assistant (PA) student is vital to your success.

In family medicine, you will encounter a broad range of patients, both in age and complexity. This rotation will therefore provide you with excellent exposure to an abundance of learning opportunities, as long as you take advantage of the experience. As a graduate, you must be prepared to provide medical care to patients of diverse populations, deliver medical care across the life span, and practice medicine as an integral member of the healthcare team. You will be expected to deliver high-quality healthcare and serve as a leader in clinical, academic, and research environments. The experience you have during the clinical rotation is what you make of it.

How to succeed in the clinical clerkship:

- Always be on time
- Be professional in both dress and demeanor
- Respect chain of command
- Address patients and staff with respect
- Take responsibility for your actions and for your learning
- Respect each patient's privacy and rights
- Be a team player
- Volunteer to help when needed
- Present and document patient information in an organized manner
- Sign, date, and time everything you are asked to document
- Be honest
- Remember that you can learn valuable lessons from everyone that you may encounter while at the clinical site

As you progress through the family medicine supervised clinical experience, you should actively seek feedback from your preceptor. In seeking this feedback, it is important to avoid generic questions such as "How am I doing?" But rather, try asking for specific suggestions for improvement such as "How can I improve upon my patient management plans?" This approach will demonstrate your ability to self-evaluate areas upon which you may need improvement and encourage preceptors to provide constructive feedback rather than nonspecific reassurance.

What Your Preceptor Wants You to Know

Tasks you will be expected to perform will include the following:

- History taking and performing complete and problem-focused physical examinations
- Clinical decision-making and reasoning
- Case integration
- Developing an appropriate therapeutic management plan
- Documentation of the patient encounter that is thorough yet succinct
- Procedures commonly performed in the primary care setting
- Provision of patient education and counseling focused on routine preventive health-care and following a healthy lifestyle
- Becoming familiar with screening tools and scoring systems specific to commonly encountered conditions in primary care. A selection of resources can be found in Appendix A of this book.

What Previous PA Students Wished They Knew Before This Rotation

- The scope of practice of the family medicine provider is broad. Not everything requires a referral to a specialist.
- You will encounter a broad range of patients, and will need to have good knowledge of specialties such as women's health and behavioral medicine.
- The pace of the day is quick; family medicine PAs often see patients every 15 minutes. This pace is in part why you should commit common entities to memory, such as preventive guidelines, immunization schedules, and treatment goals. You will not have time to look everything up.
- You can learn a lot about patients and their medical conditions by spending a little extra time talking to them, as opposed to focusing only on objective materials.

USE OF INTERPROFESSIONAL CONSULTATIONS

Physical Therapist
- Help people of all ages and stages of life overcome movement, function, and mobility challenges.
- Evaluate gait and need for ambulation assistance, prescribe exercises to improve strength and function in musculoskeletal disorders.

Occupational Therapist
- Develop and implement treatment plans to help individuals to function in self-care, home management, school, work, and play/leisure to establish a lifestyle that is optimally independent, productive, and satisfying to the individual.

Nutritionist
- Instruct patients on the appropriate diet for their underlying medical condition.
- Advise on nutrition recommended for cardiovascular disease, diabetes, chronic liver disease, chronic pulmonary disease, renal insufficiency, and genetic metabolic disorders.

Social Worker
- Help people solve and cope with problems in their everyday lives.
- Clinical social workers also diagnose and treat mental, behavioral, and emotional issues.

Pharmacist
- Aid patients with understanding of their medications and associated side effects.
- Dispense prescription medications to patients and offer expertise in their safe use.
- Conduct health and wellness screenings, provide immunizations, and provide advice on healthy lifestyles.

Respiratory Therapist
- Interview and examine patients with breathing or cardiopulmonary disorders.
- Work with physicians to develop treatment plans.
- Perform diagnostic tests (such as measuring lung capacity).
- Treat patients by using a variety of methods, including chest physiotherapy and aerosol medications.
- Teach patients how to take medications and use equipment, such as ventilators.
- Evaluate the need for ambulatory and home oxygen use.

Speech Language Pathologist
- Evaluate swallowing, aspiration risk.

Confidentiality Practices and Ethics

The American Academy of PA's *Guidelines for Ethical Conduct for the PA Profession* (established 2000, revised 2018) identify and detail the values of the PA profession. They are established under the premise that every patient encounter is unique. As a PA, it is expected you use your best judgment in any given situation, respecting patient preference, context of clinical situation, ethical concepts, and legal obligations. The practicing PA should abide by the four ethical principles of:

- Autonomy: Patient's right to make own decisions
- Beneficence: Patient's best interests
- Maleficence: Do no harm
- Justice: Fair distribution of resources, risks, and costs

Sample Documentation

History and Physical Exam

- **Chief complaint:** "In patient's own words"
- **History of Present Illness**: Chronological order of time; place of symptom onset, duration, frequency location, quality/quantity/severity, aggravating/alleviating factors, associated symptoms, treatments. Pertinent negatives, contributing habits, behaviors (alcohol use, diet, smoking, recreational drugs, exercise), clinical conditions, relevant labs, testing, and so on.

Past Medical History

- General health
- Date, time, duration, outcome, complications of childhood and adult illnesses, accidents, injuries, hospitalizations
- Immunizations
- Screening tests

Past Surgical History

- Date, type, reason, outcome, blood transfusions, complications

Family History

- Age/health/death of: Parents, siblings, children, grandparents
- Elicit a pertinent family history of:
  - Diabetes
  - Atherosclerosis, heart disease, stroke
  - Hyperlipidemia
  - Hypertension
  - Cancer
  - Bleeding disorders
  - Asthma

- Arthritis
- Mental illness
- Symptoms similar to present illness

Social History
- Birthplace, education, employment, relationship status, living situation, diet, exercise, hobbies

Medications
- Name, indication, route, dose, frequency, side effects

Allergies
- Environmental, foods, medications

Tobacco, Alcohol, Drugs
- Type, duration, frequency of use, treatment

Review of Systems
- **General:** Weight change, fatigue, weakness, fever, chills, night sweats
- **Skin:** Skin, hair, nail changes, pruritis, rashes, sores, lumps, moles
- **Head:** Trauma, headache, nausea, vomiting, visual changes
- **Eyes:** Glasses, contact lenses, blurring, tearing, itching, acute vision loss, field cuts
- **Ears:** Hearing loss, vertigo, tinnitus, discharge, earache
- **Nose/Sinuses:** Rhinorrhea, stuffiness, sneezing, allergies, epistaxis
- **Mouth/Throat/Neck:** Bleeding gums, ulcers, sore/swollen tongue, hoarseness, sore throat, tonsillar exudate, neck swelling
- **Breasts:** Skin changes, lumps, masses, tenderness, discharge, self-exams, mammograms
- **Cardiac:** Hypertension, murmurs, chest pain, palpitations, exertional dyspnea, orthopnea, paroxysmal nocturnal dyspnea, edema, most recent EKG
- **Respiratory:** Shortness of breath, wheezing, cough, sputum production, hemoptysis, pneumonia, bronchitis, asthma, emphysema, tuberculosis, most recent chest x-ray
- **GI:** Appetite, nausea, vomiting, indigestion, dysphagia, bowel movements (change, frequency, form, mucus, color, waking up at night), bleeding (hematemesis, melena, hematochezia), abdominal pain, jaundice, hepatitis
- **Urinary:** Frequency, burning, urgency, nocturia, polyuria, hematuria, incontinence, stones, flank pain, discharge, infections
- **Genital:**
  - **Male:** Discharge, sores, testicular pain, masses, hernias
  - **Female:** Menarche, regularity, frequency, duration, dysmenorrhea, last menstrual period, itching, discharge, sores, pregnancies (complications), abortions, contraception, menopause, sexually transmitted infections
- **Vascular:** Leg edema, varicose veins, claudication, clots
- **Musculoskeletal:** Muscle wasting, joint stiffness, pain, range of motion, instability, redness, swelling, arthritis, gout

- **Neurologic:** Loss of sensation, numbness, tingling, tremors, weakness, paralysis, fainting, blackouts, seizures
- **Hematologic:** Anemia, easy bruising, bleeding, petechiae, purpura, transfusions, enlarged or tender lymph nodes
- **Endocrine:** Heat/cold intolerance, excessive sweating, polyuria, polydipsia, polyphagia, thyroid disorders, diabetes mellitus, weight control
- **Psychiatric:** Mood changes, anxiety, depression, stress, memory

Physical Examination

- **General:** Sex, race, state of health, stature, development, dress, hygiene, affect
- **Vitals:** Blood pressure, pulse, respirations, weight, height, temperature, oxygen saturation
- **Skin:** Scars, rashes, bruises, tattoos, hair texture, nail pitting, stippling, jaundice
- **Eyes:** Pupil size, shape reactivity, conjunctival injection, scleral icterus, papilledema, hemorrhage, lids, extraocular movements, visual fields, visual acuity
- **Ears:** Shape, symmetry, tenderness, discharge, external canal, tympanic membrane appearance, auditory acuity
- **Nose:** Symmetry, tenderness, discharge, mucosal or nasal turbinate inflammation, sinus tenderness
- **Mouth and Throat:** Hygiene, dentures, erythema, exudate, enlarged tonsils
- **Neck:** Masses, range of motion, C-spine, tracheal deviation, thyroid size and/or masses, carotid bruits
- **Breasts:** Skin changes, symmetry, tenderness, masses, dimpling, discharge
- **Heart:** Rate, rhythm, murmurs, rubs, gallops, clicks, precordial movements
- **Lungs:** Symmetry with respiration, wheezes, crackles, vocal fremitus, whispered pectoriloquy, percussion, diaphragmatic excursion
- **Abdomen:** Contour, scars, bowel sounds, consistency (soft, firm), tenderness, rebound, guarding, spleen size, liver span, masses, percussion (tympanic, shifting dullness) costovertebral angle tenderness
- **Genitourinary:**
  - ○ **Male:** Rashes, ulcers, scars, nodules, induration, discharge, scrotal masses, hernias
  - ○ **Female:** External genitalia, vaginal mucosa and cervix (inflammation, discharge), ulcers, nodules, masses, internal vaginal support, bimanual and rectovaginal palpation of cervix, uterus, and ovaries
- **Rectal:** Sphincter tone, prostate consistency, masses, tenderness, hemorrhoids, fissures, abscess
- **Musculoskeletal:** Muscle atrophy, weakness, joint range of motion (flexion, extension, lateral bending), instability, redness, swelling, tenderness, warmth, spinal tenderness, gait
- **Vascular:** Carotid, radial, aorta, femoral, popliteal, anterior tibia, dorsalis pedis pulses, bruits, jugular venous distention, edema, varicosities
- **Lymphatics:** Cervical, supraclavicular, axillary, epitrochlear, inguinal nodes, adenopathy
- **Neurologic:** Cranial nerves, sensation, strength, reflexes, gait, cerebellar function

SOAP NOTE

Purpose

1. To improve communication among all those caring for the patient
2. To display the assessment, problems, and plans in an organized format to facilitate the care of the patient
3. To assist in record review and quality control

Subjective Data

This section of the SOAP note presents the problem from the patient's point of view. It may include the chief complaint, history of present illness, pertinent medical history, surgical history, and family histories relevant to chief complaint, current medications, diet, appetite, limitations, immunizations, and allergies.

Objective Data

This is a record of the specific objective and reproducible findings gathered by:

1. Observation of the patient
2. Physical examination
3. Laboratory studies
4. Diagnostic imaging
5. Procedures
6. Pathology

Assessment

This is a short tentative working diagnosis for each problem.

Plan

This describes your plans for the care and management of each problem. It may include one or all of the following:

1. A plan for collecting further information, such as laboratory tests or imaging
2. A plan for initial treatment with specific procedures or medications
3. Pertinent patient education discussed during the visit
4. Referral and/or consultations
5. Follow-up plan and timeline

ELECTRONIC RESOURCES

Competencies for the Physician Assistant Profession:

> https://www.aapa.org/wp-content/uploads/2017/02/PA-Competencies-updated.pdf

Guidelines for Ethical Conduct for the PA Profession

> https://www.aapa.org/wp-content/uploads/2017/02/16-EthicalConduct.pdf

1

Common Presentations in Family Medicine

Introduction

In family medicine, you will encounter a variety of clinical presentations in patients across their lifespans. It is important to develop an appropriate system for evaluating their symptoms and to determine an accurate diagnosis and proper management plan. Using patient-centered interviewing techniques, start with a chief complaint, elicit a history, and perform an appropriately focused physical examination. This information should enable you to choose the most appropriate diagnostic studies to confirm and/or rule out differential diagnoses.

When presented with a general chief complaint, there are several steps to follow in order to derive the most likely diagnosis:

1. Identify the chief complaint and pertinent past medical history
   - OPQRST (Onset, Provoking/Alleviating factors, Quality, Radiation, Severity, Timing)
   - Pertinent past medical history, surgical history, social history, family history, medication and allergy list, and a review of systems (ROS)
2. Create a problem list
   - Rank problems and identify if and how they relate to the chief complaint, and separate those problems that do not relate to the chief complaint
3. Summarize pertinent positive and negative findings, both subjective and objective
   - Performing a thorough history should help guide a focused physical examination. Putting together the findings from these two steps should help solidify the most plausible differential diagnoses

4. Formulate and prioritize appropriate differential diagnoses
   - It is helpful to list the differential diagnoses in descending order of most likely diagnosis. If this step is performed correctly, it should guide the initial management plan. Be sure to include "danger differentials," or those that carry a higher mortality risk

5. Initiate a management plan to include diagnostic evaluation and initial treatment, if indicated
   - Order diagnostic tests and laboratory studies appropriate for the differential diagnosis. Each test that is ordered should help rule in or rule out items from your differential diagnosis list
   - Initiate a care plan based on the most likely diagnosis
   - Consider referrals to other medical specialties and include other members of the interprofessional healthcare team when appropriate
   - Provide the patient with clear follow-up instructions, including indications that her or his condition may be worsening and how and when to pursue more urgent follow-up

Some of the most common general presentations you can expect to encounter in family medicine include abdominal pain, low back pain (LBP), headache, sore throat, and fatigue.

ABDOMINAL PAIN

Abdominal pain is frequently encountered in the family medicine clinic and is identified as the principal reason for seeking medical care in approximately 1.5% of all ambulatory care visits.[1-3] Abdominal pain can also be an associated symptom coexisting with many different medical conditions. The clinical evaluation of abdominal pain can be difficult due to the expansive list of plausible differential diagnoses, and due to the fact that abdominal pain can often represent referred pain from a disease state occurring in a completely separate organ system. Symptoms, occurring alone or in combination, that help support a gastrointestinal (GI) cause for abdominal pain include anorexia, jaundice, nausea, vomiting, dysphagia, odynophagia, indigestion, early satiety, constipation, diarrhea, hematochezia, hematemesis, melena, an abdominal mass, and abdominal distention.

> **CLINICAL PEARL:** Remember that many of these symptoms may also be associated with disorders NOT related to the GI tract.

The etiology of abdominal pain can range from a benign, self-limited condition requiring nothing more than reassurance and patient education, to an acute, life-threatening condition requiring emergent management in the hospital setting. Therefore, an essential component of the initial evaluation should be to determine whether the underlying cause for abdominal pain is a condition that will require hospitalization or surgical intervention. This evaluation may require close collaboration between medicine, surgery, and radiology teams.

Differential Diagnosis

Perhaps the most useful approach in developing a differential diagnosis for abdominal pain is to consider the primary location of the pain, as seen in Table 1.1. Pain located in the right upper quadrant (RUQ), left upper quadrant (LUQ), right lower quadrant (RLQ), left lower quadrant (LLQ), or pain that is epigastric or suprapubic in location can be correlated with the relevant anatomy in order to guide you to the most likely pathology. Additionally, there are some causes less likely to be associated with localized pain, but rather a more generalized pattern of pain.

> **CLINICAL PEARL:** Emergent or life-threatening causes for abdominal pain should always be included in the differential diagnosis to ensure they are not overlooked. Some of these diagnoses include bowel obstruction, GI perforation, acute cholangitis, mesenteric ischemia, myocardial infarction (MI), ruptured aortic aneurysm, and ectopic pregnancy.

TABLE 1.1 Differential Diagnosis of Abdominal Pain Based Upon Location of Pain

Right Upper Quadrant	Left Upper Quadrant
Biliary disease	Gastritis
Cholelithiasis	Gastric ulcer
Cholecystitis	Splenic injury
Cholangitis (acute, chronic, sclerosing)	Pancreatitis
Choledocholithiasis	Pneumonia (left lower lobe)
Biliary dyskinesia	
Other causes of biliary obstruction	
Hepatitis	
Pancreatitis	
Pneumonia (right lower lobe)	
Pleurisy	

Right Lower Quadrant	Left Lower Quadrant
Appendicitis	Diverticulitis
Ectopic pregnancy	Ectopic pregnancy
Pelvic inflammatory disease	Pelvic inflammatory disease
Inflammatory bowel disease	Inflammatory bowel disease
Mesenteric lymphadenitis	Irritable bowel syndrome
Nephrolithiasis	Nephrolithiasis
Inguinal hernia	Inguinal hernia
Testicular torsion	Testicular torsion
Ovarian torsion	Ovarian torsion

(continued)

TABLE 1.1 Differential Diagnosis of Abdominal Pain Based Upon Location of Pain (*continued*)

Epigastric	Suprapubic
Peptic ulcer disease	Urinary tract infection
Gastritis	Urinary retention
Gastroesophageal reflux disease	Pelvic mass
Esophagitis	
Hiatal hernia	
Functional dyspepsia	
Pancreatitis	
Myocardial infarction	
Pericarditis	
Aortic aneurysm (ruptured)	

Periumbilical	Generalized (Diffuse)
Appendicitis (upon initial presentation)	Gastroenteritis
Gastroenteritis	Bowel obstruction
Bowel obstruction	Irritable bowel syndrome
Aortic aneurysm (ruptured)	Peritonitis
	Volvulus
	Mesenteric ischemia
	Aortic aneurysm (ruptured)
	Ectopic pregnancy (ruptured)
	Diabetic ketoacidosis
	Metabolic disease
	Psychiatric disease

History

- Onset, duration, and timing: Determine whether the onset of pain was acute or gradual. Acute onset pain raises the consideration of a surgical emergency and is often associated with aortic aneurysm rupture, aortic dissection, GI perforation, ovarian or testicular torsion, and volvulus. An insidious onset of pain is more likely to occur with an infectious or inflammatory process, such as gastroenteritis or appendicitis. The duration and timing of pain also provide helpful information. Pain related to gallbladder disease is more likely to last several hours and often progresses from colicky to more constant. Irritable bowel syndrome (IBS) is unlikely to be associated with nighttime symptoms, whereas inflammatory bowel disease (IBD) can cause nighttime symptoms waking patients from sleep.
- Provoking/alleviating factors: Several factors can provoke or alleviate pain, such as food, alcohol consumption, tobacco use, body position and movement, and bowel movements.
  - Eating/Food: Cholelithiasis is often associated with worsening pain after eating a fatty meal. Peptic ulcer disease (PUD) can be aggravated *or* alleviated by eating; gastric ulcers are aggravated by eating, while duodenal ulcers are typically associated with improvement in pain after eating. Pain associated with gastroesophageal reflux disease (GERD) often worsens after eating; common dietary triggers include caffeine, spicy or acidic food, carbonated drinks, and peppermint. Patients with

IBS, IBD, functional dyspepsia, or metabolic disease may have many food triggers that aggravate abdominal pain.

○ Alcohol/tobacco: GERD and pancreatitis are aggravated by use of alcohol, while tobacco use can aggravate GERD.

○ Body position/movement: GERD symptoms are aggravated by lying supine and the pain of pancreatitis and pericarditis can be alleviated by leaning forward. Any movement can provoke the pain of peritonitis and pelvic inflammatory disease (PID), including walking, coughing, or riding in a car.

○ Bowel movements: The pain of diverticulitis or IBD is often worsened when the patient has a bowel movement, whereas pain associated with IBS is often alleviated after bowel movements.

● Quality: The patient's description of their abdominal pain can be useful as some conditions are associated with a characteristic type of pain (see Table 1.2). Frequent descriptors of abdominal pain include sharp, stabbing, burning, gnawing, boring or piercing, dull, aching, and cramping. Abdominal pain can also be colicky in nature, meaning the pain is a severe, cramping sensation that is intermittent but starts and stops rather abruptly. Colicky abdominal pain is often associated with obstruction, such as in bowel or biliary obstruction, or with nephrolithiasis.

● Radiation/Location: As is demonstrated in the differential diagnosis section earlier, the location of pain is extremely helpful for formulating differential diagnoses. Radiation of pain can also be useful in the clinical evaluation.

● Severity: Pain that is severe, wakes a patient from sleep, or becomes progressively worse should raise the suspicion of a more serious cause. Causes can include vascular emergencies or perforated intra-abdominal organs.

TABLE 1.2 Abdominal Pain Characteristics and Associated Conditions

Condition	Pain Characteristics (Quality/Radiation)
GERD	Burning
Biliary disease	Colicky or dull Radiates to right subscapular area
Irritable bowel syndrome	Crampy
Pancreatitis	Piercing Radiates to the back
Appendicitis	Pain initially periumbilical with radiation to RLQ prior to localizing in the RLQ
Intestinal obstruction	Cramping or colicky
Peptic ulcer disease	Gnawing
Splenic injury	Radiates to left shoulder
Aortic aneurysm (ruptured)	Sharp, stabbing, or tearing Radiates to sacrum, flank, or genitalia
Nephrolithiasis	Sharp, stabbing, and/or colicky Radiates to genitalia

GERD, gastroesophageal reflux disease; RLQ, right lower quadrant.

- Associated symptoms: In addition to completing a full inquiry on all GI symptoms, ROS should also include cardiovascular, pulmonary, and genitourinary assessments, at a minimum, to ensure extra-abdominal causes do not go unnoticed.

Past Medical History Specific to Complaint

- Medical illnesses/comorbidities: Ask about a past history of GI conditions that may predispose to acute or chronic abdominal pain (e.g., cholelithiasis, diverticulosis, IBS, IBD). Additionally, ask about medical diagnoses that have acute complications known to be associated with abdominal pain. For example, diabetic ketoacidosis (diabetes mellitus type 1 or 2), sickle cell crisis (sickle cell anemia), and acute adrenal insufficiency (Addison's disease) can present with abdominal pain. Hypertriglyceridemia and cholelithiasis have been associated with the development of acute pancreatitis. Immunodeficiency may predispose a patient to esophagitis. Medical history of atherosclerotic cardiovascular disease (ASCVD) should also be obtained to assess for risk of MI, aortic aneurysm rupture, or mesenteric ischemia. Atrial fibrillation can cause mesenteric ischemia from an acute thrombosis.
- Medications: A list of all prescribed and over-the-counter (OTC) medications should be obtained. Commonly used medications, such as nonsteroidal anti-inflammatory drugs (NSAIDS) and aspirin, can disrupt the gastric lining and predispose a patient to gastritis or PUD. Opioid analgesics can predispose to constipation. Acetaminophen in excess can cause hepatotoxicity. Some antidiabetic agents (e.g., dipeptidyl peptidase-4 [DPP-4] inhibitors and glucagon-like peptide-1 [GLP-1] receptor agonists) as well as thiazide diuretics have been associated with pancreatitis. Chronic corticosteroid use, especially inhaled corticosteroids, or recent antibiotic use can be associated with esophagitis. Patients may have attempted treatment on their own with antacids or OTC proton-pump inhibitors; improvement in symptoms with use of these medications may be correlated with PUD and/or GERD.
- Surgical history: Prior abdominal surgeries may be associated with adhesions, which can cause abdominal pain and intestinal obstruction.
- Social history: Ask about frequency and amount of alcohol consumption. Alcohol use disorder is a risk factor for pancreatitis. Illicit or recreational drug use, specifically cocaine, can be associated with intestinal ischemia.
- Travel history: Inquiring about a recent travel history is important for consideration of infectious etiologies, especially in the setting of co-occurring diarrhea or hematochezia.
- Sexual history: Ask about sexual partners and determine whether the patient engages in high-risk sexual behaviors. A thorough sexual history may provide information about the risk for PID and ectopic pregnancy.
- Obstetrician/gynecologist (OB/GYN) history: A thorough reproductive health history is extremely important in women experiencing abdominal pain. The risk of an ectopic pregnancy is increased in women with a prior ectopic pregnancy, history of PID, or when pregnancy occurs with an intrauterine device in place. A menstrual history, including the last normal menstrual period, should be determined for all reproductive-aged women.
- General ROS: Ask about fever, weight loss or gain, fatigue, and malaise.

- Cardiovascular ROS: Ask about chest pain or pressure, palpitations, peripheral edema, syncope, orthopnea, paroxysmal nocturnal dyspnea, risk factors for ASCVD, and whether any cardiac testing (EKG, cardiac stress test) has been completed in the past.
- Pulmonary ROS: Ask about cough, sputum production, hemoptysis, shortness of breath, dyspnea, wheezing, and pain with breathing.
- Genitourinary ROS: Ask about dysuria, urinary frequency or urgency, cloudy urine, hematuria, urinary incontinence. In women, ask about vaginal discharge and irregular vaginal bleeding.

Physical Examination

A focused physical examination should be completed in all patients being evaluated for abdominal pain (Table 1.3). The abdominal examination should be performed with the patient's hips and knees flexed in order to relax the abdominal musculature. Auscultation of the abdomen must be completed prior to percussion and palpation to ensure there is no artificial augmentation of bowel sounds. The primary goals of palpation are to localize the predominate area of tenderness, evaluate for signs of peritoneal irritation, and to identify abdominal masses or enlarged organs. Guarding may occur during palpation, which is an increase in the tone of the abdominal musculature as the patient attempts to limit evaluation of the intraperitoneal contents.

Most patients with abdominal pain should have a general assessment, cardiac, and pulmonary examinations performed. Additionally, a digital rectal examination should be completed, and women should undergo bimanual pelvic examination.

TABLE 1.3 Abdominal Pain: Correlating Physical Exam Findings With Pathologic Conditions

Body System	Physical Exam Finding	Associated Clinical Condition
Vital signs	Fever	Acute cholangitis, hepatitis, pneumonia, pancreatitis, appendicitis, PID, mesenteric lymphadenitis, diverticulitis, IBD, gastroenteritis, peritonitis
	Tachycardia, hypotension	Gastroenteritis (with concurrent dehydration), diabetic ketoacidosis, ruptured aortic aneurysm, ruptured ectopic pregnancy, gastrointestinal perforation, splenic rupture, sepsis (from appendicitis, cholangitis, bowel infarction, ischemic colitis, pancreatitis, or spontaneous bacterial peritonitis), MI, adrenal insufficiency
Skin	Jaundice	Biliary obstruction, cholangitis, hepatitis
	Poor skin turgor (tenting)	Gastroenteritis, pancreatitis, gastrointestinal cancer
HEENT	Scleral icterus	Biliary obstruction, hepatitis
Pulmonary	Crackles or signs of consolidation	Pneumonia

(continued)

TABLE 1.3 Abdominal Pain: Correlating Physical Exam Findings With Pathologic Conditions (*continued*)

Body System	Physical Exam Finding	Associated Clinical Condition
Cardiac	Irregularly, irregular rhythm	Mesenteric ischemia
Abdomen	Surgical scars	Adhesions
	Venous prominence (caput medusa)	Hepatic disease
	Ecchymosis of the flanks (Grey Turner's sign) or periumbilical area (Cullen's sign)	Acute pancreatitis (with pancreatic necrosis and retroperitoneal hemorrhage)
	Distension	Perforation (intra-abdominal air), ascites, intra-abdominal bleeding, neoplasia
	High-pitched bowel sounds	Intestinal obstruction\
	Absence of or delayed bowel sounds	Ileus
	Tympany on percussion	Intestinal obstruction
	Dullness to percussion	Ascites
	Involuntary guarding	Peritoneal inflammation, intestinal obstruction, gastrointestinal perforation
	Rigidity	Intra-abdominal bleeding
Rectal	Impacted stool	Constipation, intestinal obstruction
	Tenderness	Appendicitis
	Black, tarry stool or grossly bloody stool	PUD, bleeding diverticulum, intestinal neoplasm
Pelvic	Cervical inflammation or discharge, cervical motion tenderness	PID
	Adnexal mass or tenderness	Ectopic pregnancy, PID

HEENT, head, eyes, ears, nose, and throat; IBD, inflammatory bowel disease; MI, myocardial infarction; PID, pelvic inflammatory disease; PUD, peptic ulcer disease.

There are several specialized examination techniques that can be useful in the evaluation of abdominal pain, as seen in Table 1.4.

TABLE 1.4 Correlating Specialized Abdominal Exams Techniques With Pathologic Conditions

Special Test	Technique	Positive Finding	Associated Clinical Condition
Murphy sign	Apply deep palpation under the right costal margin	Inspiratory arrest or gasp	Cholecystitis
Rovsing sign	Apply palpation over the LLQ	Pain occurs in RLQ	Appendicitis

(*continued*)

TABLE 1.4 Correlating Specialized Abdominal Exams Techniques With Pathologic Conditions (*continued*)

Special Test	Technique	Positive Finding	Associated Clinical Condition
Psoas sign	While supine, the patient is asked to lift their thigh against the pressure of the examiner's hand	Provocation of pain	Appendicitis
Obturator sign	While supine, the examiner flexes the patient's knee to 90 degrees and passively rotates the hip internally and externally	Provocation of pain	Appendicitis
Rebound tenderness	Apply abdominal palpation followed by a quick release of the pressure	Pain occurs upon the release of palpation	Peritonitis

LLQ, left lower quadrant; RLQ, right lower quadrant.

CLINICAL PEARL: Characteristics associated with high-risk abdominal pain include the following:
- Patient age >65 years
- Comorbidities such as immunosuppression, cardiovascular disease, alcohol use disorder, cancer, diverticulosis, cholelithiasis, or IBD
- Pain that is sudden in onset, followed by vomiting
- Objective findings of rigid abdomen, involuntary guarding, or hemodynamic instability

Diagnostic Plan

LABS
- Complete blood count (CBC) with differential: Indicated when there is suspicion for an inflammatory or infectious etiology, or to evaluate for anemia. Can be useful in the evaluation of acute cholangitis, cholecystitis, hepatitis, pneumonia, pancreatitis, appendicitis, PID, mesenteric lymphadenitis, diverticulitis, IBD, gastroenteritis, and peritonitis.
  - Leukocytosis is indicative of an infectious etiology; an increased percentage of neutrophils, or a "left shift," is associated with bacterial infections. Leukopenia may be associated with viral infections.
  - Low hemoglobin and hematocrit values with microcytosis may indicate GI bleeding.
  - Macrocytosis may be associated with alcohol use disorder.
- Basic metabolic panel (BMP): Indicated for evaluation of diabetic ketoacidosis (DKA), pancreatitis, nephrolithiasis (with coexistent acute kidney injury [AKI]), dehydration, and metabolic or endocrine disease

- o Significant elevations in glucose are seen with DKA; pancreatitis may also cause glucose abnormalities.
- o Elevated creatinine levels will be seen if nephrolithiasis or dehydration is associated with AKI.
- o Gastroenteritis associated with dehydration will cause electrolyte abnormalities.
- o Abnormal calcium levels may be indicative of an endocrine etiology.
- Liver enzymes: Indicated to evaluate suspected hepatobiliary disease, such as hepatitis, biliary obstruction, cholecystitis, and cholangitis
  - o Elevations in alkaline phosphatase and/or bilirubin are suggestive of biliary obstruction.
  - o Elevations in aspartate transaminase (AST) and/or alanine transaminase (ALT) are seen with hepatitis and other liver disease.
  - o An elevated gamma glutamyltransferase (GGT) can be seen with alcohol use disorder.
- Inflammatory markers (erythrocyte sedimentation rate [ESR], CRP): Indicated when there is suspicion for an inflammatory or infectious etiology, such as cholecystitis, pancreatitis, hepatitis, IBD, appendicitis, PID, peritonitis, gastroenteritis, and pneumonia
  - o These tests are also used for monitoring regression of disease or response to treatment.
- Amylase and lipase: Indicated for evaluation of pancreatic disorders, such as acute pancreatitis
  - o Both amylase and lipase levels are elevated in acute pancreatitis; lipase is more specific than amylase.
- Urinalysis: Indicated to evaluate for urinary causes of abdominal pain (urinary tract infection [UTI], urinary obstruction, and nephrolithiasis), or for signs of biliary obstruction or ketosis
  - o UTIs may be associated with leukocytes, nitrites, or blood on a urinalysis. Blood may be seen with nephrolithiasis. Biliary obstruction or hepatitis may result in hyperbilirubinuria.
- Tissue transglutaminase IgA antibody (anti-tTG): Indicated when celiac disease is suspected of being a trigger for abdominal pain
  - o Presence of anti-tTG is highly sensitive and specific for celiac disease; however, additional testing must be completed before a diagnosis can be confirmed.
- Serum human chorionic gonadotropin: Indicated in all reproductive-aged women presenting with abdominal pain to assess for pregnancy
  - o A positive pregnancy test should be followed with a quantitative beta-human chorionic gonadotropin (HCG) test that may need to be monitored if ectopic pregnancy is suspected.

IMAGING
- Abdominal x-ray of kidney, ureter, and bladder (KUB): Indicated for evaluation of suspected obstruction, perforation, or calcifications
  - o Ileus is associated with distention and air throughout both the small and large intestines.
  - o KUB with chest x-ray is a quick way to assess for free air under the diaphragm, which is consistent with an intestinal perforation.

○ Twenty percent of gallbladder stones are radiopaque, as are 80% of renal stones.

○ Calcification of the abdominal aorta correlates with aneurysm formation.

- CT: Indicated for the evaluation of abdominal organs, especially for diseases of the liver, pancreas, bowel, spleen, and abdominal aorta. Abdominal CT will usually be ordered with contrast; evaluation for renal stones would be a notable exception to using contrast.

○ Abdominal and pelvic CT scans are usually ordered concurrently.

○ Contraindications to CT imaging include pregnancy and allergy to intravenous (IV) contrast; precautions should be taken in patients taking metformin.

○ Be judicious in your decision-making regarding ordering CT scans due to the high radiation exposure endured by the patient. Pediatric patients are especially susceptible to the risks of radiation, and CT scans should not be completed unless absolutely medically necessary.

○ Abdominopelvic MRI may be considered for some liver or pelvic diseases (e.g., further evaluation of liver hemangioma), but in most cases CT is more appropriate.

- Ultrasound: Indicated for evaluation of the liver, gallbladder, pancreas, bile ducts, spleen, kidneys, ureters, bladder, and abdominal aorta

○ Ultrasound is a useful initial study that is generally regarded as safe and without contraindications. This is a particularly useful test in children and pregnant women.

- Hepatobiliary iminodiacetic acid (HIDA) scan: Nuclear scan of the gallbladder that allows for visualization of the biliary tree; gallbladder ejection fraction can be determined when the test is completed with cholecystokinin (CCK) stimulation.

○ Cholecystitis is associated with a reduced ejection fraction or reproduction of symptoms with CCK administration. This test is usually performed if there is a high suspicion for cholecystitis with negative findings on abdominal ultrasound.

- Upper GI series: Indicated for the evaluation of dysphagia, reflux, or dyspepsia

○ Filling defects identified on an upper GI series may indicate a benign or malignant space-occupying lesion.

○ If perforation is suspected, use a water-soluble contrast medium; NEVER use barium in this situation.

○ If PUD is suspected but no ulcers are appreciated on an upper GI series, endoscopy should be completed as a next step in evaluation.

PROCEDURES

- Esophagogastroduodenoscopy (EGD) and colonoscopy: Indicated for direct visualization of the GI tract, and can serve both diagnostic and therapeutic roles in the management of GI disorders

○ Evaluate for hiatal hernia, tumors, esophageal varices, PUD, mucosal inflammation, and mechanical obstruction (e.g., strictures, polyps, esophageal webs, or rings)

Initial Management

- Determine whether the pain is suggestive of an emergent disease process. If the evaluation revealed any "red flag" findings, such as fever, hypotension, abdominal rigidity or involuntary guarding, or peritoneal irritation, then the patient should be referred to the ED for further management.
- A CBC with differential, BMP, liver enzymes, and urinalysis will be indicated in most patients with acute abdominal pain. A pregnancy test should be ordered in all women of childbearing age. Amylase and lipase should be ordered if pancreatitis is expected. Chronic abdominal pain may indicate the need for celiac disease antibody testing, gastrointestinal tumor markers, or allergy testing.
- The need for diagnostic imaging should be determined and appropriate imaging ordered; abdominal x-rays, ultrasound, or CT will usually be the initial imaging test of choice. In more chronic cases of abdominal pain or in cases suspicious for malignancy or IBD, EGD and/or colonoscopy should be ordered.
- Determine whether the pharmacotherapeutic treatment is necessary and prescribe appropriate medication. For example, antibiotics for UTI, PID, or other bacterial infections; antacids or proton-pump inhibitors for GERD; appropriate medications (e.g., osmotic laxatives, antidiarrheal agents, antispasmodics, or antidepressants) for IBS; or, possibly, alpha-blockers to help facilitate passage of urinary stones. Pain management should be considered in treating patients with abdominal pain, with special care to avoid NSAIDS if gastritis or PUD is in the working differential. Opioids should be used judiciously, and should be avoided in cases of chronic abdominal pain.
- Patients with acute, self-limiting causes for abdominal pain, such as viral gastroenteritis, should be provided with reassurance and appropriate patient education regarding conservative treatment (e.g., dietary modifications and increased consumption of clear fluids).
- Recommend dietary restrictions or modifications that may help improve symptoms. It may be necessary for the patient to start a food and/or bowel movement diary to help identify causes of abdominal pain.
- Abdominal pain of unknown etiology after an appropriate diagnostic evaluation should be considered for referral to a gastroenterologist. Behavioral medicine or psychiatry referrals may be appropriate for chronic, functional abdominal pain.

Key Points ...

- Identifying the specific location of the abdominal pain (RUQ, LUQ, RLQ, LLQ, epigastric, suprapubic, periumbilical, or diffuse) is an essential step for developing the initial, most plausible differential diagnoses.
- Remember to consider non-GI etiologies for abdominal pain, such as acute coronary syndrome, abdominal aortic aneurysm, ectopic pregnancy, and pneumonia.

(continued)

(continued)

- Patients at increased risk for intestinal ischemia (e.g., history of ASCVD, hypercoagulability, atrial fibrillation) who present with severe abdominal pain should be evaluated emergently.
- Findings associated with obstruction, perforation, vascular compromise, or peritoneal irritation warrant hospital admission and immediate surgical consultation.
- Abdominal ultrasound is a useful test for initial diagnostic imaging; it does not have contraindications and is low-risk for complications.

REFERENCES

1. Jacobs DO. Abdominal pain. In: Jameson J, Fauci AS, Kasper DLet al, eds. *Harrison's Principles of Internal Medicine*. 20th ed. New York, NY: McGraw-Hill; 2018.
2. McQuaid KR. Gastrointestinal disorders. In: Papadakis MA, McPhee SJ, Rabow MW, eds. *Current Medical Diagnosis & Treatment*. New York, NY: McGraw-Hill; 2019.
3. Rui P, Okeyode T. National ambulatory medical care survey: 2015 state and national summary tables. http://www.cdc.gov/nchs/ahcd/ahcd_products.htm. Accessed December 1, 2018.

ELECTRONIC RESOURCES

American College of Radiology Diagnostic Appropriateness Criteria:

https://acsearch.acr.org/list

FATIGUE

Fatigue is an extremely common symptom encountered in family medicine. It accounts for up to 3% of office visits in primary care medicine when it is the sole presenting symptom, and it is a contributing symptom in up to 20% of visits.[1,2] Fatigue can be a challenging symptom to evaluate, even for experienced clinicians, because it is a nonspecific complaint that has a wide range of possible differential diagnoses, spanning nearly every organ system, as seen in Table 1.5. Additionally, patients may confuse fatigue with other symptoms, such as weakness or sleepiness. Unfortunately, in many cases, no definite cause for the fatigue can be identified; this can be a source of frustration for both the patient and the clinician. It is critical that the family medicine physician assistant (PA) identify whether there is a secondary cause for the fatigue that can be treated, and if no discrete etiology can be identified, the PA should provide extensive support and education to help the patient manage their symptom.

Differential Diagnosis

TABLE **1.5** Differential Diagnosis of Fatigue

Endocrine	Neurologic	Rheumatologic/Immune	Other
Thyroid disorders	Multiple sclerosis	Systemic lupus erythematosus	Anemia
Diabetes mellitus	Myasthenia gravis	Rheumatoid arthritis	Malignancy
Obesity	Parkinson's disease	Sarcoidosis	Physical inactivity
Chronic kidney disease	Secondary to stroke	Sjögren's syndrome	Pregnancy
Pituitary disorders	Secondary to traumatic brain injury	Vasculitic disorders	Chronic fatigue syndrome
Hypercalcemia		Fibromyalgia	Medication adverse effects
Adrenal insufficiency			
Hypogonadism			
Vitamin D deficiency			

Psychiatric Disorders	Infectious	Gastrointestinal	Cardiopulmonary
Depressive	Lyme disease	Inflammatory bowel disease	Heart failure
Anxiety	HIV infection	Celiac disease	COPD
Somatic symptom	Hepatitis	Liver failure	Sleep apnea
Sleep–wake	Infectious mononucleosis	Malnutrition	
Substance-related	Endocarditis		
	Tuberculosis		

COPD, chronic obstructive pulmonary disease.

History

- Onset, duration, and timing: Ask about the duration of symptoms; fatigue lasting longer than 6 months is considered chronic. Determine whether the fatigue started in relation to other symptoms, diseases, major stresses, or life events, or whether it coincided with the initiation of a new medication. Ask whether the symptoms are constant, intermittent, or if they worsen throughout the day or with activity.[2,3]
- Provoking/alleviating factors: Determine whether there are any aggravating or alleviating factors that impact the patient's fatigue. This information can be particularly useful in identifying whether it is actually muscle weakness or sleepiness that the patient is experiencing but describing as fatigue.
- Quality: Try to have the patient describe what he or she is actually experiencing. Fatigue may be described as a general sense of weakness (without any actual muscle weakness), a lower level of energy throughout the day, decreased concentration, or even emotional instability.[4]
- Severity: A critical component in the evaluation and management of a patient with fatigue is to understand the impact on his or her daily functioning. Ask the patient whether symptoms are interfering with work, interpersonal relationships, or his or her ability to care for him- or herself.

- Associated symptoms: Fatigue is a chief complaint that warrants a complete medical history and comprehensive ROS in order to adequately evaluate for secondary causes.

Past Medical History Specific to Complaint

- Medical illnesses/comorbidities: Determine whether the patient has any chronic medical illnesses, such as kidney or liver disease, endocrinopathies, ASCVD or heart failure, chronic obstructive pulmonary disease (COPD), neurodegenerative or CNS disorders, rheumatologic or autoimmune disease, or psychiatric disorders.
- Medications: Ask the patient about all medications (prescription and OTC) and supplements taken on a regular basis; many medications are known to be associated with fatigue, particularly first-generation antihistamines, antidepressants, benzodiazepines, antipsychotics, sedatives/hypnotics, opiates, some antiepileptics, and some antihypertensives (e.g., beta-blockers).
- Family history: Determine whether there is a family history of any chronic medical conditions, including cancer, cardiovascular disease, autoimmune or rheumatologic disorders, endocrine disorders, and neurologic disease.
- Health maintenance: Determine whether the patient has received all relevant preventive medicine screenings based upon her or his demographic information (e.g., breast/cervical/colon cancer screening, hepatitis C, and HIV screening), and if she or he is up-to-date on all recommended immunizations.

> **CLINICAL PEARL:** It is critical to assess for up-to-date screening for various cancers in order to assess the possibility of an occult malignancy.

- Social history: Ask about use of tobacco, alcohol, and illicit drugs. It is particularly important to inquire about the use of injection drugs, which may predispose to hepatitis, HIV infection, and endocarditis. Inquire about the patient's relationship status, occupation, and any recent stresses or major life events.
- Travel history: If there is concern for an infectious etiology, travel history may be pertinent for determining risk.
- Sexual history: Ask about sexual partners and determine whether the patient engages in high-risk sexual behaviors, which could increase the risk of HIV infection.
- OB/GYN history: Menstrual history should be obtained in reproductive-aged women to assess for possible pregnancy.
- General ROS: Ask about fever, chills, night sweats, weight loss or gain, weakness, and malaise.

> **CLINICAL PEARL:** Fatigue accompanied by weight loss and/or unexplained fevers is concerning for a possible malignancy.

- Skin: Ask about rashes, hair or nail changes, and photosensitivity.
- HEENT: Ask about changes in vision, red eyes, dry eyes, URI symptoms, mouth lesions/sores, hoarseness, and frequent infections.
- Pulmonary: Ask about shortness of breath or dyspnea, cough, hemoptysis, wheezing, recurrent bronchitis, and pleurisy.
- Cardiovascular ROS: Ask about chest pain or pressure, palpitations, peripheral edema, syncope, orthopnea, paroxysmal nocturnal dyspnea, risk factors for ASCVD, and whether any cardiac testing (EKG, cardiac stress test) has been completed in the past.
- GI ROS: Ask about abdominal pain, nausea, vomiting, diarrhea, constipation, hematochezia, melena, hematemesis, dysphagia, and heartburn.
- Genitourinary ROS: Ask about urinary frequency, hematuria, and obstructive urinary symptoms (e.g., hesitancy, straining).
- Musculoskeletal: Ask about myalgias, arthralgias, and joint deformities.
- Hematologic/lymphatic ROS: Ask about swollen lymph nodes, bleeding, bruising, and blood clots.
- Endocrine ROS: Ask about heat or cold intolerance, polyuria, polyphagia, polydipsia, and flushing.
- Neurologic ROS: Ask about headaches, numbness, paresthesias, muscle weakness, and difficulty with concentration.
- Psychiatric: Ask about depression, anxiety, insomnia or other sleep difficulty, alcohol or substance use, and stress levels.

Physical Examination

Similar to the medical history obtained in the evaluation of fatigue, the physical examination should also be fairly comprehensive. The information obtained in the medical history can occasionally be utilized to help focus the necessary components of the physical exam; however, oftentimes the medical history does not provide a lot of clarity about the most likely etiology. In the absence of a narrowed differential, the physical exam should be thorough in order to further exclude the presence of organic disease. Table 1.6 is a thorough, yet not exhaustive, list of possible physical examination findings which may help to identify a pathophysiologic cause for fatigue.

Diagnostic Plan

Since there is such a broad differential diagnosis for fatigue, the history and physical examination should guide the diagnostic evaluation. In the absence of any significant findings on history and physical examination, only a handful of laboratory studies are recommended for further diagnostic evaluation, especially since laboratory results only affect management in 5% of patients presenting with fatigue.[2]

- CBC with differential: Indicated to evaluate for anemia, inflammatory or metabolic disorders, infection, or malignancy
- Comprehensive metabolic panel (CMP): Indicated to evaluate for kidney or liver disease, diabetes mellitus, hypercalcemia, electrolyte abnormalities, or signs of metabolic disease or malnutrition
- ESR: Indicated when there is suspicion for an inflammatory or infectious etiology

TABLE 1.6 Fatigue: Correlating Physical Exam Findings With Pathologic Conditions

Body System	Physical Exam Finding	Associated Clinical Condition
Vitals	Elevated blood pressure	Hypothyroidism, chronic kidney disease, heart failure
	Elevated body mass index	Obesity
	Fever	Acute HIV infection, acute hepatitis, infectious mononucleosis, endocarditis, tuberculosis
General	Masked facies	Parkinson's disease
	Moon facies, "buffalo hump"	Cushing's disease
Skin	Pale	Anemia
	Hyperpigmentation	Adrenal insufficiency
	Erythema migrans	Lyme disease
	Purple striae	Cushing's disease
	Dry skin, thinning and/or coarse hair, brittle nails	Hypothyroidism
	Rash	Systemic lupus erythematosus, inflammatory bowel disease, celiac disease, vasculitic conditions
	Jaundice	Acute hepatitis, liver failure
	Janeway lesions, Osler nodes, Roth spots	Endocarditis
HEENT	Exophthalmos, extraocular muscle weakness	Hyperthyroidism
	Edematous tonsils with exudate	Infectious mononucleosis
Neck	Thyroid enlargement	Hypothyroidism, hyperthyroidism
Pulmonary	Adventitious breath sounds	Tuberculosis, COPD
	Decreased breath sounds, hyperresonance to percussion, "barrel" chest	COPD
Cardiovascular	New murmur	Endocarditis
	Extremity edema	Heart failure
Gastrointestinal	Hepatomegaly	Acute hepatitis
	Abdominal mass	Intrabdominal cancer
Genitourinary	Prostate nodule	Prostate cancer
Musculoskeletal	Joint swelling or nodules	Rheumatoid arthritis
Hematologic/ immunologic	Lymphadenopathy	HIV, infectious mononucleosis, malignancy
Neurologic	Decreased sensation	Multiple sclerosis
	Muscle weakness	Multiple sclerosis, myasthenia gravis
	Muscle fatigability	Myasthenia gravis
	Gait disturbance, cogwheel rigidity, bradykinesia	Parkinson's disease
Psychiatric	Flat affect	Depressive disorders

COPD, chronic obstructive pulmonary disease.

- Thyroid-stimulating hormone (TSH): Indicated as an initial test to evaluate for hypo- or hyperthyroidism
- Urinalysis: Indicated to screen for signs of kidney disease, biliary disease, or ketosis
- Serum human chorionic gonadotropin: Indicated in all reproductive-aged women presenting with fatigue to assess for pregnancy

Additional tests that may be considered based on information obtained in the medical history and/or physical examination include the following:

- Hemoglobin A1C
- Iron studies
- 24-hour urine protein, creatinine, albumin
- Follicle-stimulating hormone, luteinizing hormone, testosterone, and/or estrogen levels
- 25-OH vitamin D level
- Hepatitis antibodies
- HIV antibody
- Polysomnogram (sleep study)
- Spirometry (pulmonary function test)
- Blood cultures
- Purified protein derivative (PPD) test for tuberculosis
- Echocardiogram
- Antinuclear antibody
- Rheumatoid factor
- Cyclic citrullinated peptide (CCP) antibody
- Tissue transglutaminase IgA antibody (anti-tTG)
- Acetylcholine receptor antibody
- Lyme disease antibodies/enzyme-linked immunosorbent assay (ELISA) test

Initial Management

- The initial steps in management should be to attempt to identify whether the fatigue is secondary to another condition that can be treated or managed.
- Initial diagnostic evaluation should include CBC, ESR, CMP, TSH, urinalysis, and pregnancy test. Additional tests should be directed toward specific information elicited during the history and physical examination.
- If an underlying psychiatric condition is identified, the patient should be referred for cognitive behavioral therapy, and pharmacotherapeutics should be considered along with a determination of whether referral to psychiatry is warranted.
- It is important to validate the patient's symptoms even when an underlying cause is not able to be identified. You must then establish realistic expectations for the patient regarding the likelihood of symptom resolution, especially in cases of chronic fatigue (nearly two-thirds experience limited improvement and it is extremely rare to have complete resolution).[2]
- Ensure the status of all chronic medical conditions has been optimized through appropriate treatment and management plans.

- Exercise therapy should be incorporated into the management plans of most patients experiencing chronic fatigue.
- Patients with chronic fatigue, as with many functional disorders, respond well to regularly scheduled office visits during which progress can be evaluated and the management plan can be reinforced.

Key Points ...

- Fatigue is associated with many acute and chronic medical conditions, but it is often difficult to clearly identify the specific etiology.
- Evaluation of a patient with fatigue as the chief complaint demands that you complete a comprehensive medical history and physical examination.
- Diagnostic tests should be limited and focused to information elicited during the history and physical examination.
- Management of the patient should include validation of symptoms, patient education regarding expectations for improvement, and a focus on exercise, coping mechanisms, and psychological health.

REFERENCES

1. Nadler PL, Gonzales R. Common symptoms. In: Papadakis MA, McPhee SJ, Rabow MW, eds. *Current Medical Diagnosis & Treatment 2019*. New York, NY: McGraw-Hill; 2019.
2. Rosenthal TC, Majeroni BA, Pretorius R, Malik K. Fatigue: an overview. *Am Fam Physician*. 2008;78(10):1173–1179.
3. Gelfand JM, Douglas VC. Fatigue. In: Jameson J, Fauci AS, Kasper DL, et al., eds. *Harrison's Principles of Internal Medicine*. 20th ed. New York, NY: McGraw-Hill; 2018.
4. Fosnocht KM, Ende J. Approach to the adult patient with fatigue. In: Post TW, ed. *UpToDate*. Waltham, MA: UpToDate Inc; 2019. http://www.uptodate.com

HEADACHE

Headaches are one of the most common reasons for patients to seek medical care, with approximately half of the worldwide adult population having been symptomatic with a headache at least once in the previous year.[1] Headaches range in severity from minor inconveniences to life-threatening emergencies. Headaches of various etiologies are associated with typical clinical presentation patterns that can help aid the clinician in determining the underlying pathology. Clinicians treating patients for headache disorders must be vigilant to evaluate for red flag symptoms or signs indicating an emergent situation with a serious underlying cause for the headache.

Differential Diagnosis

The International Headache Society (IHS) classifies headaches into primary and secondary types, many of which are outlined in Table 1.7. Primary headaches are those for which the headache itself is the core condition; tension-type headaches are the most common type of primary headache, accounting for 69% of cases. Migraine headaches account for 16% of primary headaches. Secondary headaches are headaches caused by other underlying conditions; the majority (63%) of secondary headaches are attributed to infection. Head injury or trauma accounts for only 4% of secondary headaches.[2,3]

The differential diagnosis for primary headaches includes the following:

- Tension-type headache
- Migraine headache
- Trigeminal autonomic cephalalgias (includes cluster headaches)
- Other (includes new daily persistent headache)

History

- Onset, duration, and timing: Determine when the headache began, including whether this is an isolated headache or whether there has been a pattern of repetitive headaches. Inquire about duration of the headache(s);

TABLE 1.7 Differential Diagnosis for Secondary Headaches

Category	Examples
Substance use, exposure, or withdrawal	Carbon monoxide exposure Cocaine-induced headache Medication overuse headache Withdrawal from caffeine, opioids, estrogen
Nonvascular intracranial disorder	High or low cerebrospinal fluid Postlumbar puncture headache Intracranial neoplasm
Headache or facial pain due to disorder of the HEENT structures	Cervicogenic Acute angle-closure glaucoma Sinusitis Temporomandibular joint disorder
Disorder of homeostasis	Hypoxia Hypertension Hypertensive emergency Pheochromocytoma
Trauma/injury to head and/or neck	Traumatic head injury Whiplash
Infection	Bacterial or viral meningitis Localized infection/abscess Systemic viral, bacterial, fungal, or parasitic infection
Cranial/cervical vascular disorder	Temporal arteritis Transient ischemic attack Cerebrovascular accident Subarachnoid hemorrhage

HEENT, head, ears, eyes, nose, and throat.

tension-type headaches can last 30 minutes to 7 days, whereas migraines typically last 4 to 72 hours. The onset of the headache is critical for determining risk for a more serious etiology; thunderclap, or sudden-onset headaches that become severe within seconds to minutes, are typical of a subarachnoid hemorrhage or other intracranial bleeding. More benign causes for headache(s) usually have a more insidious onset. Ask the patient about the timing of the headache(s); early morning headaches are associated with increased intracranial pressure or hypoxia related to sleep apnea. Also inquire about the events surrounding the onset of the headache(s), such as whether the patient had just sneezed or coughed or had been exerting themselves.[2,3]

- Provoking/alleviating factors: Provoking and alleviating factors can be extremely useful in working through a differential diagnosis list. Migraine headaches have many possible triggers and aggravating factors, such as bright lights, loud noise, certain foods, menstruation, stress, or certain odors. Migraines are often alleviated by sleep or by resting in a cold, dark room. Headaches that are aggravated by coughing or lifting can indicate increased intracranial pressure from a mass or neoplasm.
- Quality: The patient's description of their headache can be useful as some conditions are associated with a characteristic type of pain. Migraine headaches are often throbbing or pulsating, whereas tension-type headaches may be described as tightness. Cluster headaches are classically described as a sharp or piercing pain. Other headaches may be described as dull, aching, pressure, or squeezing. In cases of a primary headache, the clinician should inquire about the presence of an aura (reversible visual, sensory, or speech symptoms that last 5 to 60 minutes and occur before or at the onset of the headache).
- Radiation/location: Determine the location and laterality of the headache. The most common presentation for migraines is unilateral. Tension headaches are usually bilateral or band-like around the entire head, and cluster headaches are usually unilateral and located in the orbital or temporal areas. Temporal arteritis will have pain over the temporal artery, which may radiate to the jaw or teeth. Secondary headaches from meningitis may have pain that radiates down the neck or spine.
- Severity: Ask patients to rate the severity of their headache on a 10-point scale; a higher severity headache should cause higher suspicion for a serious cause. The "worst headache of [the patient's] life" should raise suspicion for an intracranial hemorrhage, and progressively worsening pain may indicate an intracranial mass, subdural hematoma, or medication overuse.
- Associated symptoms: In addition to completing a full inquiry on all neurologic symptoms, ROS should also include components from general, head, eyes, ears, nose, and throat (HEENT), cardiovascular, GI, and psychiatric components.
- An essential component of the medical history in patients presenting with a headache includes an assessment for red flag symptoms that may indicate a more serious cause. These include the following:
  - ○ Abrupt or sudden in onset, thunderclap onset
  - ○ New onset headaches in a patient older than 50 years
  - ○ New onset or severe headache in a pregnant or postpartum patient

○ Worst or first severe headache of life
○ Change in the pattern or severity of chronic headaches
○ Medical history of cancer, immunocompromised, or increased risk of coagulopathy
○ Awakes patient from sleep or persistent morning headaches with nausea
○ Brought on by exertion or with postural changes, or worsens with coughing, lifting, or bending
○ Weight loss

Past Medical History Specific to Complaint

- Medical illnesses/comorbidities: Determine whether the patient has a history of neurologic disorders, specifically a known history of headaches. If the patient has an established headache diagnosis, it is critical to establish the patient's normal characteristics, patterns, and frequency of headaches to determine whether the current headache deviates from the patient's established headache disorder. Ask about a medical history of hypertension, new-onset or poorly controlled. Hypertension itself can cause headaches or could increase risk for other serious etiologies, such as cerebrovascular accident (CVA). Medical history of immunosuppression, such as with HIV infection, can predispose the patient to an increased risk of meningitis or intracranial abscess. Lyme disease is associated with possible encephalitis. Medical history of cancer can indicate risk of metastasis to the brain.[3–5]
- Accidents/injuries: Ask about recent head trauma, which can be associated with underlying structural damage or bleeding.
- Medications: Aspirin and anticoagulants can increase the risk of intracranial bleeding. Chronic use of NSAIDS, opioids, or migraine abortifacient medications can be associated with medication overuse headaches.
- Family history: Inquire about a family history of headache disorders, especially migraines.
- Social history: Illicit drug use, specifically cocaine, and excessive consumption of caffeine can induce headaches.
- OB/GYN: Take a menstrual history in all reproductive-aged women; migraine headaches can be associated with hormonal fluctuations.
- Neurologic ROS: Ask about numbness, paresthesias, weakness, seizures, confusion, altered level of consciousness, or difficulty with speech or gait.
- General ROS: Ask about fever, weight loss or gain, fatigue, and malaise.
- HEENT ROS: Ask about recent or current infections of the ear, nose, throat, or facial skin as these can be complicated by extension into the central nervous system (CNS), causing meningitis or intracranial abscess.
- Cardiovascular ROS: Ask about chest pain or pressure, palpitations, peripheral edema, syncope, orthopnea, paroxysmal nocturnal dyspnea, risk factors for ASCVD, and whether any cardiac testing (EKG, cardiac stress test) has been completed in the past.
- GI ROS: Ask about nausea and vomiting.
- Psychiatric ROS: Ask about depression, anxiety, sleep difficulty, personality or behavior changes, stress, or recent trauma.

Physical Examination

Perform a thorough physical examination and correlate pertinent positives with clinical conditions when present, as seen in Table 1.8. Include a neurologic examination in patients presenting for a headache, especially patients presenting with new-onset headache, changes in headache patterns, or with any other red flag symptoms. The neurologic examination should be comprehensive, including cranial nerves, sensory and motor components, deep tendon reflexes, cerebellar function, gait, and mental status. Additionally, vital signs, general assessment, and HEENT examinations should also be completed.[3–5]

TABLE 1.8 Headache: Correlating Physical Exam Findings With Pathologic Conditions

Body System	Physical Exam Finding	Associated Clinical Condition
Vital signs	Severely elevated blood pressure	Hypertensive urgency or emergency, CVA, intracranial pathology
	Fever	Meningitis, encephalitis, intracranial abscess
General	Photosensitivity	Migraines
Skin	Rash or cellulitis of head, face, or neck	Encephalitis, meningitis
HEENT	Papilledema	Encephalitis, meningitis, intracranial mass, pseudotumor cerebri
	Cotton wool spots, flame hemorrhages	Hypertensive retinopathy
	Decreased visual acuity	Glaucoma, temporal arteritis, optic neuritis
	Red eye with cloudy cornea, nonreactive pupil	Acute angle-closure glaucoma
	Unilateral ptosis, lacrimation, conjunctival injection, rhinorrhea	Cluster headache
	Tenderness over temporal artery	Temporal arteritis
Neurologic	Altered mental status/level of consciousness	Infection, intracerebral bleed, intracranial mass
	Focal neurologic signs	Arteriovenous malformation, intracranial mass
	Nuchal rigidity	Meningitis
	Kernig sign (resistance to knee extension that occurs when the hip is flexed at 90 degrees)	Meningitis
	Brudzinski sign (spontaneous flexion of the hips that occurs when the examiner performs passive flexion of the neck)	Meningitis

CVA, cerebrovascular accident; HEENT, head, eyes, ears, nose, and throat.

CLINICAL PEARL: Abnormal findings on physical examination may help narrow the diagnosis, but the clinician must remember that headaches can have serious or life-threatening causes even in the presence of all normal findings.

CLINICAL PEARL: The following findings on physical examination are considered red flags that may indicate a more serious cause: altered mental status or confusion, fever, focal neurologic deficits, nuchal rigidity, globe tenderness, papilledema, tender temporal artery, severe hypertension.

Diagnostic Plan

LABS

- CBC with differential: Indicated for evaluation of infectious causes of headache[3-6]
  - ○ Leukocytosis may be seen with meningitis or encephalitis
- Inflammatory markers (ESR, CRP): Indicated when there is suspicion for an inflammatory or infectious etiology
  - ○ Temporal arteritis is associated with significantly high ESR levels
- Lumbar puncture for cerebrospinal fluid (CSF) analysis: Indicated to evaluate for subarachnoid hemorrhage, neoplasm, and infectious or inflammatory etiologies. CSF analysis includes a Gram stain, white blood cell count, red blood cell count, glucose, total protein, culture, and a measure of opening pressure.
  - ○ An elevated opening pressure, which correlates with increased intracranial pressure, can be seen with infectious etiologies, bleeding, or with a mass. All of these causes can also cause an elevated protein level to be seen on CSF analysis.
  - ○ Red blood cells are associated with subarachnoid hemorrhage or other bleeding.
  - ○ White blood cell counts will be mildly elevated with viral infections. Bacterial infections typically have a significantly elevated white blood cell count, which is usually associated with a low glucose level.

IMAGING

- CT or MRI: Indicated for evaluation of the head and brain for a mass or intracranial bleed. If the headache is suspected of extending from an underlying sinusitis, sinus CT would be appropriate

---

CLINICAL PEARL: If an intracranial bleed is suspected, CT imaging should be performed WITHOUT contrast.

> **CLINICAL PEARL:** Whether CT or MRI is utilized depends on the suspected underlying etiology. Consult the American College of Radiology Appropriateness Criteria or with a radiologist directly if you are uncertain of the preferred diagnostic neuroimaging for a given suspected diagnosis.

OTHER

- Polysomnogram (sleep study): Indicated for chronic, recurrent, early morning headaches which may be associated with hypoxia as a result of obstructive sleep apnea
- Intraocular pressure measurement: Indicated to evaluate for glaucoma

Initial Management

- Determine whether there are any red flag symptoms or signs that would indicate the need for emergent evaluation and treatment. These patients should be referred to the ED for further management.
- Determine whether there is a need for neuroimaging. In patients without any red flag symptoms or signs and without a clinical presentation suggestive of a secondary headache, there is usually not a need for neuroimaging.
- Nonpharmacologic treatment options for nonemergent headaches include physical therapy, acupuncture, dental treatment (in cases of malocclusion), relaxation therapy, stress reduction, and biofeedback techniques.
- Provide patient education regarding common triggers of primary headache disorders
  - ○ If the underlying etiology for the headache cannot be determined at the initial visit, the patient should keep a headache diary to help identify potential triggers or patterns.
- For primary headache disorders, target the cause of the headache. Abortive and/or prophylactic treatment regimens may be followed for pharmacologic management of migraine headaches. There are many medication options, such as acetaminophen, NSAIDS, caffeine, triptans, ergot alkaloids, beta-blockers, antiepileptics, and botulinum toxin. Cluster headaches may be treated with oxygen therapy, triptans, or other agents. For more detailed information on specific therapies that are indicated based on the underlying cause of the primary headache, see Chapter 2, Common Disease Entities in Family Medicine.
- For secondary headache disorders, identify and treat the underlying cause:
  - ○ Acute bacterial meningitis: Perform head CT and lumbar puncture for CSF analysis, blood cultures, and start the patient on bactericidal antibiotics that penetrate the blood brain barrier.
  - ○ Cervicogenic: Consider imaging of the cervical spine with x-ray or MRI. Nonpharmacologic management options include neck-strengthening

exercises, physical therapy, spinal manipulation, or acupuncture. Treatment may include acetaminophen, NSAIDS, tricyclic antidepressants, local nerve blocks, trigger point injections, or epidural steroid injections.

○ Mass lesion: Order MRI with gadolinium and refer for tissue biopsy
○ Medication overuse: Avoidance of trigger medication for 2 months
○ Subarachnoid hemorrhage: Order noncontrast CT of the brain and/or lumbar puncture and initiate emergent neurosurgical evaluation
○ Temporal arteritis: Perform temporal artery biopsy and start high-dose prednisone

Key Points ...

- Tension-type headaches are the most common primary headache disorder, followed by migraines. Infectious causes are the most common reason for a secondary headache.
- In patients with recurrent headaches presenting to the clinic for evaluation, it is critical to identify the typical pattern and characteristics of their headaches to identify changes from their normal clinical presentation.
- A complete neurologic examination must be completed in all patients presenting to the clinic for evaluation of an acute onset headache.
- Neuroimaging with CT or MRI and CSF analysis is indicated in most patients with a headache associated with red flag symptoms or signs.
- Treatment of primary headache disorders is dependent on identification of the underlying cause of the headache.

REFERENCES

1. World Health Organization website. Headache disorders. April 8, 2016. https://www.who.int/news-room/fact-sheets/detail/headache-disorders. Accessed December 9, 2018.
2. Headache Classification Committee of the International Headache Society (IHS). The international classification of headache disorders, 3rd edition. *Cephalalgia.* 2018;38(1):1–211. doi:10.1177/0333102417738202
3. Hainer BL, Matheson EM. Approach to acute headache in adults. *Am Fam Physician.* 2013;87(10):682–687.
4. Nadler PL, Gonzales R. Common symptoms. In: Papadakis MA, McPhee SJ, Rabow MW, eds. *Current Medical Diagnosis & Treatment 2019.* New York, NY: McGraw-Hill; 2019.
5. Goadsby PJ. Headache. In: Jameson J, Fauci AS, Kasper DL, et al., eds. *Harrison's Principles of Internal medicine.* 20th ed. New York, NY: McGraw-Hill; 2018.
6. Seehusen DA, Reeves MM, Fomin DA. Cerebrospinal fluid analysis. *Am Fam Physician.* 2003;68(6):1103–1109.

LOW BACK PAIN

LBP is an exceedingly common symptom encountered in family medicine clinics. It is a leading cause of disability in the United States[1] and is the second most common reason for patients to seek treatment at a primary care office.[2] At any given time, 30% of adults in the United States will report having experienced back pain in the prior 3 months.[3] It is estimated that the lifetime prevalence for experiencing significant back pain in the United States is at least 80%.[4] Primary care providers are often the first practitioners seen for diagnosis and management of this condition. The primary objective in the evaluation of the patient with back pain should be to distinguish mechanical back pain from other more serious causes, such as fracture, infection, malignancy, autoimmune disease, or neurologic pathology (Table 1.9).

> **CLINICAL PEARL:** Known risk factors for mechanical back pain include increasing age, inactivity, overweight or obesity, genetic predisposition, stress, heavy lifting or pushing, and smoking.

> **CLINICAL PEARL:** Mechanical causes are the most prevalent (>95%) underlying reason for a patient to experience LBP, with lumbar strains or sprains accounting for the highest percentage of mechanical etiologies.[5]

TABLE 1.9 Differential Diagnosis of Low Back Pain

Mechanical	Nonmechanical, Spinal	Nonmechanical, Nonspinal
Musculoskeletal strain	Neoplasm	Abdominal aortic aneurysm
Degenerative disc disease	Metastatic malignancy	Abdominopelvic mass
Herniated disc	Multiple myeloma	Renal
Spinal stenosis	Infection	Pancreas
Facet joint disease	Osteomyelitis	Ovarian
Spondylosis	Epidural abscess	Pyelonephritis
Spondylolisthesis	Inflammatory arthritis	Nephrolithiasis
Vertebral fracture	Cauda equina syndrome	Pancreatitis
		Pelvic pathology
		Endometriosis
		Pelvic inflammatory disease
		Prostatitis
		Shingles

Source: Herndon CM, Zoberi KS, Gardner BJ. Common questions about chronic low back pain. *American Family Physician. 2018;* 91(10):708–714; Engstrom JW. Back and neck pain. In: Jameson J, Fauci AS, Kasper DL, et al., eds. *Harrison's Principles of Internal Medicine.* 20th ed. New York, NY: McGraw-Hill; 2018; Kinkade, SK. Evaluation and treatment of acute low back pain. *American Family Physician. 2007;* 75(8):1182–1188.[5]

History

- Onset, duration, and timing: Information about the onset and timing of LBP can help determine the underlying etiology. Sudden, progressive pain may be associated with a fall or injury. Insidious pain is more likely with degenerative disease or nonmechanical causes. Pain that occurs at night may be associated with malignancy, and pain that is worse in the morning with improvement throughout the day may be associated with an inflammatory arthritis. The duration of LBP will help to categorize it as acute, subacute, or chronic. Acute back pain lasts <4 weeks, subacute lasts 4 to 12 weeks, and chronic back pain lasts >12 weeks.[6]

> **CLINICAL PEARL:** A high percentage of patients with acute LBP will have resolution of symptoms within one week, and 95% of patients will never progress to chronic LBP (i.e., symptoms resolve within 12 weeks).[5]

- Provoking/alleviating factors: Several factors can have an effect on LBP, such as body positon or movements. Pain associated with a herniated disc worsens with Valsalva maneuvers and with coughing or sneezing. Spinal stenosis characteristically worsens with standing upright or walking, but improves with leaning forward or sitting. Pain associated with degenerative causes, such as spondylosis, worsens with movement and improves with rest. Inflammatory arthritis is often worse at rest, and there is alleviation of pain with activity. Spinal infections may be aggravated by palpation of the vertebrae.
- Quality: Patients should be asked to describe the pain, and a variety of descriptors may be utilized (e.g., deep, superficial, aching, boring, throbbing, sharp, burning, shooting, or cramping). Musculoskeletal strains are often described as dull, aching pain, or as tightness. Radicular pain (e.g., from nerve root impingement associated with a herniated disc) may be described as sharp, burning, tingling, or numb.
- Radiation/location: Determine whether the pain radiates from the primary location. There may be some radiation of pain from musculoskeletal sprains or strains, but radiation rarely extends beyond the buttocks. Pain that radiates down the leg beyond the knee (i.e., sciatica) is associated with a herniated disc.
- Severity: Severity of pain is helpful to assess in order to monitor progress and response to treatment; however, differences in pain tolerance can make it difficult to determine the likelihood of various differentials based on severity of pain alone. Additionally, there are significant variances in how conditions can present; vertebral compression fractures and herniated discs are examples of conditions that can be asymptomatic in some cases, or can cause severe pain associated with significant disability.
- Associated symptoms: In addition to completing a full inquiry on all musculoskeletal symptoms, a neurologic ROS should be completed in all patients. Consider completing cardiovascular, abdominal, and urinary ROS.

Past Medical History Specific to Complaint

- Medical illnesses/comorbidities: Ask about a prior history of musculoskeletal, rheumatologic, or autoimmune disorders. Osteoporosis and malignancy are associated with an increased risk for vertebral compression fractures. Metastasis to the bone should be considered if there is a medical history of cancer, particularly of the breast, lung, prostate, or GI. Cardiovascular disease (or risk factors for cardiovascular disease [CVD]) and collagen vascular disease (e.g., Marfan syndrome) can indicate risk for an aortic aneurysm or dissection.

> **CLINICAL PEARL:** Back pain and syncope in a patient with known vascular disease should prompt the PA to consider the possibility of aortic involvement.

- Medications: Corticosteroids are known to accelerate bone loss and can lead to an earlier onset or worsening of osteoporosis, which can predispose the patient to fractures.
- Surgical history: Inquire about any recent procedures involving instrumentation of the epidural space as this may indicate risk for an epidural abscess or other infectious etiology.
- Social history: History of IV drug use can lead to osteomyelitis through hematogenous spread of infection.
- Sexual history: High-risk sexual behaviors or a new sexual partner may be associated with nonmechanical, nonspinal back pain occurring as a result of PID or prostatitis.
- OB/GYN history: A thorough gynecologic history may be appropriate if there is suspicion for endometriosis or an ovarian cyst.
- General ROS: Ask about fever, weight loss or gain, fatigue, night sweats, and malaise.
- Neurologic ROS: Ask about paresthesias, numbness, weakness, and urinary or bowel incontinence.
- Cardiovascular ROS: Ask about chest pain or pressure, palpitations, peripheral edema, syncope, orthopnea, paroxysmal nocturnal dyspnea, risk factors for ASCVD, and whether any cardiac testing (EKG, cardiac stress test) has been completed in the past.
- Abdominal ROS: Ask about abdominal pain, nausea, vomiting, constipation, diarrhea, dysphagia, heartburn, loss of appetite, or early satiety.
- Urinary ROS: Ask about dysuria, urinary frequency or urgency, urinary retention, and hematuria.

Physical Examination

Complete a focused physical examination in all patients with LBP (Table 1.10). Examination of the spine should include inspection for deformities, abnormal curvature, and for skin abnormalities. Palpation and percussion of the spine and paravertebral muscles should be performed to evaluate for step-off deformities and pain. Evaluate range of motion, including flexion, extension, lateral bending, and rotation; it is helpful to document the degree to which the patient is able to move in each of these directions, and whether pain is elicited with

TABLE **1.10** Low Back Pain: Correlating Physical Exam Findings With Pathologic Conditions

Body System	Physical Exam Finding	Associated Clinical Condition
Vital signs	Hypotension, tachycardia	Ruptured aortic aneurysm, aortic dissection
Skin	Erythema, warmth, soft-tissue swelling (signs of infection)	Osteomyelitis
	Vesicular lesions on an erythematous base	Shingles
Cardiac	New murmur	Endocarditis (may be sign of osteomyelitis if there has been hematogenous spread of infection)
	Diminished peripheral pulses	Ruptured aortic aneurysm
Abdomen	Mass or distention	Aortic aneurysm, malignancy
	Epigastric pain	Pancreatitis
	Costovertebral angle tenderness	Pyelonephritis
Musculoskeletal	Soft-tissue swelling	Sprain, strain, fracture
	Bruising, contusion	Fracture
	Positive straight leg raise (radicular pain with raising the extended leg of the affected side 30–70 degrees, while the foot is in dorsiflexion)	Herniated disc
Neurologic	Decreased sensation, decreased motor strength, hyporeflexia (see Table 1.11 for more specific nerve root findings)	Mass effect, cord compression, nerve impingement
Rectal	Decreased anal sphincter tone	Cauda equina syndrome
	Enlarged or tender prostate	Prostatitis
Pelvic	Cervical discharge, cervical motion tenderness, adnexal tenderness	PID

PID, pelvic inflammatory disease.

such movements. A normal range for lumbar flexion is 75 to 90 degrees, 30 degrees for extension and rotation, and 35 degrees for lateral bending.[2,5]

Patients being evaluated for LBP must also have a focused neurologic examination completed by the examining provider, including an assessment of strength, sensation, and deep tendon reflexes (Table 1.11). Depending on the most likely differential diagnoses, patients may also need a cardiovascular, abdominal, pelvic, and/or rectal examination completed.

CLINICAL PEARL: Red flag findings suggestive of an urgent or emergent cause of LBP include fever, unexplained weight loss, recent infection, history of cancer, progressive or profound neurologic deficit, signs of sacral nerve root compression, urinary retention, saddle anesthesia, difficulty walking, and loss of bowel or bladder function.

TABLE **1.11** Correlating Nerve Root Involvement With Neurologic Exam Findings

Nerve Root	Reflex Affected	Motor Deficits	Sensory Deficits
L3	Patellar	Hip flexion, knee extension	Knee
L4	Patellar	Knee extension, ankle dorsiflexion	Medial foot
L5	None	Great toe/ankle dorsiflexion	Dorsal foot
S1	Achilles	Plantar flexion	Lateral foot

Diagnostic Plan

LABS

- CBC with differential: Indicated for evaluation of infectious causes of LBP or if malignancy is suspected

> **CLINICAL PEARL:** Fever and leukocytosis may NOT be present with osteomyelitis; if there is a high suspicion for this condition, imaging must be performed despite a normal CBC.

- Inflammatory markers (ESR, CRP): Indicated when there is suspicion for an inflammatory or infectious etiology
  - ESR and CRP may be elevated with the spondyloarthropathies
- Human leukocyte antigen (HLA)-B27: Indicated for evaluation of suspected spondyloarthropathy, specifically ankylosing spondylitis
- Serum protein electrophoresis: Indicated in the evaluation of suspected multiple myeloma, in which case an M-spike may be seen with this test
- Tumor markers (e.g., alpha fetoprotein, CA 19-9, CA 15-3, carcinoembryonic antigen [CEA], prostate-specific antigen [PSA], beta-2 microglobulin): May be indicated if there is concern for a specific type of malignancy

IMAGING

- Plain radiograph (x-ray): X-ray is an appropriate first-line imaging study to evaluate for compression fracture, tumor, or infection

> **CLINICAL PEARL:** In the absence of red flag findings, imaging is rarely indicated as a component of the initial evaluation. A trial of conservative treatment is most appropriate, and imaging should only be considered after 4 to 6 weeks of persistent symptoms.

- MRI without contrast: Indicated for patients with LBP requiring advanced or follow-up imaging. MRI may be appropriate as initial imaging in some situations, but the cost and time can be prohibitive in some situations.
  - Evaluate for all conditions for which plain radiograph evaluates and for disc disease, herniated disc, facet joint disease, spinal stenosis, spondylosis, spondylolisthesis, and cauda equina syndrome.

> **CLINICAL PEARL:** Judicial utilization of imaging with careful clinical correlation is required given the high rates of abnormal findings, even in asymptomatic individuals. For example, anywhere from 9% to 76% of asymptomatic patients will have a herniated disc on lumbar MRI.[5]

- CT imaging is rarely indicated for the evaluation of LBP, but may be utilized if MRI cannot be performed, or if a nonspinal etiology is suspected (e.g., aortic dissection, abdominal mass, or nephrolithiasis).

Initial Management

- The majority of cases of acute back pain are self-limited and will resolve with conservative, noninvasive treatment, including heat, exercise, physical therapy, acupuncture, massage, or spinal manipulation.[7]
- Patients should be educated to avoid heavy lifting, bending, twisting, or strenuous exercise during the acute phase; however, complete bed rest should also be avoided. Rather, patients should continue normal activities, as tolerated.
- Patient education should include information about the high rate of recurrences associated with LBP. Clinicians should encourage lifestyle changes that may help prevent these recurrences, such as maintaining a healthy weight and increasing the strength of core muscles (abdominal and back muscle groups).
- Pharmacologic treatment that can be considered for acute or subacute LBP includes NSAIDS and skeletal muscle relaxants. For persistent symptoms, pharmacologic options may include tramadol or duloxetine.[6]
- Short-term treatment with opioid analgesics may be appropriate for cases of severe discogenic pain that is refractory to treatment with NSAIDS. However, patients should be informed of the risks for dependence and addiction. Severe radicular pain may also be responsive to epidural corticosteroid treatment.
- Patients with chronic LBP may benefit from referral to a spine specialist/surgeon, cognitive behavioral therapy, or pain management.

Key Points ...

- Mechanical causes are the most common reason for a patient to experience LBP.
- Imaging is not necessary in most patients with acute, localized LBP without signs or symptoms of a serious underlying condition.
- Patients with a clinical presentation suspicious for infection, malignancy, or cauda equina syndrome as the underlying etiology for LBP should be emergently evaluated and treated.

(continued)

(continued)

- Pharmacologic management of acute LBP should include NSAIDS and/or skeletal muscle relaxants.
- Opioids should be avoided for the treatment of acute LBP except in cases of contraindications, intolerance, or unresponsiveness to NSAIDS.

REFERENCES

1. Maher C, Underwood M, Buchbinder R. Non-specific low back pain. *Lancet.* 2017;389:736–747. doi:10.1016/S0140-6736(16)30970-9
2. Luke A, Ma C. Sports medicine & outpatient orthopedics. In: Papadakis MA, McPhee SJ, Rabow MW, eds. *Current Medical Diagnosis & Treatment 2019.* New York, NY: McGraw-Hill; 2019.
3. Herndon CM, Zoberi KS, Gardner BJ. Common questions about chronic low back pain. *Am Fam Physician.* 2015;91(10):708–714.
4. Engstrom JW. Back and neck pain. In: Jameson J, Fauci AS, Kasper DL, et al., eds. *Harrison's Principles of Internal Medicine.* 20th ed. New York, NY: McGraw-Hill; 2018.
5. Kinkade SK. Evaluation and treatment of acute low back pain. *Am Fam Physician.* 2007;75(8):1182–1188.
6. Qaseem A, Wilt TJ, McLean RM, et al. Noninvasive treatments for acute, subacute, and chronic low back pain: a clinical practice guideline from the American college of physicians. *Ann Intern Med.* 2017;166:514–530. doi: 10.7326/M16-2367
7. Barreto TW, Lin KW. Noninvasive treatments for low back pain. *Am Fam Physician.* 2017;96(5):324–327.

SORE THROAT

Sore throat, or pharyngitis, is an extremely common reason for patients to seek medical care in the family medicine setting. Often, sore or irritated throats occur as a result of an infectious process; viral infections (e.g., adenovirus, rhinovirus, Epstein–Barr virus, herpes simplex virus) account for an estimated 60% to 90% of cases of pharyngitis.[1] Bacterial infections are the second leading cause for infectious pharyngitis, accounting for 5% to 30% of cases, depending upon the age of the population and the season of the year.[2] Pharyngitis is at the highest prevalence during the winter and early spring, and the highest incidence of cases occurs in children between 4 and 7 years of age.

In addition to infectious causes of sore throat, there are various other etiologies, including disease processes that originate from within and outside of the throat, as seen in Table 1.12. While there are many relatively benign reasons for a sore throat, there are also life-threatening conditions associated with sore throat; therefore, as with all chief complaints, a thorough evaluation is essential for the identification and appropriate management of more serious conditions.

Differential Diagnosis

TABLE **1.12** Differential Diagnosis of Sore Throat

Bacterial Infections	Viral Infections	Other
Group A beta-hemolytic streptococcus	Upper respiratory infection	Allergic rhinitis/postnasal drip
Nonstreptococcus, bacterial pharyngitis	Laryngitis	Gastroesophageal reflux
Corynebacterium diphtheria	Infectious mononucleosis	Inflammatory causes
	Herpetic gingivostomatitis	Dry mucosa
Neisseria gonorrhoeae	Hand, foot, and mouth disease	Chemical exposure
Fusobacterium necrophorum	Aphthous ulcer	Kawasaki disease
	Acute HIV infection	Behçet's syndrome Stevens–Johnson syndrome Foreign body Referred pain from extrapharyngeal source
Other anaerobic bacteria		
Epiglottitis		Dental abscess
Retropharyngeal abscess		Otitis media
Peritonsillar abscess		Otitis externa
Lateral pharyngeal abscess		Oral candidiasis
		Head/neck cancer
		Psychogenic cause

CLINICAL PEARL: Group A beta-hemolytic streptococcal (GABHS) infection is the most common bacterial cause of a sore throat. GABHS accounts for 5% to 10% of pharyngitis in adults and 15% to 30% in children.[2]

History

- Onset, duration, and timing: Determine whether the onset of the pain was acute or gradual. Acute onset pain is more likely with GABHS infections or epiglottitis, whereas viral infections typically have a more insidious onset. Determine the duration of the pain; chronic or recurrent pain may suggest a noninfectious etiology. Pain that is worse lying supine may be associated with gastric reflux, and pain worse in the mornings may be associated with postnasal drip.
- Provoking/alleviating factors: Ask about increased pain with swallowing or talking, or if symptoms worsen with exposure to common allergens, certain foods, or noxious chemicals (e.g., smoke inhalation). Determine whether the patient has attempted any medication (e.g., antihistamines, antacids, proton-pump inhibitors) and whether the pain was alleviated with use.
- Quality: Ask the patient about the quality of the pain. Often the pain will be described as sharp, burning, or scratching.
- Radiation/location: Pain isolated to one side of the throat may be associated with a peritonsillar abscess. Radiation to the ears, jaw, or chest may indicate an extrapharyngeal source of pain (e.g., GERD with chest radiation).
- Severity: Pain high on the severity scale is often associated with bacterial infections.

> **CLINICAL PEARL:** Patients with epiglottitis or peritonsillar abscess characteristically have pain so severe that they are drooling on examination due to being unwilling to swallow because of the pain.

- Associated symptoms: In addition to completing a full inquiry of all HEENT and general symptoms, it may also be pertinent to complete a ROS for GI symptoms and to evaluate for symptoms associated with autoimmune, rheumatologic, or vasculitic conditions.

Past Medical History Specific to Complaint

- Medical illnesses/comorbidities: Determine whether the patient has a medical history of recurrent GABHS infections, GERD, allergic rhinitis, or if they are immunocompromised.
- Medications: Inquire about recent use of medications, particularly medications associated with Stevens–Johnson syndrome, such as NSAIDS or sulfonamides. Determine whether the patient has taken antibiotics in the past 3 months.
- Family history: Determine whether there is a family history of any malignancies or respiratory conditions.
- Social history: Ask about tobacco or drug use, and about recent exposure to sick contacts.
- Travel history: Ask the patient whether they have traveled recently.
- Sexual history: Ask about high-risk sexual behaviors that may increase risk of acquiring sexually transmitted infections. Oral sex may be associated with acquiring HIV, herpes simplex virus, gonococcal pharyngitis, human papillomavirus, and syphilis.
- Vaccinations: Inquire about vaccination status.
- HEENT ROS: Ask about red eye, eye drainage, ear pain or discharge, ear swelling, dizziness, nasal congestion or drainage, sneezing, sinus pain, mouth sores, dental problems, hoarseness, headache, and increased or recurrent infections.
- General ROS: Ask about fever, weight loss or gain, fatigue, and malaise.
- Pulmonary ROS: Ask about cough, shortness of breath, wheezing, and dyspnea.
- GI ROS: Ask about gastric reflux, heartburn, nausea, and vomiting.

Physical Examination

Complete a focused physical examination in all patients being evaluated for sore throat (Table 1.13). Perform a complete HEENT examination with the primary purpose being to identify if the sore throat is infectious in nature, and if it is more likely a viral or bacterial etiology. Most patients being evaluated for sore throat should have a general assessment, cardiac, and pulmonary examinations performed. Consider skin and abdominal examinations based on information obtained in the medical history.

TABLE 1.13 Sore Throat: Correlating Physical Exam Findings With Pathologic Conditions

Body System	Physical Exam Finding	Associated Clinical Condition
Vitals	Fever	Bacterial pharyngitis, epiglottitis, retropharyngeal abscess, peritonsillar abscess, or lateral pharyngeal abscess
General	Drooling, muffled voice, distressed appearance, tripod posturing	Epiglottitis
Skin	Viral exanthem (maculopapular rash)	Viral pharyngitis
	Scarlatiniform rash	GABHS
	Vesicular lesions of hands/feet	Hand, foot, and mouth disease
HEENT	Conjunctivitis, coryza	Viral pharyngitis
	Tonsillopharyngeal erythema and edema +/− exudate	Infectious mononucleosis, GABHS
	Palatal petechiae	GABHS
	Oropharyngeal vesicles or ulcers	Herpangina, hand, foot, and mouth disease
	White plaques of oropharyngeal mucosa	Oral candidiasis
	Deviation of uvula (to contralateral side), bulging of soft palate	Peritonsillar abscess
	Gray pseudomembrane	Diphtheria
	Erythema or bulging of the tympanic membrane	Otitis media
	Erythema, edema, or exudate of the external ear canal	Otitis externa
	Gingival erythema, edema, or abscess	Dental abscess
Neck	Anterior cervical lymphadenopathy	GABHS
	Posterior cervical lymphadenopathy	Infectious mononucleosis
	Neck asymmetry or mass	Retropharyngeal, peritonsillar, or lateral pharyngeal abscess
	Trismus, submandibular swelling	Lateral pharyngeal abscess
Pulmonary	Cough	Viral pharyngitis
	Respiratory distress	Deep neck infection (causing obstruction of airway)
	Stridor	Epiglottitis
Gastrointestinal	Hepatosplenomegaly	Infectious mononucleosis

GABHS, Group A beta-hemolytic streptococcal.

CLINICAL PEARL: Life-threatening causes of sore throat include epiglottitis, retropharyngeal abscess, lateral pharyngeal abscess, peritonsillar abscess, and diphtheria.

Diagnostic Plan

LABS

- Rapid antigen detection test (RADT; "rapid strept"): Indicated to evaluate for GABHS infections at the point of care. This test is useful for evaluating patients at intermediate risk for GABHS based on their clinical presentation.
  - A positive RADT is considered diagnostic for GABHS infection.

> **CLINICAL PEARL:** A negative RADT may need to be followed by a throat culture for confirmation, especially in children, who are at higher risk of complications from GABHS infection, including peritonsillar abscess, rheumatic fever, and poststreptococcal glomerulonephritis.

- Heterophile antibody test ("monospot"): Indicated to evaluate for infectious mononucleosis. Some facilities offer this test at the point of care.
  - Limitations of this test include a high false-negative rate early in disease, and other viral infections besides Epstein–Barr virus can cause a positive result.[3]
- Throat culture: Indicated to evaluate for a bacterial cause of pharyngitis
- CBC with differential: Indicated when there is suspicion for an infectious etiology. Leukocytosis with a left shift is consistent with bacterial causes, whereas leukopenia may occur with viral etiologies.

> **CLINICAL PEARL:** Atypical lymphocytosis is often seen with infectious mononucleosis.

- HIV antigen/antibody testing: Indicated to evaluate for an acute HIV infection

> **CLINICAL PEARL:** It can take several weeks for HIV antibody tests to be positive with a newly acquired infection. If a new infection is suspected, it is critical to order antigen testing along with antibody testing.

  - Liver enzymes: May be useful in cases of suspected infectious mononucleosis as liver enzymes frequently rise with this infection

IMAGING

- Lateral neck x-ray: Indicated in the evaluation of ill-appearing patients with difficulty swallowing. A "thumb sign" may be appreciated in patients with epiglottitis.
- CT neck with IV contrast: Indicated for further evaluation of suspected deep neck infections

OTHER

- Centor criteria:[4] While not a diagnostic test per se, the Centor criteria are commonly utilized to help guide clinical decision-making in the diagnosis of GABHS pharyngitis. There are four main criteria, with each factor earning a score of one point: (a) fever, (b) anterior cervical lymphadenopathy, (c) tonsillar swelling or exudate, and (d) the absence of cough. Age is sometimes utilized as a fifth criterion since GABHS infections are more common in children. If using age as an additional factor, children aged 3 to 14 years earn one additional point, and adults over 45 years have one point subtracted from their Centor score.
  - ○ Patients with a Centor score of 2 to 3 points should have a RADT or throat culture performed as a component of their diagnostic evaluation.

> **CLINICAL PEARL:** A Centor score of ≤1 point indicates symptomatic treatment and monitoring are most appropriate, without a need for diagnostic tests or antibiotics. A score of ≥4 points indicates that empiric treatment with antibiotics should be initiated.

Initial Management

- Determine whether the pain is suggestive of an infectious or noninfectious etiology. If infection is suspected, determine whether the infection is more likely viral or bacterial.
- Consider inpatient management if epiglottitis or a deep neck infection is suspected, or if the patient is clinically unstable.
- In a distressed patient exhibiting signs of airway obstruction do not attempt physical examination or any procedures (e.g., throat swab) unless you are prepared to perform emergent airway management.
- Complete appropriate point-of-care testing to further the evaluation and diagnosis (e.g., RADT, monospot testing).
- If GABHS is suspected, empirical treatment with penicillin is indicated. In patients allergic to penicillin, cephalosporins, clindamycin, and macrolides are all reasonable alternatives. If the allergic reaction to penicillin involved an IgE-mediated anaphylactic-type reaction, cephalosporins should be avoided due to the risk of cross-reactivity.

> **CLINICAL PEARL:** Instruct patients to complete the entire prescription of antibiotics even though symptoms will begin to improve, if not resolve, after 48 to 72 hours.

- Antibiotic treatment for patients with viral infections or noninfectious etiologies is completely inappropriate, despite patient requests. Time should be spent on patient education emphasizing the disease process and the implications of inappropriate antibiotic prescribing, as well as recommendations for appropriate symptomatic treatment.

- In cases of severe edema causing oropharyngeal obstruction, such as with infectious mononucleosis, corticosteroid treatment may be appropriate.
- Consider other appropriate treatment options for noninfectious etiologies of sore throat, such as antihistamines and/or intranasal corticosteroids for allergic rhinitis and postnasal drip, antacids or proton-pump inhibitors for GERD, or topical antifungals for oral candidiasis.
- Symptomatic treatment in the form of rest, liquids, and analgesics should be encouraged. Analgesia may be provided in the form of acetaminophen or NSAIDS. Medicated throat lozenges and topical anesthetics can also be utilized.

Key Points ...

- Viruses are the most common cause of infectious pharyngitis; of bacterial causes for pharyngitis, GABHS is most common.
- The following features are suggestive of a bacterial cause for pharyngitis: age 5 to 15 years, fever, tonsillopharyngeal inflammation and/or exudates, palatal petechiae, anterior cervical lymphadenopathy, history of exposure to streptococcal pharyngitis, scarlatiniform rash.
- The following features are suggestive of a viral cause for pharyngitis: conjunctivitis, coryza, diarrhea, hoarseness, ulcerative stomatitis, viral exanthem.
- Diagnostic algorithms, such as Centor criteria, are useful for developing evaluation and management plans for patients presenting with an infectious etiology for sore throat.
- Complications from GABHS infection can include poststreptococcal glomerulonephritis and rheumatic fever.
- Remember to consider and appropriately manage noninfectious etiologies for sore throat.

References

1. Williams BD, Usatine RP, Smith MA. Pharyngitis. In: Usatine RP, Smith MA, Chumley HS, et al., eds. *The Color Atlas of Family Medicine.* 2nd ed. New York, NY: McGraw-Hill; 2013.
2. Choby BA. Diagnosis and treatment of streptococcal pharyngitis. *Am Fam Physician.* 2009;79(5):383–390.
3. Marshall-Andon T, Heinz P. How to use ... the monospot and other heterophile antibody tests. *Arc Dis Child Educ Pract Ed.* 2017;102:188–193. doi:10.1136/archdischild-2016-311526
4. McIsaac WJ, White D, Tannenbaum D, Low DE. A clinical score to reduce unnecessary antibiotic use in patients with sore throat. *Can Med Assoc J.* 1998;158(1):75–83.

2

Common Disease Entities in Family Medicine

CARDIOLOGY

CORONARY ARTERY DISEASE: CHRONIC STABLE

Etiology

Chronic stable coronary artery disease (CAD) is defined as the existence of a reversible myocardial perfusion defect, previous infarction, or the objective evidence of plaques confirmed through coronary artery catheterization and/or CT angiography.

Epidemiology

Coronary heart disease remains the leading cause of cardiovascular death in the United States, accounting for one in seven deaths (>366,800). The incidence of CAD increases with age and is more common in men. The mortality rate has continued to decline over the past decade secondary to medical advances and the aggressive patient education campaigns that focus on lifestyle changes and risk factor modification.[1] Risk factors for the development of CAD include hypertension (HTN), hyperlipidemia, diabetes, and tobacco use.

Clinical Presentation

Patients may complain of chest discomfort, pain, or pressure that is associated with increased activity, cold, large meals, or stress. The pain is described as a tightness, burning, or squeezing centered behind the sternum. This pain may radiate into the neck, jaw, shoulder, or arm. The pain/discomfort may also be accompanied by difficulty breathing, nausea, diaphoresis, or vomiting. Patients with diabetes mellitus (DM), elderly patients, and women can present with atypical symptoms such as difficulty breathing without chest pain or discomfort. The patient's medical and/or family histories are often positive for

HTN, hyperglycemia, hyperlipidemia, obesity, and smoking. Family history of premature CAD may be considered when quantitative risk-based assessment is uncertain.

> **CLINICAL PEARL:** Unstable angina (UA) differs from stable disease in that it occurs with increased frequency and duration and is severe, unprovoked, and/or occurs at rest.

Physical examination may be normal. General findings of obesity and HTN are common. Examination of the eyes can reveal diabetic or hypertensive retinopathy. Jugular venous distension (JVD) may be present secondary to right ventricular overload/failure. Pulmonary edema (crackles) and diminished breath sounds at the lung bases due to fluid can be present on auscultation. The cardiovascular exam may identify arrhythmias, heart murmurs, gallops, or a shift of in the point of maximal impulse (PMI). Carotid, aortic, renal, and/or femoral bruits and diminished peripheral pulses may be found on examination. On the abdominal exam, ascites and hepatomegaly secondary to passive congestion may be present. Peripheral edema may be found secondary to heart failure (HF).

Diagnosis
Laboratory findings can reveal elevated lipid and serum glucose levels. On electrocardiography pathologic Q waves, left ventricular hypertrophy (LVH), arrhythmias, and conduction defects may be present. The chest x-ray (CXR) may show cardiomegaly, pulmonary edema, and aortic calcifications. Echocardiography can also show LVH, reduced ejection fraction, and wall motion abnormalities. Exercise stress testing can also confirm the presence of CAD. Positive findings include poor exercise capacity, exercise-induced angina, abnormalities in systolic blood pressure (BP), chronotropic incompetence, >2-mm ST depression, multiple leads with ST depressions, ST segment elevation, and ventricular ectopy.

Management
Risk reduction:

- BP control: Maintain levels <130/80[2]
- Lipids
  - Robust evidence exists that lipid-lowering drugs (statins) have benefit for primary and secondary prevention of atherosclerotic cardiovascular disease (ASCVD) events. The evidence is strongest for statins. Moderate- to high-intensity statin is indicated if the risk for an ASCVD event is 7.5% or greater. An ASCVD risk calculator can be found at www.cvriskcalculator.com.
  - Guidelines recommend checking lipid levels 1 to 3 months after starting statins. Recommendations for further follow-up laboratory testing vary.[3]
  - American College of Cardiology/American Heart Association (ACC/AHA) 2018 guidelines recommend assessing a patient's 10-year CVD risk every 4 to 6 years in adults 40 to 75 years old and

without CVD, DM, not yet on lipid therapy, and those with low-density lipoprotein (LDL) 70 to 189 mg/dL.

○ Lipid-lowering therapy is recommended for the following populations:

- Patients with any form of clinical ASCVD
- Patients with primary LDL-C levels of 190 mg/dL or greater
- Patients with DM, 40 to 75 years of age, with LDL-C levels >70 mg/dL
- Patients without diabetes, 40 to 75 years of age, with an estimated 10-year ASCVD risk ≥7.5%
- Specific recommendations include the following:
  - High-intensity statin in those with CVD and age ≤75
  - High-intensity statin in those with LDL-C >190
  - Moderate- or high-intensity statin for type 1 DM (DM-1) or type 2 DM (DM-2) aged 40 to 75
  - Moderate- to high-intensity statin for 40 to 75 years olds with >7.5% 10-year CVD risk[3]

- Glucose control: Goal A1C <7%[4]
- Weight control: Nutritional counseling on how to follow a heart healthy diet, maintain a body mass index (BMI) <25 (at least 10% baseline)
- Smoking cessation: Referral for active participation in support groups, counseling, and pharmacologic treatment combined
- Physical activity as tolerated: Participation in a structured cardiopulmonary rehabilitation program, maintaining or increasing (30–60 minutes) of moderate-intensity aerobic activity 5 days a week
- Annual flu vaccine

Medical therapy is detailed in Table 2.1. Daily antianginal medication options include beta-blockers, calcium channel blockers, long-acting nitrates, and ranolazine. Sublingual nitroglycerin is indicated for immediate relief of chest pain.

TABLE 2.1 Medical Therapy for Coronary Artery Disease

	Lipid Lowering Drugs (Based on ASCVD Risk)	Antiplatelet Drugs	Antianginal Drugs
First-Line Therapy	High intensity: Atorvastatin 40–80 mg daily Rosuvastatin 20–40 mg daily	Aspirin	Metoprolol Atenolol Bisoprolol **In heart failure use:** Metoprolol Carvedilol
Alternative/ Adjunctive Therapy	Moderate intensity: Atorvastatin 10–20 mg daily Rosuvastatin 5–10 mg daily Simvastatin 20–40 mg daily Pravastatin 40–80 mg daily Lovastatin 40 mg daily	Clopidogrel Ticagrelor Prasugrel	Amlodipine Nifedipine Isosorbide mononitrate or dinitrate Verapamil[a] Diltiazem[a] Ranolazine[b]

ASCVD, atherosclerotic cardiovascular disease.
[a] Contraindicated in patients with left ventricular dysfunction.
[b] Prolongs QTI, contraindicated with liver impairment.

> **CLINICAL PEARL:** There are no data to support the use of nonstatin medications to reduce the risk of mortality in patients with cardiovascular disease.[5]

Cardiology referral should be considered if the patient's symptoms are refractory to medical treatment; history and/or noninvasive testing is positive for left ventricular dysfunction, multivessel disease, left main disease, or disease involving the proximal left anterior descending artery.

REFERENCES

1. Benjamin EJ, Virani SS, Callaway CW, et al. Heart disease and stroke statistics—2018. A report from the American Heart Association. *Circulation*. 2018;137:e67–e492. doi:10.1161/CIR.0000000000000573
2. Whelton PK, Carey RM, Aronow WS, et al. ACC/AHA/AAPA/ABC/ACPM/AGS/APhA/ASH/ASPC/NMA/PCNA guideline for the prevention, detection, evaluation, and management of high blood pressure in adults. *Hypertension*. 2018;71(6):1269–1324. doi:10.1161/HYP.0000000000000066
3. Last AR, Ference JD, Rollmann ME. Hyperlipidemia: drugs for cardiovascular risk reduction in adults. *Am Fam Physician*. January 15, 2017;95(2):78–87B.
4. ACCORD Study Group. Nine-year effects of 3.7 years of intensive glycemic control on cardiovascular outcomes. *Diabetes Care*. 2016;39(5):701–708. doi:10.2337/dc15-2283
5. Braun MM, Stevens WA, Barstow CH. Stable coronary artery disease: treatment. *Am Fam Physician*. 2018;97(6):376–384.

EDEMA: LOWER EXTREMITY

Etiology

Edema occurs as a result of increased extracellular volume in conditions where:

- Hydrostatic pressure exceeds colloid oncotic pressure
- There is an increase in capillary permeability
- Lymphatic obstruction is present

Bilateral lower extremity edema is a common finding in the elderly population and the underlying etiology can range from benign, such as venous insufficiency, to serious, such as venous thrombosis. Lower extremity edema should be classified as acute if present <72 hours or chronic if present >72 hours. Note whether the edema is unilateral or bilateral, as the etiology and treatment will differ.[1] Common causes of edema are outlined in Table 2.2. Less common causes of lower extremity edema include Baker's cyst rupture, reflex sympathetic dystrophy, liver disease, nephrotic syndrome, constrictive pericarditis, myxedema, and malnutrition.

Epidemiology

The most common causes include venous insufficiency, HF, medication adverse effects, and pulmonary hypertension. The sudden onset of unilateral edema is concerning for a deep venous thrombosis and requires prompt assessment.

TABLE 2.2 Common Causes of Lower Extremity Edema

Bilateral Edema	Unilateral Edema
Venous insufficiency	Venous insufficiency
Heart failure	Deep venous thrombosis
Pulmonary hypertension	Lymphedema
Hypoalbuminemia	
Medications	

Source: Trayes, K. P., Studdiford, J. Sl, Pickle, S., et al. (2013). Edema: diagnosis and management. *American Family Physician,* 88(2):102–110.

Clinical Presentation

When obtaining the patient's history, be sure to clarify the timing of edema. Sudden onset of edema may occur with conditions such as thrombus or cellulitis. Edema that worsens throughout the day as the patient is ambulating is suggestive of venous insufficiency and may cause stasis changes. Edema secondary to venous inefficiency typically improves after the patient is supine at night, while edema of HF will persist despite elevation of the legs. Chronic, generalized edema is more likely to represent HF, renal insufficiency, or end stage liver disease. Conditions such as obstructive sleep apnea, chronic obstructive pulmonary disease (COPD), thyroid disorders, cancer, trauma, previous pelvic surgery, inguinal lymphadenectomy, or previous radiation therapy can contribute to the edema. Vasodilators, such as calcium channel blockers, can lead to swelling while nonsteroidal anti-inflammatory drug (NSAID) or steroid use can be associated with fluid retention.

> **CLINICAL PEARL:** During the history, identify any risk factors for DVT such as malignancy, estrogen therapy, recent travel, recent surgery, and immobilization.

On the physical examination, search for signs suggestive of the underlying cause. Positive skin findings may include ulcerations and weeping, which can be seen with venous insufficiency. Thickened, dough-like, dorsal foot swelling with squared off toes, jaundice, and spider angiomata are associated with underlying liver disease. Shiny, atrophic skin is seen with reflex sympathetic dystrophy. Exophthalmos, a diffusely enlarged or a nodular thyroid, is suggestive of thyroid pathology. JVD can be seen with HF, in addition to pulmonary crackles or rales, extra heart sounds, and a new murmur. Key physical exam findings of DVT include differences in calf circumference, tenderness along deep veins, prominence of collateral veins, a palpable cord, and pitting edema.

When examining the lower extremities, pay attention to bony architecture, including the tibia, medial malleolus, and dorsum of foot. A brawny, nonpitting edema that is unilateral or bilateral is more likely to be associated with lymphedema, while pitting edema is associated with DVT, HF, or iliac vein compression. Increased temperature is more consistent with cellulitis or DVT. Pretibial myxedema is associated with Graves' disease. Resting tremors or asterixis can be noted on the neurological exam in patients with cirrhosis.

Diagnosis

Laboratory studies may include a D-dimer and/or a hypercoagulable workup (protein C, S, antithrombin III, lupus anticoagulant, Factor V Leiden, prothrombin variant, fibrinogen, activated protein C [APC] resistance) to support a diagnosis of thrombus formation. A complete blood count (CBC) may reveal leukocytosis with neutrophilia suggesting infection/inflammation. A metabolic panel should be ordered to evaluate renal function and sodium levels. A hepatic profile showing an elevation in aminotransferases and bilirubin is consistent with liver disease. Low serum albumin can be seen in liver disease, renal disease, and malnutrition states. A urinalysis with proteinuria can be seen with renal insufficiency. Imaging studies along with their diagnosis are included in Table 2.3.

Management

Primary therapy should address the underlying cause:

- General management when associated with an increase in hydrostatic pressure: restrict salt intake, avoid long periods of standing or sitting, leg elevation, use of support stockings, avoid tight-fitting garments
- Venous insufficiency: Leg elevation, compression stockings, pneumatic compression devices, which are contraindicated in patients with peripheral artery disease
- Lymphedema: Physiotherapy with manual massage and multilayer bandages, compression stockings, and pneumatic compression devices
- Venous thrombosis: Low-molecular-weight heparin, or an alternative anticoagulant, and compression stockings. Cases of proximal DVT should be treated with catheter-directed thrombolysis.
- Medication related: Discontinue the offending medication

TABLE 2.3 Diagnostic Evaluation of Lower Extremity Edema

Diagnostic Test	Indication
Ankle-brachial index testing: findings may impact treatment options (i.e., compression therapy in venous insufficiency)	Risk factors for peripheral arterial disease
CT venography	Unilateral edema and suspected pulmonary embolus
Duplex ultrasonography	Chronic venous insufficiency, thrombus
Echocardiogram	Evaluate ventricular function, valvulopathy, evidence of pulmonary hypertension
MR venography	Pelvic or distal DVT
MR lymphangiography	Signs and symptoms suggestive of lymphatic obstruction
Polysomnography	Signs and symptoms of sleep apnea such as excessive daytime somnolence, snoring
Radiography	Evaluate for trauma
Venous compression ultrasound with doppler	Signs and symptoms of DVT such as unilateral erythema, edema, risk factors for venous stasis

DVT, deep venous thrombosis; MR, magnetic resonance.

Source: Trayes, K. P., Studdiford, J. S., Pickle, S., et al. (2013). Edema: diagnosis and management. *American Family Physician, 88*(2):102–110.

REFERENCES

1. Trayes KP, Studdiford JS, Pickle S, et al. Edema: diagnosis and management. *Am Fam Physician.* 2013;88(2):102–110. doi:10.1097/ACM.0b013e318277d5b2

HEART FAILURE

Etiology

HF is a condition that occurs when the cardiac muscle is no longer able to pump blood to deliver the oxygen and nutrients required to meet the body's metabolic demands, resulting in the principal symptoms of dyspnea and fatigue. Heart failure can occur from ischemic and nonischemic causes. HF is categorized using the following physiological patterns:

- High output: Occurs due to decreased systemic vascular resistance, decreased arterial–venous oxygen gradient, and an elevated cardiac output (CO). Examples include aortic insufficiency, mitral regurgitation, ventricular septal defect, arteriovenous (AV) fistulas, anemia, sepsis, thyrotoxicosis, Paget's disease, and Beriberi.
- Low output: Impairment of left ventricular pumping results in decreased CO and end-organ hypoperfusion
- Left sided: Occurs due to a reduction in left ventricular function and CO, secondary to ischemic and nonischemic causes
- Right sided: Occurs due to a reduction in right or left ventricular function, characterized by a low output syndrome. Right-sided HF is most often due to left-sided HF.
- Systolic: Inability to eject sufficient blood
- Diastolic: Impaired relaxation and filling

HF can be classified into two major subtypes:

- HF with preserved ejection fraction (HFpEF) or left ventricular ejection fraction (LVEF) $\geq$50%
- HF with reduced ejection fraction (HFrEF) or LVEF <50%

Epidemiology

In order to better identify and manage patients with or who are at high risk for developing HF, the American College of Cardiology Foundation and American Heart Association (ACCF/AHA) have identified several stages of disease progression, as outlined in Table 2.4. Identifying those patients who are at risk for HF (Stages A and B), educating them about how to manage modifiable risk factors, and arranging for close follow-up can result in a reduction in patient morbidity and mortality.[1] The majority of HF patients fall in Stage B.

TABLE 2.4 Heart Failure Stages

Stage	Definition
A	Patients with risk factors but no evidence of structural heart disease
B	Patients with structural heart disease but have no presenting signs or symptoms
C	Patients with a history of or current signs or symptoms of heart failure
D	Patients with refractory failure requiring specialty treatments

HF is a major cause of morbidity and mortality nationwide. Americans over the age of 40 years have a 20% lifetime risk for developing HF. Data from the Framingham Study revealed that the incidence of HF is 10 per 1,000 in patients >65 years of age. According to a 2012 National Center for Health Statistics brief, it is estimated that there are 5.7 million adults in the United States living with HF and one million annual hospitalizations for HF. The prevalence continues to increase due to the improved survival of those diagnosed and treated with this disease; however, the median survival time once the patient becomes symptomatic is 5 years. Men and women are affected equally.[2,3] The most common risk factor for developing HF is CAD. Additional risk factors include hypertensive heart disease, valvular heart disease, and cardiomyopathies.

Those patients with HFpEF are more likely to be older, white, female, and have a history of atrial fibrillation or flutter, mitral or aortic valvular disease, pericardial diseases that impact diastolic function, or chronic lung disease in addition to the classic risk factors of underlying cardiovascular disease. They may present with a milder form of HF and have a lower risk of cardiovascular mortality. Epidemiologic studies during recent years have suggested that the prevalence of HFpEF is increasing over time relative to that of HFrEF in the United States.[4] Patients with HFrEF are those with underlying left ventricular systolic dysfunction. HFrEF can be due to ischemic causes such as myocardial infarction (MI) or nonischemic causes including alcohol use, tachycardia induced, viral related, and idiopathic causes.

Clinical Presentation

A complete personal and family medical history of CAD, diabetes, and HTN is critical to determine the patient's severity of illness and risk factors. Additional comorbidities can alter the clinical presentation of HF. Patients may present with signs and symptoms related to inadequate coronary perfusion or volume overload. General symptoms can include fatigue, weakness, decreased exercise tolerance, and sleep disorders. Cardiac and pulmonary symptoms that are associated with elevated filling pressures and passive congestion include shortness of breath, orthopnea, paroxysmal nocturnal dyspnea (PND), peripheral edema, chest pain, and palpitations. Patients who have right-sided HF can complain of right upper quadrant (RUQ) discomfort secondary to passive liver congestion. Patients may complain of reduced urinary output. Neurological complaints can include confusion, disorientation, and memory lapses. The extremities may appear mottled, cool, and have diminished pulses, and associated peripheral edema.

Precipitating causes of an acute decompensation of HF may include acute coronary syndrome, acute valvular disease such as aortic/mitral regurgitation secondary to infective endocarditis, thrombosed prosthetic valve, progressive chronic valvular disease, arrhythmias, uncontrolled HTN, or aortic dissection. Decompensation of chronic HF is commonly due to poorly controlled HTN, rhythm disturbances, infections, or nonadherence to medications and/or diet.

CLINICAL PEARL: Patients who have a history of chronic HF may adjust to their symptoms and may not recognize, or they may even minimize, their symptoms.

Routine examination with each encounter should include vital signs, weight, estimates of jugular venous pressure (JVP), and peripheral edema. General findings on exam are often reflective of volume overload and can include hypo- or HTN, orthostatic changes, narrowed pulse pressure, tachycardia, irregular pulse, and increased weight. Findings on skin exam can include jaundice, diaphoresis, and cyanosis. Examination of the lungs may reveal rales, tachypnea, and dullness to percussion of the lung bases secondary to effusion. Cardiac exam findings may include extra heart sounds such as S_3 and/or S_4, heart murmur, and/or elevated JVP. Abdominal findings can include hepatomegaly, ascites, jaundice, and/or hepatojugular reflux. Extremity exam may reveal peripheral edema, cool extremities, mottling, or reduced capillary refill. Neurological findings can include mental status changes, confusion, and disorientation.

Patients presenting with acute pulmonary edema are often tachypneic, exhibit the use of accessory muscles, have an abnormal lung exam (crackles), and room air oxygen saturation <90%. Those patients considered to be in cardiogenic shock have systolic BP <90 mmHg, a drop in mean arterial pressure (MAP) >30 mmHg, and urine output <0.5 mL/kg/hr. Exam findings of high output failure include tachycardia, warm extremities, pulmonary edema, and hypotension. Specific findings seen with right HF include increased JVP, RUQ tenderness, hepatomegaly, edema, and hypotension.

> **CLINICAL PEARL:** The most useful clinical findings that increase the diagnosis of HF are a prior history of HF, presence of PND, S_3 gallop, CXR with pulmonary venous congestion, and atrial fibrillation.

> **CLINICAL PEARL:** The differential diagnosis of acute decompensated HF should include other noncardiac conditions that can cause acute respiratory distress such as pulmonary embolism, pneumonia, and asthma.

Diagnosis

Laboratory evaluation should be individualized based on the patient history and exam findings and may include the following:

- CBC: Evaluate for dilutional anemia due to volume overload, secondary erythrocytosis from chronic lung disease
- Blood glucose: To identify hyperglycemia
- Arterial blood gas or end tidal CO_2: Can be seen with early respiratory failure and acidosis with hypoperfusion
- D-dimer: May be elevated with hemodynamically significant pulmonary embolus
- Arterial saturation: To assure adequate oxygenation ≥94%
- Complete metabolic panel: To evaluate metabolic, hepatic, and renal function
- Lipid profile: For ASCVD risk stratification

- Thyroid-stimulating hormone (TSH): To rule out hypo- or hyperthyroidism as a contributing factor
- Urinalysis: To evaluate for proteinuria, hematuria
- Brain natriuretic peptide: When elevated can be useful to support the diagnosis of HF
- Cardiac troponin: Can identify myocardial injury/necrosis, acute decompensated HF, and guide risk stratification, prognosis
- In selected patients, levels of the following may be indicated: ferritin, human immunodeficiency virus (HIV), plasma metanephrines, protein electrophoresis, antinuclear antibodies (ANA) if the clinical picture is suggestive of a secondary etiology

Imaging can be fairly extensive in order to appropriately diagnose the patient and should be individualized:

- 12 lead EKG: Indicated in all patients who present for evaluation of HF to evaluate for ST-T wave ischemic changes, LVH, pathologic Q waves indicative of previous infarction, arrhythmias
- CXR: To evaluate for cardiomegaly, pulmonary edema, bilateral effusions R>L, pneumonia
- Echocardiogram: Initial evaluation with echo should be performed in all patients presenting with HF in order to assess ventricular function. Increased chamber size, presence of hypertrophy can be seen with HFrEF. Abnormal valve function, such as the abnormal flow across mitral valve, can be seen with HRpEF. Estimates of pulmonary pressures, stroke volume, and the presence of wall motion abnormalities can also be identified.
- Right heart catheterization: May be indicated in the acutely ill patient, resistant to therapy, patients with multiorgan system failure (MOSF), can measure the pulmonary capillary wedge pressure (PCWP), which may be elevated, reduced CO, and an elevated systemic vascular resistance (SVR)
- Magnetic resonance imaging: If echo is nondiagnostic, this can be helpful in evaluating right ventricular size and function and uncommon conditions such as infiltrative diseases and myocarditis
- Nuclear medicine stress test: Assess for ischemia and viable heart muscle
- Coronary angiography: When ischemia is suspected and percutaneous intervention may be pursued

Management

General recommendations as guided by HF stage are outlined in Table 2.5. The initial pharmacologic management should include beta-blockers, angiotensin-converting enzyme inhibitors (ACE-I)/angiotensin II receptor blockers (ARBs), with loop diuretics as needed. Additional medications that may be added if symptoms persist include aldosterone receptor antagonists, digoxin, and a neprilysin inhibitor/ARB combination, such as sacubitril/valsartan. A neprilysin inhibitor/ARB combination compared to an ACE inhibitor alone has been found to reduce the occurrence of cardiovascular death or hospitalization for HF by 20% along with a 16% reduction in all-cause mortality. These findings suggest that sacubitril/valsartan should replace ACE inhibitors or angiotensin receptor blockers as the foundation of treatment of symptomatic patients with HFrEF.[5] A summary of the medication options for HF is presented in Tables 2.6 through 2.9.

TABLE 2.5 Treatment Guide Using Heart Failure Progression Stages A to D

Stage	Management
A	Maximize treatment for underlying risk factors (hypertension, diabetes, hypercholesterolemia)
	Smoking cessation, alcohol cessation, routine exercise plan
	ACE/ARB especially in those patients with coexisting vascular disease and DM
	Statins when indicated for other causes
B	As earlier plus beta-blockers in all patients with reduced EF, risk for malignant ventricular arrhythmias, ischemia/infarction, decompensated heart failure with ICD placement, coronary revascularization, valve repair/replacement
C	Neprilysin inhibitor/ARB, beta-blockers, diuretics, aldosterone antagonists for volume retention, digitalis, isosorbide, hydralazine
D	End of life care. Selected patients: transplantation, chronic inotropes, mechanical support, clinical trials for experimental therapies (surgical, medical)

ACE/ARB, Angiotensin-converting enzyme/Angiotensin II receptor blockers; DM, diabetes mellitus; EF, ejection fraction; ICD, implantable cardioverter-defibrillator.

> **CLINICAL PEARL:** Patients with acute decompensated HF should not be treated with beta-blockers until they have stabilized. Nondihydropyridine calcium channel blockers are contraindicated in patients with reduced LVEF.

> **CLINICAL PEARL:** Caution with use of diuretics when managing diastolic dysfunction.

TABLE 2.6 ACE Inhibitors for Use in Heart Failure Patients With Left Ventricular Systolic Dysfunction

Medication	Starting Dose Daily	Maximum Daily Dose
Captopril	6.25 mg three times daily	50 mg three times daily
Enalapril	2.5 mg twice daily	10–20 mg twice daily
Fosinopril	5–10 mg once daily	40 mg once daily
Lisinopril	2.5–5.0 mg once daily	20–40 mg once daily
Perindopril	2 mg once daily	8–16 mg once daily
Quinapril	10 mg twice daily	40 mg twice daily
Ramipril	1.25–2.5 mg once daily	10 mg once daily
Trandolapril	1 mg once daily	4 mg once daily

ACE, angiotensin-converting enzyme.

TABLE 2.7 ARBs for Use in Heart Failure Patients With Intolerance to ACE Inhibitors

Medication	Starting Dose	Maximum Daily Dose
Candesartan	4–8 mg once daily	32 mg once daily
Losartan	25–50 mg once daily	150 mg once daily
Valsartan	20–40 mg twice daily	160 mg twice daily

ARB, angiotensin II receptor blocker.

TABLE 2.8 Diuretics to Manage Volume Overload in Heart Failure Patients

Medication	Starting Dose	Maximum Daily Dose
Bumetanide	0.5–1.0 mg once or twice daily	10 mg
Furosemide	20–40 mg once or twice daily	600 mg
Torsemide	10–20 mg once daily	200 mg
Chlorothiazide	250–500 mg once or twice daily	1000 mg
Chlorthalidone	12.5–25 mg once daily	100 mg
Hydrochlorothiazide	25 mg once or twice daily	200 mg
Indapamide	2.5 mg once daily	5 mg
Metalozone	2.5 mg once daily	20 mg
Amiloride	5 mg once daily	20 mg
Spironolactone	12.5–25 mg once daily	25 mg twice daily
Triamterene	50–75 mg twice daily	200 mg
Eplerenone	25 mg once daily	50 mg once daily

TABLE 2.9 Beta-Blockers for Blood Pressure and Rate Control, Decreasing Workload of the Heart in Heart Failure Patients

Medication	Starting Dose	Maximum dose
Bisoprolol	1.25 mg once daily	10 mg once daily
Carvedilol	3.125 mg twice daily	50 mg twice daily
Metoprolol CR	12.5–25 mg once daily	200 mg once daily

Additional Treatment Indications:

- Aldosterone receptor antagonist: For patients with LVEF <35% and glomerular filtration rate (GFR) >30 mL/min/1.73 m^2 and K+ <5.0 mEq/L
- Hydralazine and/or nitrates: In black patient population with ACE/beta-blocker (BB) refractory HF
- Digoxin: Can be used in patients with reduced left ventricular function to improve symptoms
- Anticoagulation: If documented mural thrombi by echo or MRI, or in patients who have permanent/persistent and paroxysmal atrial fib and an additional risk factor (age >75 years old, history of stroke (h/o) stroke or transient ischemic attack, HTN, DM)

- Supplemental oxygen, noninvasive ventilatory support to maintain saturations >94%
- Routine use of invasive hemodynamic monitoring in patients with acutely decompensated HF is not recommended

Nonpharmacological management:
- Primary prevention: Identifying and maximizing therapy in those patients with known risk factors for HF, especially HTN, CAD, and diabetes, smoking, dyslipidemia, and family history
- Fluid restriction: 1.5 to 2 L/d with volume overload, especially in patients with hyponatremia
- Referral dietary education on heart healthy diet: Reduced sodium <2 g/d, limited fats
- Cardiac rehabilitation, exercise training
- Clinical: Daily weighing to monitor for rapid weight gain
- Monitor electrolytes, renal function with diuretic therapy
- All patients who are discharged from the hospital should see the provider within 7 to 14 days for follow-up

> **CLINICAL PEARL:** Acute decompensated HF is associated with high post-discharge readmission rates.

Surgical options:
- Cardiac resynchronization therapy with implantable defibrillator
- Mechanical circulatory support
- Cardiac transplantation

REFERENCES

1. Hunt SA, Abraham WT, Chin MH, et al. 2009 focused update incorporated into the ACC/AHA 2005 guidelines for the diagnosis and management of heart failure in adults: a report of the American College of Cardiology Foundation/American Heart Association task force on practice guidelines: developed. *Circulation.* 2009;119:e391–479. doi:10.1161/CIRCULATIONAHA.109.192065
2. Hall MJ, Levant S, DeFrances CJ. *Hospitalization for Congestive Heart Failure: United States, 2000–2010.* NCHS data brief, no 108. Hyattsville, MD: National Center for Health Statistics; 2012.
3. Ventura HO, Silver MA. Observations and reflections on the burden of hospitalizations for heart failure. *Mayo Clin Proc.* 2017;92:175–178. doi:10.1016/j.mayocp.2016.12.009
4. Goldberg RJ, Gurwitz JH, Saczynski JS, et al. Comparison of medication practices in patients with heart failure and preserved versus those with reduced ejection fraction. *Am J Cardiol.* 2013;111:1324–1329. doi:10.1016/j.amjcard.2013.01.276
5. Jhund PS, McMurray JJV. The neprilysin pathway in heart failure: a review and guide on the use of sacubitril/valsartan. *Heart.* 2016;102:1342–1347. doi:10.1136/heartjnl-2014-306775

HTN: PRIMARY

Etiology

HTN is a chronic state of elevation of BP beyond the normal range, with a complex etiology that occurs as a result of disturbances in hemodynamic parameters. Precipitating factors for primary HTN include an increase in peripheral vascular resistance, an enhanced sympathetic tone, and disruptions in the renin–angiotensin–aldosterone axis. Consider secondary hypertension as a cause in the initial evaluation and treatment of patients who present with new-onset HTN, particularly if they have severe or resistant HTN, present at a young age, and if they have severely high BP or evidence of end-organ damage.[1] Possible causes of secondary HTN include the following:

- Primary renal disease (parenchymal or vascular)
- Pheochromocytoma
- Hyperthyroidism
- Hyperaldosteronism
- Cushing's syndrome
- Coarctation of the aorta
- Obstructive sleep apnea
- Medications (stimulants, decongestants, oral contraceptives)

Epidemiology

HTN is common, affecting approximately 78 million people in the United States.[2] Primary HTN is responsible for 90% to 95% of cases.[1] Although the prevalence of HTN generally increases with age, in Blacks it has an earlier onset and tends to be more severe.[2] HTN has a familial tendency, and it is thought that it is caused by a mix of environmental and genetic factors.[2]

Risk Factors for Primary HTN:

- Family history of HTN
- Obesity
- Smoking
- Sedentary lifestyle
- Excessive alcohol consumption
- Older age

Clinical Presentation

New-onset primary HTN is often asymptomatic and detected on routine measurement of vital signs during an office visit. Patients may present with symptoms ranging from a mild headache, or less commonly, to life-threatening presentations such as encephalopathy. A comprehensive history and physical examination is necessary for a patient who presents with new-onset HTN.

Inquire about symptoms suggestive of HF, such as dyspnea, orthopnea, and lower extremity edema. Ischemic heart disease symptoms include chest pain or discomfort and palpitations. Because of the strong association of sleep apnea and HTN, ask about snoring and excessive daytime somnolence. Focal neurologic deficits should be elicited.

During the physical examination, review the current vital signs, including BMI, as well as personally measuring BP, in both arms, using proper technique with a cuff of the appropriate size. A thorough physical examination is necessary, and particular attention should be directed to the following areas of examination:

- Skin: Purple striae or other dermatologic signs of an endocrine disorder
- Eyes: Pupils for symmetry and reactivity, fundoscopic exam to evaluate for papilledema, and hypertensive retinopathy
- Neck: Circumference as a risk factor for obstructive sleep apnea; thyroid exam; evaluation for distended veins
- Lungs: Auscultate for signs of HF
- Cardiac: Auscultate heart for rate and rhythm, evaluation for murmurs, and carotid bruits; palpate for PMI, strength, timing and symmetry of peripheral pulses; assess for leg edema
- Abdomen: Palpate abdominal aorta; auscultate for renal bruits; CVA tenderness, or other renal abnormalities
- Neurologic: General neurologic examination

> **CLINICAL PEARL:** Proper technique and appropriate cuff size is imperative to accurately assess BP

Diagnosis

The diagnosis of HTN is based on two or more readings on two or more occasions; if systolic and diastolic BP are in two different categories, the higher category is used. Table 2.10 outlines the American College of Cardiology/American Heart Association (ACC/AHA) classification of HTN.

Appropriate testing at the time of diagnosis can screen for a secondary cause of HTN, evidence of end-organ damage, and can help stratify cardiovascular risk. To assess for a renal cause, or end-organ damage, perform:

- CBC
- Glomerular filtration rate (GFR)
- Blood urea nitrogen (BUN) and creatinine
- Electrolytes
- Urinalysis for microalbumin

An EKG and lipid panel can help to stratify cardiovascular risk. Consider a fasting glucose to assess for metabolic syndrome and a TSH level to assess for a thyroid cause.

TABLE 2.10 American College of Cardiology/American Heart Association Hypertension Classifications

Normal blood pressure	<120 and <80
Elevated blood pressure	120–129 and <80
Stage 1 hypertension	130–139 or 80–89
Stage 2 hypertension	140–149 or 90–99
Stage 3 hypertension	≥160 or ≥100

Source: Whelton PK, Carey RM, Aronow WS, et al. 2017 high blood pressure clinical practice guideline, a report of the American College of Cardiology/American Heart Association Task Force on clinical practice guidelines. *Hypertension.* 2018;71(6). doi:10.1161/HYP.0000000000000065

Management

Effective treatment of HTN often includes both lifestyle modifications (nonpharmacologic therapy) as well as pharmacologic therapy. Lifestyle modification should be implemented at the time of diagnosis and continue despite initiation of pharmacologic therapy.

Recommendations for lifestyle modifications include weight reduction if the patient is overweight or obese; dietary changes such as adherence to a diet of fruits, vegetables, nuts, low-fat dairy, fish, poultry, and whole grains; regular aerobic exercise; smoking cessation; and limiting alcohol intake. Dietary sodium restriction of less than 2,400 mg of sodium per day is helpful.[4]

> **CLINICAL PEARL:** When discussing lifestyle modifications and treatment of HTN with patients, it is important to take into consideration the patient's social determinants of health (socioeconomic situation, safety of neighborhood, food security) and how those may affect the patient's ability to adhere to treatment recommendations.

HTN management can be summarized as follows:[3]

- Normal: <120/80 mmHg: Recommend lifestyle modifications, reassess in 1 year
- Elevated: 120 to 129/<80 mmHg: Recommend lifestyle modifications, reassess in 3 to 6 months
- Stage 1: 130–139/80–89 mmHg: Determine the 10-year ASCVD risk:
  - ≥10%: Lifestyle modifications and initiate pharmacologic therapy, reassess in 1 month
  - <10%: Lifestyle modifications, reassess in 3 to 6 months
- Stage 2: ≥140/90 mmHg: Initiate two agents in different classes if BP is >20/10 mmHg above their goal (can be combination drug)

Additional pertinent clinical information:

- For adults with confirmed HTN and known CVD or 10-year ASCVD event risk of 10% or higher a BP target of <130/80 mmHg is recommended
- For adults with confirmed HTN, without additional markers of increased CVD risk, a BP target of <130/80 mmHg may be reasonable
- Diabetes, chronic kidney disease in adults ≥65 years of age: Initiate treatment for SBP ≥130 or DBP ≥80 with a goal <130/80

Table 2.11 summarizes common medications used to treat HTN, and blood pressure goals to ensure adequate treatment.

> **CLINICAL PEARL:** Consider the clinical picture. CAD or HF may alter the first-line drug therapy.

Generally, patients with HTN will require lifelong pharmacologic treatment. In some patients, weight reduction may normalize BP without the need for pharmacologic treatment. These patients should still be monitored regularly to ensure their BP remains normal. Explain the importance of BP control to reduce the risk of complications, such as renal disease, cardiovascular

TABLE 2.11 Selection of Pharmacologic Treatment for Patients With Hypertension

Population	Race	Medication Choices
Patients *without* diabetes or CKD	Black	Thiazide diuretic or CCB; either alone or in combination
	Non-Black	Thiazide diuretic or ACEI or ARB or CCB; either alone or in combination
Patients *with* diabetes, no CKD	Black	Thiazide diuretic or CCB; either alone, or in combination
	Non-Black	Thiazide diuretic or ACEI or ARB or CCB; either alone or in combination
Patients *with* CKD, *with* or *without* diabetes	All races	ACEI or ARB; either alone or in combination with a different class of drugs

Note: ACEI and ARB should not be used in combination.

ACEI, ACE inhibitor; ARB, angiotensin II receptor blocker; CCB, calcium channel blocker; CKD, chronic kidney disease.

Source: Whelton PK, Carey RM, Aronow WS, et al. 2017 high blood pressure clinical practice guideline, a report of the American College of Cardiology/American Heart Association Task Force on clinical practice guidelines. *Hypertension.* 2018;71(6):e13–e115. doi:10.1161/HYP.0000000000000065

disease, and retinopathy. Patients should be encouraged to take their medications as prescribed even though they may not have any symptoms of HTN.

REFERENCES

1. Charles L, Triscott J, Dobbs B. Secondary hypertension: discovering the underlying cause. *Am Fam Physician.* 2017;96:453–461.
2. Kotchen TA. Hypertensive vascular disease. In: Jameson J, Fauci AS, Kasper DL, et al., eds. *Harrison's Principles of Internal Medicine.* 20th ed. New York, NY: McGraw-Hill; 2018.
3. Whelton PK, Carey RM, Aronow WS, et al. 2017 high blood pressure clinical practice guideline, a report of the American College Of Cardiology/American Heart Association Task Force on clinical practice guidelines. *Hypertension.* 2018;71:e13–e115. doi:10.1161/HYP.0000000000000065
4. American Academy of Family Physicians. Clinical practice guideline hypertension. https://www.aafp.org/patient-care/clinical-recommendations/all/highbloodpressure.html

INFECTIOUS ENDOCARDITIS: PROPHYLAXIS

Etiology

Infectious endocarditis (IE) is an uncommon but life-threatening condition. The most common pathogen cultured from patients who are diagnosed with this condition is Streptococcus viridans (SV; alpha-hemolytic streptococci). The incidence of SV and culture negative IE appears to be decreasing, while the frequency of staphylococcal and enterococcal infections has increased.

Epidemiology

The mean age of patients with IE is 55 years old. Over half of the patients are male. Risk factors include dental procedures that involve manipulation of gingival tissue or the periapical region of the teeth, and perforation of the oral mucosa. Additional risk factors for IE include valvulopathies and congenital heart defects.

Management

There is no supportive evidence for IE prophylaxis in gastrointestinal (GI) procedures or genitourinary procedures, absent a known active infection. Protection from endocarditis in patients undergoing high-risk procedures is not guaranteed. Systematic reviews have demonstrated that antibiotic prophylaxis does not eliminate the presence of bacteremia. There is, however, general consensus that antibiotic prophylaxis is reasonable in patients who are deemed to be at increased risk of infective endocarditis or at a greater risk of experiencing adverse events from it. Refer to Box 2.1.

In general, those individuals who are identified to be at risk for developing bacterial IE should be encouraged to maintain good oral hygiene to reduce their risk of bacterial seeding. They should be instructed to seek regular professional dental care and to use appropriate dental products, such as manual, powered, and ultrasonic toothbrushes; dental floss; and other plaque-removal devices as recommended by their dental provider. Antibiotic prophylaxis is reasonable to consider for respiratory tract procedures such as tonsillectomy and adenoidectomy and drainage of an empyema as well as surgical procedures that involve infected skin, skin structure, or soft tissues. Treatment regimens are outlined in Table 2.12.

Box 2.1 Recommendations for infectious endocarditis prophylaxis

Indication: All dental procedures that involve the manipulation of gingival tissue or periapical area of the tooth and perforation of the oral mucosa in patients with:

1. Prosthetic cardiac valves
2. Transcatheter implanted prosthesis and homografts
3. Prosthetic material used with cardiac valve repair, annuloplasty rings, chords
4. Previous infective endocarditis
5. Unrepaired cyanotic congenital heart disease
6. Repaired congenital heart disease with:
   a. Residual shunts
   b. Valvular regurgitation at the site of or adjacent to the site of a prosthetic patch or prosthetic device
7. Cardiac transplant with valve regurgitation from an abnormal valve

Source: Nishimura RA, Otto CM, Bonow RO, et al. 2017 AHA/ACC focused update of the 2014 AHA/ACC guideline for the management of patients with valvular heart disease: A report of the American College of Cardiology/American Heart Association Task Force on Clinical Practice Guidelines. 2017;135:e1159–e1195. doi:10.1161/CIR.0000000000000503

CLINICAL PEARL: Cephalosporins should not be prescribed in patients with a history of anaphylaxis, angioedema, or urticaria with penicillin or ampicillin.

TABLE **2.12** Treatment Regimens for Infectious Endocarditis Prophylaxis

	Agent	Route: Oral	Route: IM or IV
First line	Amoxicillin	2 g as a single dose 30–60 minutes prior to procedure	
	Ampicillin		2 g IM or IV
	Cefazolin or ceftriaxone		1 g IM or IV
Allergy to penicillin	Cephalexin	2 g as a single dose 30–60 minutes prior to procedure 600 mg	1 g IM or IV
	Cefazolin or ceftriaxone		600 mg IM or IV
	Clindamycin		
	Azithromycin; clarithromycin	500 mg	

IM, intramuscular; IV, intravenous.

Source: Nishimura RA, Otto CM, Bonow RO, et al. 2017 AHA/ACC focused update of the 2014 AHA/ACC guideline for the management of patients with valvular heart disease: A report of the American College of Cardiology/American Heart Association Task Force on Clinical Practice Guidelines. *Circulation. 2017*;135:e1159–e1195. doi:10.1161/CIR.0000000000000503

ELECTRONIC RESOURCES

American College of Cardiology/American Heart Association Guideline for the Management of Patients With Valvular Heart Disease:

http://circ.ahajournals.org/content/135/25/e1159#sec-44

Slipczuk L, Codolosa JN, Davila CD, et al. Infective endocarditis epidemiology over five decades: a systematic review. *PLOS ONE*. 2013;8(12):e82665. doi:10.1371/journal.pone.0082665

Wilson W, Taubert KA, Gewitz M, et al. Prevention of infective endocarditis: Guidelines from the American Heart Association. *JADA*. 2008;139(1):3S-24S. doi:10.14219/jada.archive.2008.0346

DERMATOLOGIC SYSTEM

ACNE AND RELATED DISORDERS

ACNE VULGARIS

Etiology

Acne is a follicular skin disease that arises due to a disorder in the pilosebaceous unit. It is characterized by plugged follicles and sebum retention, leading to excessive bacterial growth and release of fatty acids. The key factors in the pathogenesis of acne are follicular keratinization, androgens, and bacteria (propionibacterium acnes). Acne can be inflammatory and noninflammatory and occurs mostly on the face, chest, and back. Common contributory factors include emotional stress, drugs such as lithium, oral contraceptives, and androgens.

> **CLINICAL PEARL:** Although many patients associate acne with some foods, there is no conclusive evidence that acne is caused by food.

Epidemiology

Acne is the most common chronic skin disease of adolescents and young adults. It affects about 85% of young people (men and women) and usually begins around puberty.[1] It tends to be more severe in men. There is also familial predisposition, as most individuals with a history of cystic acne have relatives with a history of severe acne.

Clinical Presentation

- Acne manifests as comedones, papules, pustules, nodules, or cysts
- It can present as open comedones (blackheads) or it can be closed comedones ("white heads") with flesh-colored, 1-mm papules
- Open or closed comedones can become erythematous papules, pustules, nodules, or cysts ranging from 1 to 5 mm
- Acne inflammatory lesions can lead to hyperpigmentation and hypertrophic scarring
- Common affected areas are the face, neck, chest, back, rarely buttocks
- Lesions may be associated with pain and can persist for months. Most episodes are worse in the fall or winter.

Diagnosis

A diagnosis of acne vulgaris is made based on history and physical examination findings. The presence of comedones are required to make the diagnosis. Laboratory studies may be ordered if other conditions such as hyperandrogenism or polycystic ovary syndrome (PCOS) are suspected.

The severity of acne can be staged as:

- Mild (few localized comedones, papules, pustules)
- Moderate (many comedones, papules, pustules, with or without a few scars)
- Severe (numerous or extensive superficial lesions, several nodules/cysts, and scars)

Management

Acne treatment should be aimed at unblocking the hair follicle, reducing sebum production, and stopping bacterial colonization. The long-term goal is to prevent scarring and the associated psychosocial trauma. Generally, the treatment depends on the stage of acne.

- For mild acne: Use topical antibiotics and benzoyl peroxide gels. The commonly used topical antibiotics are clindamycin and erythromycin. If there is no improvement, add topical retinoids. Patients must be instructed regarding the gradual increases in concentration. Start with a low concentration (0.01%), then medium (0.025%) to high 0.05% cream/gel or liquid.

- For moderate acne: Add an oral antibiotic to the above regimen. The commonly used oral antibiotics are minocycline and doxycycline at 50 to 100 mg twice daily.
- For severe (nodulocystic) acne: Systemic treatment with isotretinoin is indicated in addition to topical treatment.

> **CLINICAL PEARL:** Isotretinoin is teratoagenic and is contraindicated in pregnancy. Patients must be on effective contraception.

- Isotretinoin should never be used concurrently with tetracycline as this combination has been reported to cause benign intracranial swelling.
- Instruct patients to avoid triggers and exacerbating factors such as emotional stress and comedogenic oils.

> **CLINICAL PEARL:** When managing a patient with acne, it is important to address the psychosocial trauma that can be associated with this disease. Acne can lead to maladjustment between parent and children, general insecurity and feelings of inferiority, impaired self-image, altered body image, decreased self-esteem, embarrassment, shame, social impairment, preoccupation, anger, and depression.

ACNE ROSACEA

Etiology

Rosacea is a chronic follicular acneiform disorder of the facial pilosebaceous units. It is an inflammatory disorder that is characterized by an increased reactivity of capillaries leading to flushing and telangiectasia.

Epidemiology

Rosacea is a common skin disorder affecting about 10% of fair-skinned people, mainly women between 30 and 50 years old.[1] It is more common in people with Celtic ancestry and those from southern Mediterranean regions.

Clinical Presentation

- Insidious onset of reddening of the face (flushing), malar erythema, red papules, and pustules
- Outbreaks are episodic, triggered by heat, exposure to sun, hot liquids, alcohol, and spicy foods
- In the late stages, patients have red faces, papules, nodules, telangiectasia, sebaceous hyperplasia, lymphedema, and facial disfigurement
- Rosacea presents with a symmetrical distribution on the face, rarely in the neck, trunk, and scalp
- Rosacea may also be present with nasal and ocular symptoms. Patients may have enlarged nose (rhinophyma), swollen eye lids (blepharophyma), swollen ear lobes (otophyma), and swelling of the chin (gnathophyma)

Diagnosis

Rosacea is a clinical diagnosis based on history and physical examination findings. Laboratory examination may involve bacterial culture to rule out *Staphylococcus aureus*. The differential diagnosis of rosacea includes acne vulgaris, perioral dermatitis, bacterial folliculitis, seborrhea, and systemic lupus erythematosus.

The severity of rosacea can be staged as:

- Stage 1: Persistent erythema with telangiectasia
- Stage 2: Persistent erythema with telangiectasia, papules, tiny pustules
- Stage 3: Persistent deep erythema, dense telangiectasia, papules, pustules, nodules

Management

- Patients should be advised to avoid triggers such as alcohol, hot beverages, spicy foods, and sunlight.
- Use topical treatment (initial treatment) with metronidazole gel or cream (0.75% or 1%) once or twice daily. Erythromycin gel is also used but is less effective.
- Oral antibiotics are more effective than topical treatment. Commonly used oral antibiotics include minocycline, doxycycline, tetracycline, and metronidazole.
- Facial disfigurement, swollen nose (rhinophyma), and telangiectasia can be treated by surgery.

> **CLINICAL PEARL:** A low-dose regimen of oral isotretinoin may help patients with severe rosacea that does not respond to antibiotics and topical treatments.

◼ FOLLICULITIS

Etiology/Epidemiology

Folliculitis is an inflammatory reaction in the hair follicle usually caused by *S. aureus* but can also be caused by other organisms. It occurs mostly in young adults.

Clinical Presentation

- Red papule/pustule with central hair
- Often asymptomatic, pruritic, or tender
- It can be chronic and/or recurrent
- Distribution is mostly on the buttocks, thighs, scalp, arms
- Carbuncles (boils) can present as red, tender, pus-filled fluctuant nodule in hair-bearing areas of the head, neck, body
- Risk factors include occlusion, perspiration, and tight clothes

Diagnosis

Laboratory examination may involve bacterial culture and Gram staining to confirm the causative organism, such as *S. aureus*. Bacterial culture is also performed for antibiotic susceptibility testing.

Management

- Patients should be advised to limit occlusion and maceration.
- Use antibacterial cleansers and topical treatments, such as mupirocin 2%, on nares for 1 to 2 weeks to reduce seeding of *S. aureus*.
- For systemic treatment, the commonly used antibiotics are cephalexin and dicloxacillin. Treat for about 1 to 4 weeks.
- For abscess (boils), incision and drainage is recommended.

CLINICAL PEARL: Cloths and materials used for warm compresses need to be handled with care to avoid the spread of resistant bacteria (infection control).

■ HIDRADENITIS SUPPURATIVA

Etiology/Epidemiology

Hidradenitis suppurativa results from occlusion of pilosebaceous units within intertriginous zones and secondary inflammation of apocrine glands. It can co-occur with cystic acne and obesity. This condition has a genetic predisposition, particularly nodulocystic acne. It is most common in adults and affects women more than men.

Clinical Presentation

- In the early phase, patients may present with pain and point tenderness.
- As the disease progresses, the affected area may develop draining, purulent nodules, sterile abscesses, and comedones (double headed). Sinus tracts or fistulae, along with hypertrophic scars, may occur later in the disease.
- Most affected areas are axillae, breasts, groin, and anogenital areas, as seen in Figure 2.1.

Diagnosis

Laboratory examination is recommended to rule out secondary bacterial infection. Otherwise, the diagnosis is often clinical.

Management

It is recommended to use combination therapy with intralesional glucocorticoids, surgical excision, oral antibiotics, and isotretinoin.

- Oral antibiotics: Tetracycline, doxycycline, erythromycin
- Topical antibiotics: Clindamycin
- Steroids: Prednisone
- Oral retinoids: Accutane

Be cognizant of the potential psychosocial impact this condition may have on patients. Surgical excision is often required to drain abscesses, fibrotic nodules, or sinus tracts.

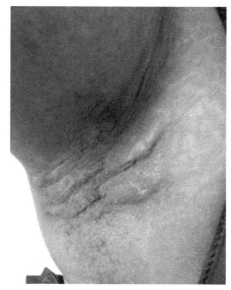

FIGURE 2.1 Hidradenitis suppurativa on the axilla.
Source: Lyons F, Ousley L. *Dermatology for the Advanced Practice Nurse.* New York, NY: Springer Publishing Company; 2014.

REFERENCES

1. Wolff K, Johnson RA. *Fitzpatrick's Color Atlas and Synopsis of Clinical Dermatology.* New York, NY: McGraw Hill; 2009.
2. Lyons F, Ousley L. *Dermatology for the Advanced Practice Nurse.* 1st ed. Springer Publishing Company; 2014.

DERMATITIS/ECZEMATOUS DISORDERS

▧ DERMATITIS: ATOPIC

Etiology

Atopic dermatitis (atopic eczema) is a chronic inflammatory skin condition that presents with pruritic, erythematous, and scaly skin lesions often localized to the flexural surfaces of the body. It can be acute, subacute, or chronic relapsing and is often associated with other atopic disorders such as hay fever, allergic rhinitis, and asthma. The disease results from a combination of genetic and environmental factors. A genetic defect in the filaggrin protein may be involved through disrupting the epidermis, in addition to alterations in immunologic responses.[1]

> **CLINICAL PEARL:** The terms atopic dermatitis, atopic eczema, and IgE dermatitis are used synonymously to refer to the same disease.

Epidemiology

Atopic dermatitis is highly prevalent in both children and adults. It usually starts in infancy and affects about two out of 10 children. It is a leading nonfatal health burden attributable to skin diseases.[2] It is estimated that 1% to 5% of adults have atopic dermatitis. It is slightly more common in men than women and is commonly seen in the children of those affected. Lesions can be exacerbated by exposure to allergens, irritants, and bacteria, as well as winter conditions, wool clothing, and emotional stress.

Clinical Presentation

- Atopic dermatitis is characterized by epidermal barrier dysfunction, immune responses, and pruritus,
- Pruritus and scratching leads to a cycle of increased inflammation and lichenification,
  - Complications include chronic postinflammatory skin changes, scarring, and secondary skin infections from *Staphylococcus, Streptococcus*, and herpes species,
- Common features include skin dryness, erythema, oozing, crusting, and lichenification,
- Pruritus is a hallmark of atopic dermatitis and is responsible for most of the disease burden to patients and families,
- The most commonly affected anatomical sites (distribution) are flexures, neck, eyelids, forehead, face, wrists, and dorsum of the hands and feet,
- In infants, the lesions may present as red skin, confluent erythema, or tiny vesicles on an edematous face. It may also be associated with scaling and crusting,
- The lesions may be exacerbated by winter conditions, wool clothing, and emotional stress,

Diagnosis

A diagnosis of atopic dermatitis is made clinically based on history and physical examination findings. Blood studies may show elevated IgE in serum and eosinophilia. Laboratory investigations are usually carried out to rule out herpes simplex virus (HSV) in crusted lesions and to rule out secondary colonization with *S. aureus*.

- Atopic dermatitis can be acute, subacute, or chronic relapsing.
- Acute and subacute lesions generally have poorly defined erythematous patches, papules, and plaques with or without scaling.
- Common features in chronic atopic dermatitis include pruritus, xerosis, thickening of the skin (lichenification), painful fissures, alopecia, periorbital pigmentation, and infraorbital fold below eyelids.

Management

- The goals of treatment are to reduce pruritus and dermatitis, prevent exacerbations and secondary complications, as well as to minimize therapeutic risks such as steroid-induced thinning of the skin (atrophy) or Cushing's syndrome.
- Prevention and treatment of dermatitis should focus on restoration of epidermal barrier function, which is best achieved using emollients. Therefore, moisturizing agents should be an essential part of atopic

dermatitis management, applied after bathing to improve hydration. Non-soap cleansers with a low pH and those without fragrances should be recommended. If the atopic dermatitis is not responding to nonpharmacological interventions (good skin care and moisturizers), recommend corticosteroids. If steroids are not effective or if they cause side effects such as atrophy, then topical calcineurin inhibitors should be recommended.

- Topical therapy is the mainstay of treatment. Topical corticosteroids are the first-line therapy for acute flares but should be combined with systemic therapy in severe cases.
- Oral antihistamines are useful in reducing itching. Hydroxyzine, 10 to 100 mg four times daily, is sufficient for pruritus.
- If secondary infection with *S. aureus* is suspected, oral antibiotics such as dicloxacillin or erythromycin are indicated according to drug sensitivity.
- Patients with severe refractory dermatitis may benefit from second-line therapies such as phototherapy and cyclosporine (5 mg/kg/d for not more than 6 months due to systemic side effects). There is also growing evidence that severe refractory dermatitis can be improved by omalizumab, a recombinant humanized monoclonal antibody targeting the high-affinity Fc receptor of Ig.[3]

> **CLINICAL PEARL:** When managing patients with atopic dermatitis, prioritize skin hydration, control of pruritus, topical anti-inflammatory therapies, and management of infection. Educate patients to avoid rubbing and scratching of the skin. Encourage the use of moisturizers, especially glycerol-containing creams. These agents help in restoring epidermal barrier function, prolong time to flare, and reduce the number of flares and the amount of topical corticosteroids needed.

■ DERMATITIS: CONTACT

Etiology

Contact dermatitis is a generic term that refers to acute or chronic inflammatory skin conditions that appear after contact with a foreign substance. It is characterized by erythematous and pruritic skin lesions. There are two forms of contact dermatitis. Allergic contact dermatitis is caused by an antigen that elicits a delayed hypersensitivity reaction. Irritant contact dermatitis occurs after contact with a chemical irritant (nonimmune-modulated irritation of the skin). Irritant contact dermatitis may occur after a single exposure to the offending agent; the skin lesion is dependent on the concentration of the irritant and is generally confined to the area of exposure. Allergic contact dermatitis is dependent on sensitization, occurs only in sensitized individuals, and is an immune reaction that may spread beyond affected sites. Substances that commonly cause contact dermatitis include poison ivy, nickel, fragrances, soaps, industrial solvents, wool.

Epidemiology

Irritant contact dermatitis accounts for about 80% of all occupational skin disorders, making it the most common form of occupational skin disease.

Allergic contact dermatitis accounts for about 7% of occupationally associated illness in the United States.[4] There are more cases of nonoccupational allergic contact dermatitis compared to those associated with occupation.[4]

Clinical Presentation

- Clinical presentation of contact dermatitis varies according to the etiology (allergen or irritant) and according to the affected site of the body (Table 2.13). Generally, contact dermatitis manifests as erythema, scaling, and relatively well-demarcated visible borders.
- Acute irritant contact dermatitis may start as a burning or stinging sensation. Lesions may range from erythema and vesiculation to vesicles and blisters.
- Chronic irritant contact dermatitis develops slowly after repeated exposure to offending agents. Common chronic features include skin dryness, chapping, erythema, hyperkeratosis, scaling, fissures, and crusting.
- The most commonly affected anatomical site for irritant contact dermatitis is the hands.
- Acute allergic contact dermatitis manifests as a well-demarcated erythema and edema. Lesions range from papules and vesicles to bullae and plaques. In chronic cases, plaques may turn into lichenification.
- A common cause of allergic contact dermatitis is exposure to urushiol, a substance in the sap of some plants, such as poison ivy and oak. When in contact with skin, it causes linear streaks of erythema and vesicles. Other common causes of allergic contact dermatitis include jewelry (nickel) and topical products such as medicine causing reactions with demarcated borders. An example of contact dermatitis is seen in Figure 2.2 A through C.

Diagnosis

A diagnosis of contact dermatitis is made clinically based on history and physical examination findings. Patch tests may be useful in confirming a causative agent in allergic contact dermatitis.

TABLE 2.13 Differentiating Allergic From Irritant Dermatitis

	Allergic	Irritant
Location	Usually exposed areas of the skin	Usually hands
Symptoms	Pruritus	Burning, pruritus, pain
Surface appearance	Papules, vesicles, and bullae	Dry and fissured skin
Lesion borders	Distinct angles, lines, and borders, but spreads in the periphery	Distinct borders confined to site of exposure
Evolution	Less rapid than irritant	A few hours after exposure (rapid)
Incidence	Occurs only in the sensitized patient	May occur in any person exposed to the irritant
Dose dependence of causative agents	Relatively independent of amount applied, depends on degree of sensitization	Concentration dependent

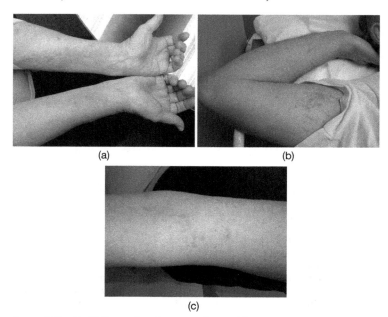

(a)   (b)

(c)

FIGURE 2.2 (A–C) Example of contact dermatitis.
Source: Lyons F, Ousley L. *Dermatology for the Advanced Practice Nurse.* New York, NY: Springer Publishing Company; 2014.

Management

- Priority should include identification of and avoiding the causative agent. Patients should be encouraged to wear protective clothing or use barrier creams. For patients with nickel allergy, it is helpful to cover the metal tab of jeans with an iron-on patch or a few coats of clear nail polish.
- For acute contact dermatitis, cool compresses, calamine lotion, and colloidal oatmeal baths may help to reduce symptoms.
- For localized acute allergic contact dermatitis, treat with mid- to high-potency topical glucocorticoids such as betamethasone dipropionate or clobetasol propionate.
- Systemic steroid therapy is often required if the dermatitis is severe or if it involves large areas of the skin (>20%).

▋ DERMATITIS: PERIORAL

Etiology

The etiology of perioral dermatitis is unknown but it is exacerbated by topical steroids.

Epidemiology

Perioral dermatitis occurs mainly in young women, adolescents, and preschoolers.

Clinical Presentation

- Insidious onset of subacute lesions occurs over weeks to months.
- The lesions (rash) are characterized by erythematous papulopustules on an erythematous background. The papules are irregularly grouped and symmetrical.
- Lesions are generally distributed around the mouth, nasolabial folds, and cheeks. Occasionally, tiny papules and a few pustules can be found around the lower eyelids.
- Unlike acne vulgaris, there are no comedones in perioral dermatitis.

Diagnosis

The diagnosis is clinical, based on history and physical examination findings. Laboratory examination may involve bacterial culture to rule out *S. aureus*. The differential diagnosis of perioral dermatitis includes contact dermatitis, atopic dermatitis, acne vulgaris, seborrhea, and rosacea

Management

- Patients should be advised to avoid triggers such as topical glucocorticoids.
- Use topical treatment (initial treatment) with metronidazole gel 0.75% two times daily or 1% once daily. Erythromycin gel (2% twice daily) can also be used.
- For systemic treatment, the commonly used oral antibiotics are minocycline or doxycycline, 100 mg daily until clear, and then taper to 50 mg daily for another 8 weeks. Tetracycline can also be used. Start with 500 mg twice daily until clear and then taper to 500 mg daily for 4 weeks, followed by 250 mg daily for 4 weeks.

REFERENCES

1. Maintz L, Novak N. Getting more and more complex: the pathophysiology of atopic eczema. *Eur J Dermatol.* 2007;17(4):267–283.
2. Weidinger S, Novak N. Atopic dermatitis. *Lancet.* 2016;387:1109. doi:10.1016/S0140-6736(15)00149-X.
3. Holm JG, Agner T, Sand C, et al. Omalizumab for atopic dermatitis: case series and a systematic review of the literature. *Int J Dermatol.* 2017;56(1):18–26. doi:10.1111/ijd.13353.
4. Wolff K, Johnson RA. *Fitzpatrick's Color Atlas and Synopsis of Clinical Dermatology.* New York, NY: McGraw Hill; 2009.

INFECTIONS AND INFESTATIONS

▪ NEOPLASMS OF THE SKIN: BENIGN

Skin cancers are the most common form of human cancers, with one in every five Americans likely to develop skin cancer at one point in their lives.[1] The incidence is rising due to the increased occupational and recreational UV light exposure, as well as the aging population. Skin neoplasms can be benign, malignant, or premalignant. The vast majority of malignant skin cancers falls into three categories: basal cell carcinoma (BCC), SCC, and melanoma. In people with AIDS, other skin cancers such as Kaposi sarcoma are also common. This section discusses benign neoplasms, with malignant neoplasms to follow.

Most skin cancers are curable if caught early, which is why regular total body skin physical examinations are imperative. The use of noninvasive optical technologies, such as dermatoscopy, may be helpful to improve diagnostic accuracy in some skin cancers. If the diagnosis is unclear based on history and physical examination, refer for biopsy and histopathologic examination to rule out malignancy.

Etiology

Benign skin lesions may result from genetic mutations and can be inherited. They may be associated with systemic diseases and can be acquired from external factors such as chronic trauma and sun exposure. For example, seborrheic keratosis arises from benign proliferation of immature keratinocytes.[2] Melanocytic nevi (moles) result from the proliferation of cutaneous melanocytes. Skin tags are frequently associated with insulin resistance and metabolic syndrome (diabetes and obesity). Epidermal cysts can arise from implantation of the follicular epithelium in the dermis following a traumatic event to the skin. Cherry angiomas are acquired capillary proliferations.

Epidemiology

Seborrheic keratosis is the most common benign epithelial tumor and its incidence increases with age.[2] Lipomas are the most common subcutaneous soft-tissue tumors, occurring in one per 1,000 persons annually.[3] Skin tags (acrochordons) and cherry angiomas are also common, affecting up to 50% of adults.[4] Mongolian spots are more common in infants of Asians and American Indians than in any other racial groups. Port-wine stain occurs in about three out of 10 newborns and never disappear spontaneously.

Clinical Presentation

- Benign skin neoplasms present in a variety of ways and are categorized in Table 2.14. **Dermal tumors** such as **skin tags** (acrochordon) are an outgrowth of normal skin and attached by narrow and thin stocks (pedunculated). They are about 1 mm to 1 cm in diameter and are commonly found in the axilla, neck, inframammary, and inguinal regions.
- **Dermatofibromas** appear as firm hyperpigmented nodules and will characteristically dimple when pinched (retraction or Fitzpatrick's sign). They occur mostly in adults and are generally localized to the lower extremities.
- Epidermal benign skin tumors include **seborrheic keratosis** (most common), which is papular, hyperpigmented, sessile, and rough with a typical stuck-on appearance. Seborrheic keratoses appear as warty hyperkeratotic lesions and are often located on the trunk, face, and upper extremities. An example of this is seen in Figure 2.3.

CLINICAL PEARL: Differentiating seborrheic keratosis from melanoma can be difficult as they both have irregularities and variable dark colors. Keratoses tend to have rougher surfaces compared to melanoma lesions.

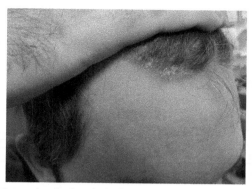

FIGURE 2.3 Example of seborrheic dermatitis.
Source: Lyons F, Ousley L. *Dermatology for the Advanced Practice Nurse.* New York, NY: Springer Publishing Company; 2014.

- Appendageal tumors include subepidermal keratin cysts such as **milia** and **epidermal cysts** such as epidermoid cysts. Milia are multiple tiny white papules frequently located in the face. Epidermoid cysts can occur anywhere on the body and typically appear as round, skin-colored dermal nodules with a central punctum.
- Vascular benign skin tumors include cherry angioma and pyogenic granuloma. **Cherry angioma** present with dilated capillaries are round, bright to dark red, and have well-demarcated vascular papules in middle-aged and older adults.
- **Pyogenic granulomas** are rapidly growing, red, dome-shaped, friable papules that bleed profusely after minor trauma. They can occur in all ages and anywhere on the body, but frequently occur on the gingiva during pregnancy.
- **Melanocytic nevi (moles)** present as small (<6 mm) irregularly pigmented macules, papules, or plaques. They can be acquired or congenital and are concentrated on sun-exposed areas of the face, trunk, extremities, and scalp. Occasionally, they can be found on the palms, soles, and nail matrix. Atypical nevi share some of the clinical features of melanoma (asymmetry, border irregularities, color variability, and diameter >6 mm).

> **CLINICAL PEARL:** Patients are at increased risk of melanoma if they have multiple atypical nevi (>6 mm in diameter), history of sun exposure, and family and/or personal history melanoma.

- **Solar lentigo** are commonly referred to as age spots, or liver spots, and typically present as small, well-circumscribed brown macules on sun-exposed areas. Solar lentigo should be differentiated from lentigo maligna melanoma, a gradual type of melanoma with irregular borders and variable pigmentation.

TABLE 2.14 Benign Skin Neoplams

Dermal	Epidermal	Appendageal
Skin tags (acrochordon)	Seborrheic keratosis	Usually hands
Dermatofibroma	Dermatosis papulosa nigra	Milium
Neurofibroma		

Vascular	Melanocytic Disorders	Subcutaneous fat tumors
Cherry angioma	Melanocytic nevi	Lipoma
Pyogenic granuloma	Solar lentigo	Angiolipoma
Port-Wine stain	Mongolian spot	Angiolipoma

- Subcutaneous fat tumors such as **lipomas** develop superficially in the subcutaneous tissues and present as soft, painless subcutaneous nodules most frequently on the trunk and upper extremities.

Diagnosis

Diagnosis is based on lesion features and clinical history. If the diagnosis is inconclusive based on history and physical examination, skin biopsy and histopathological examinations should be performed. You should always apply the ABCDE rule for pigmented lesions. The ABCDE rule refers to asymmetry, border irregularity, color variability, diameter >6.0 mm, elevation, and evolving.[5]

Management

Benign skin neoplasms that are symptomatic or cosmetically bothersome can be managed with simple procedures, such as excision, cryotherapy, pharmacotherapy, and curettage with or without electrodessication. The choice of treatment depends on the type, size, and location of the tumor.

- Acrochordons (skin tags) and seborrheic keratoses can be managed with cryotherapy and shave excision.
- Epidermoid cysts, lipomas, dermatofibromas, and pyogenic granulomas are also managed by excision.
- Cherry angioma are often removed by laser therapy and electrodessication.
- Melanocytic nevi are treated surgically through a combination of freezing liquid nitrogen therapy and shaving. Melanocytic nevi have the potential of turning into malignant melanoma and need to be monitored closely. Indications for removal include (a) location on scalp, mucous membrane, or anogenital area, (b) rapid changes in size, (c) irregular border, (d) if lesion becomes eroded without much trauma, (e) if lesion becomes persistently itchy or bleeds, or (f) if there is a high suspicion for melanoma.[1] In all cases, educate patients on the use of sunscreen and sun protection.

■ NEOPLASMS OF THE SKIN: PREMALIGNANT AND MALIGNANT

Etiology

Environmental and genetic factors can cause genetic mutations, leading to rapid multiplication of skin cells and subsequent formation of malignant tumors. Contributing factors may include immunosuppressive therapy, chronic arsenic exposure, chemotherapy, and radiation therapy.

The vast majority of malignant skin cancers fall into melanoma and the nonmelanoma skin cancers (BCC and SCC). Melanomas arise from melanocytic cells in the epidermis. BCC arises from the basal layer of the epidermis. SCC arises from the squamous cells of the epidermis. Both genetic and environmental factors contribute to the development of malignant skin cancers.

Epidemiology

Actinic keratosis is the most common form of precancerous skin lesion. It starts in middle age and is most often found in men and Caucasians. Outdoor workers and sportspersons are at higher risk for developing actinic keratosis. BCC is the most common form of skin cancer. According to the Skin Cancer Foundation, more than four million cases of BCC are diagnosed in the United States each year. It is more common in Caucasians compared to dark-skinned populations. The incidence in men is higher than in women. Sunny areas, in addition to those close to the equator, have more cases compared to other regions, such as the Midwestern United States. The incidence increases with age. SCC is the second most common form of skin cancer, with more than one million cases being diagnosed each year in the United States. Malignant melanoma is the most dangerous form of skin cancer and is the sixth most common cancer in both men and women in the United States.[6]

Clinical Presentation

- **Actinic keratosis** presents as multiple dry, rough, adherent scaly lesions on sun-exposed skin, such as the face, scalp, ears, shoulders, neck, back of hands, and forearms. An example of this is seen in Figure 2.4.
- They are often elevated, 2 to 6 mm in diameter, rough in texture, and resemble warts. They may appear white, red, dark tan, pink, or flesh-toned. On palpation, lesions have a sandpaper texture. On dermatoscopy, a honeycomb pattern may be observed. Actinic keratosis on the lip (actinic cheilitis or solar cheilitis) often appears as fragile, bleeding, and crusty lesions. It is usually found on the lower lip and is a persistent rough or scaly area. It is painless, but patients may complain of a consistent dry sensation and cracking of the lips.
- **BCC** is a slow-growing skin cancer commonly found on sun-exposed skin (face more frequently involved than trunk). BCC lesions appear like open sores, red patches, pink growths, shiny bumps, or scars. They can be nodular, superficial, and morpheaform. Nodular BCC is the most common type of BCC and typically are found on the face as pink- or flesh-colored papules with ulceration, telangiectasia, and raised borders. BCC lesions do not normally metastasize beyond the original tumor site.
- **SCC** lesions are raised, firm, skin-colored, or pink in appearance. They often present as keratotic papules or plaques on sun-damaged skin.
  - ○ Lesions are characterized by skin depression with raised edges that are indurated, inflamed, and often crust or ooze.[7]
  - ○ The majority of SCC lesions arise from lesions previously diagnosed clinically as actinic keratosis. Similar to BCC, SCC is a slow-growing cancer, although some variants of SCC, such as the spindle cell type, enlarge rapidly.

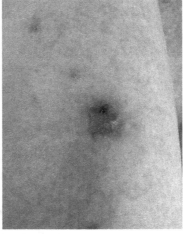

Figure 2.4   Example of actinic keratosis.
Source: Lyons F, Ousley L. *Dermatology for the Advanced Practice Nurse.* 1st ed. New York, NY: Springer Publishing Company.

- **Melanoma** lesions are typically asymmetrical in shape, have irregular borders and mottled colors with different shades of brown, tan, black, grey, blue, red, and white. The lesion diameters are >6.0 mm, the lesion is elevated, and there is a history of increasing in size over time. Melanoma presents in various forms, including superficial spreading melanoma, lentigo maligna melanoma, acral lentiginous melanoma, nodular melanoma, desmoplastic melanoma, and other variants. Superficial spreading melanoma is the most common, accounting for over 70% of all melanomas.[1] Nodular melanomas are the second most common type, accounting for over 15% of all melanomas.[1] The clinical feature of the various melanoma subtypes are shown in Table 2.15. Figure 2.5 details the clinical appearance of malignant melanoma.

Diagnosis

The main goal is to identify skin cancers early before tumor invasion and metastases occur.

The entire skin surface from head to toe, mucous membranes, nails, and lymph nodes should be examined in each patient. Ensure adequate illumination, and if needed, utilize hand lenses to evaluate lesions and variations in pigment patterns. Magnification of the epidermis by dermatoscopy allows a more precise examination of skin pigmentation and lesion morphology. Suspicious lesions should be biopsied and referred to specialists. In general, the diagnosis of skin cancer is made clinically and confirmed by histopathology. Once a diagnosis of skin cancer has been made, it should be staged to determine prognosis, metastatic risk, and treatment options. Sentinel lymph

TABLE **2.15** Melanoma Types, Anatomical Sites, and Characteristics.

Type	Anatomical Site(s)	General Characteristics
Superficial spreading	Upper back, lower legs, but can occur at any site	Most common—about 70% of all melanomas Average age at diagnosis: 40–50 years Variably pigmented macules or thin plaque with irregular borders Lesions may have multiple shades of red, blue, black, gray, and white Delayed vertical growth Months to 2 years radial growth
Nodular	Trunk, head, neck, but can occur at any site	About 15% of all melanomas Average age at diagnosis: 40–50 years Discrete nodules, with dark pigmentation, but may be amelanotic, with symmetric borders, and relatively small diameter Immediate vertical growth
Lentigo maligna	Face, neck, dorsa of hands	About 5% of all melanomas Average age at diagnosis: 70 years Predominantly brown to tan when flat Reddish brown, bluish black when nodules Delayed vertical growth. Lesion gradually enlarges over years and may develop darker, asymmetric foci of pigmentation, color variegation, and raised areas
Acral lentiginous	Palmar, plantar, and subungual surfaces	About 5%–10% of all melanomas Average age of diagnosis: 60 years First appear as dark brown to black irregularly pigmented macules or patches Occasionally amelanotic or hypomelanotic Raised areas, ulceration, and bleeding Early vertical growth Radial growth months to years Very common type of melanoma among dark-skinned individuals
Desmoplastic	Chronically sun-exposed areas of older patients. Head, neck, and other sites	Average age of diagnosis: 60 years Amelanotic (pigmentation frequently absent) Slowly growing plaque, nodule, or scar-like growth

node biopsy is recommended for evaluating lymph node involvement, staging, and assessing prognosis.

For BCC, dermatopathology will show atypical basal cells. Lesions that have changed in size or shape or have other features suggestive of malignant melanoma should be biopsied. The most important prognostic factor for a newly diagnosed melanoma is its staging classification, and the best predictor of its metastatic risk is the lesion's thickness.[8,9]

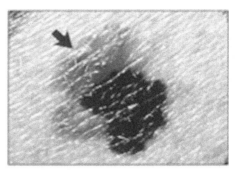

FIGURE 2.5 Example of malignant melanoma.
Source: Courtesy of National Cancer Institute.

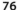 **CLINICAL PEARL:** Patients with atypical moles and those at high risk for skin cancer should be advised to perform regular self-examinations and should have other family members screened.

Less common subtypes of melanoma, such as nodular melanomas or those that involve the nail unit, and melanomas occurring in children lack the typical melanoma features and are likely to be missed by the ABCDE criteria. These may be more difficult to diagnose clinically and dermoscopically. In this scenario, alternative criteria such as EFG (Elevation, Firm on palpation, continuous Growth for 1 month) may be used.

MANAGEMENT
In general, the management of skin neoplasms depends on type, stage, and location. Mohs surgery is considered the most effective treatment modality for many BCCs and SCCs. Other options include cryosurgery or electrosurgery for very small lesions, particularly in less-sensitive sites such as the scalp. Very small superficial lesions can also be managed with photodynamic therapy, topical treatment with 5-floururacil, and imiquimod. Secondary treatment includes radiation therapy and electrocautery with curettage. Treatment of melanoma depends on the stage. For clinically localized melanoma (stages 1 and 2) surgical excision is recommended. Systemic adjuvant therapy is indicated in patients with metastatic disease.

▪ SKIN INFECTIONS: BACTERIAL

Etiology
Cutaneous bacterial infections result from microbial invasion of the skin and its supporting structures. They present as acute inflammation of skin and subcutaneous tissue. They can be classified as simple (uncomplicated) or complicated (such as necrotizing fasciitis) or as suppurative or nonsuppurative. The most common bacteria responsible for community-acquired skin infections are methicillin-resistant *S. aureus* (MRSA) and beta-hemolytic

Streptococcus. Key risk factors include puncture wounds, insect bites, preexisting skin infections, intravenous (IV) drug use, and a compromised immune system.

Lyme disease is caused by *Borrelia burgdorferi* spirochete and is transmitted by *Ixodes* (deer) ticks. Rocky Mountain spotted fever is caused by the *Rickettsia* family and is spread by several species of ticks, including the American dog tick (*Dermacentor variabilis*), Rocky Mountain wood tick (*Dermacentor andersoni*), and the brown dog tick (*Rhipicephalus sanguineus*).

CLINICAL PEARL: Whereas simple skin infections are usually caused by a single organism with localized clinical findings, complicated skin infections can be mono- or polymicrobial and may manifest with a systemic inflammatory response syndrome (SIRS). Staphylococcus aureus is the leading cause of both complicated and noncomplicated skin infections.

Epidemiology

Bacterial skin infections are a major cause of morbidly, ranging from cellulitis, impetigo, folliculitis, erysipelas, and abscesses to necrotizing fasciitis. The greatest incidence is among adults, men, and Blacks.[10,11] Lyme disease is the most commonly reported vector-borne illness in the United States. Each year, approximately 30,000 cases of Lyme disease are reported to the Centers for Disease Control and Prevention (CDC), and most cases are concentrated in the Northeast and Upper Midwest of the United States where infected ticks are common. Cases have also been reported in some areas of Northern California, Oregon, and Washington. Lyme disease is most common in spring and mid-fall.

Rocky Mountain spotted fever (RMSF) cases have been reported throughout the United States, although five states, North Carolina, Oklahoma, Arkansas, Tennessee, and Missouri, account for over 60% of the cases. According to the CDC, the incidence of RMSF (also categorized as Spotted Fever Rickettsiosis—SFR) has increased during the last decade, from less than two cases per million persons in 2000 to over 11 cases per million in 2014. American Indians report higher number of SFR infections than other race groups, and the majority of reported cases are among people at least 40 years old.

Clinical Presentation

- **Cellulitis** manifests with redness, pain, tenderness, swelling, and warmth of the affected area. It is a spreading infection and the affected person may develop a fever and swollen lymph nodes. Cellulitis can occur anywhere on the skin but frequently affects the legs.
- **Impetigo** presents as red papules to honey-crusted erosions secondary to superficial infection of *S. aureus* and *Streptococcus pyogenes*. The golden yellow crusts are arranged as scattered, discrete lesions and may become confluent over time.
- **Bullous impetigo** presents with blisters filled with clear yellow or turbid fluid with erythematous halo.
- **Necrotizing fasciitis** is characterized by a rapid progression of infection along fascial planes and is usually associated with redness, edema, warmth,

and extensive cutaneous soft-tissue necrosis. The affected area may have crepitus, indicating gas in the soft tissue. Patients with necrotizing fasciitis may have fever and pain disproportionate to the physical findings. Necrotizing fasciitis can be distinguished from nonnecrotizing infections by the tense edema and bullous changes.

- **Staphylococcal scalded skin syndrome (SSSS)** results from systemic exfoliative toxin from *S. aureus* and is very common in neonates and young children. The infection manifests with erythema, tenderness, exfoliation, perioral, and periorbital crusting. The epidermis appears wrinkled and can be removed by gentle pressure (Nikolsky sign).
- **Lyme disease** first presents as erythematous plaque at the tick bite site, accompanied by fever, chills, myalgia, headache, weakness, photophobia, and lymphocytosis.
  - ○ The initial erythematous macule or papule expands centrifugally within days with a distinct red border at the bite site (erythema migrans). Lesions can be solitary, multiple, or appear as concentric rings (bull's eye or target lesion). Disseminated disease presents with secondary lesions, neuritis, carditis, migratory musculoskeletal pain, and arthralgias. If untreated, Lyme disease presents with a sequelae of systemic complications.
- **Rocky Mountain spotted fever** manifests with a sudden onset of macules and papules after a tick bite. Fever, chills, severe headache, and myalgia are common. The rash characteristically begins on wrists, forearms, and ankles. The rash later spreads on the arms, thighs, trunk, and face. The lesions may later become hemorrhagic and will not blanch.

Diagnosis

A diagnosis of bacterial skin infections is predominantly clinical. In situations of uncertain diagnosis or in severe infections, laboratory investigations should be considered to rule out sepsis and to determine the need for inpatient care. Commonly ordered labs are CBC, C-reactive protein, and liver and kidney function tests. Elevated C-reactive protein, creatinine, glucose, and total white blood count in a setting of low serum sodium and hemoglobin are indicative of necrotizing fasciitis.

Blood cultures are useful for patients with severe infections, signs of systematic involvement, in immunocompromised hosts, and when surgery is indicated. Tissue biopsies are the preferred diagnostic test for necrotizing soft-tissue infections. Although imaging is not indicated for simple soft-tissue infections, it may be useful in assessing the extent and depth of infection.

For the diagnosis of Lyme disease and Rocky Mountain spotted fever, clinical and epidemiological consideration are very important, especially in the early phases of the diseases. Suspect these diseases in patients living in or visiting endemic areas who present with a triad of rash, fever, and a history of tick bite during the first 3 days of the illness. The diagnosis of late disease is confirmed by serological tests.

Management

The initial management of skin infection should be determined by severity, location, comorbidities, type of infection, and presence or absence of purulence.

- For mild and localized infections, such as **impetigo,** with no systemic involvement and no uncontrolled comorbidities, start with topical antibiotics, such as mupirocin.
- Mild purulent and localized infections in easily accessible sites can be treated with incision and drainage alone.
- Infections with systemic spread or infections in uncontrolled comorbidities, such as diabetes, require inpatient management, and/or parenteral antibiotics.
- Serious infections, such as sepsis and necrotizing fasciitis, require parenteral antibiotics, inpatient management, often with critical care, and surgery.
- In general, antibiotic therapy should be considered for **abscesses involving extensive cellulitis**, rapid progression, poor responders to drainage, or those abscesses involving specific sites, such as face, hands, and genitalia. Also consider antibiotics in patients with significant comorbid conditions.
- Commonly used antibiotics for mild to moderate skin infections include penicillin G, amoxicillin/clavulanate (Augmentin), clindamycin, cefazolin, cephalexin, and dicloxacillin.
- Treatment of **necrotizing fasciitis** involves surgical debridement of necrotic tissue combined with empiric high-dose IV broad-spectrum antibiotics. Antibiotic choices for necrotizing and other complicated skin infections depend on susceptibility and may include penicillin G, clindamycin, and carbapenems.
- Management of **Lyme disease** requires amoxicillin in young children and doxycycline in older children and adults.
- **Rocky Mountain spotted fever** can be treated by tetracycline, doxycycline, or chloramphenicol.

> **CLINICAL PEARL:** Immunocompromised patients are at high risk for skin or soft-tissue infection and may not exhibit classic clinical or laboratory findings because of their attenuated inflammatory response. Initiate diagnostic testing and broad-spectrum antimicrobial therapy early.

■ SKIN INFECTIONS: FUNGAL

Etiology

Fungal infections of the skin, hair, and nails can result either from superficial or deep cutaneous infections or from systemic dissemination. Superficial fungal infections are the most common and are usually caused by overgrowth of mucocutaneous microbiomes. Candidiasis is mainly caused by the yeast *Candida albicans* and other candida species that require warm, humid microenvironments. Dermatophytosis is caused by a unique group of fungi (dermatophytes) that require keratin for growth. Examples include onychomycosis or *tinea unguium* (dermatophytosis of the nails) and *Tinea pedis* (dermatophyte of the feet). Skin fungal infections can also be caused by Malassezia species such as tinea versicolor. Malassezia species require humid microenvironments and lipids for growth. Fungal infections can be spread from person to person, animal to humans, or from the environment (such as dust).

Epidemiology

Candida species are present on about 20% of healthy individuals, but the incidence is increased by antibiotic therapy, pregnancy, estrogen-containing oral contraception, host defense defects, diabetes, and obesity. Dermatophytosis occurs most frequently in children as scalp or intertriginous infections. Onychomycosis is more prevalent in older adults.

Clinical Presentation

- **Cutaneous candidiasis** occurs in moist sites and occluded areas such as *intertriginous* areas and the diaper area. Patients will have pruritus, tenderness, and pain. The rash manifests with bright erythematous glistening skin in folds, pustulovesicular *satellite* lesions, and red macules with collarette of scale. Chronic infection of the nail apparatus (*paronychia*) can lead to nail dystrophy.
- Candida interdigital occurs as maceration in the webspaces of fingers and feet.
- Diaper dermatitis occurs in the genital, perianal inner aspect of the thigh and buttocks regions. It presents with irritability and discomfort, with erythema, edema, and papular and pustular lesions. There is scaling at the margins.
- **Oropharyngeal candidiasis** patients may develop white cottage cheese-like flecks on mucosal surfaces of the mouth. In candidal leukoplakia, white plaques that cannot be wiped off are notable on the buccal mucosa, tongue, and/or hard palate.
- In **dermatophytosis**, the lesions are characterized by redness, scaling at the edges, and central clearing. **Tinea capitis** (caused by Trichophyton species) is the most common dermatophytosis in children, affecting the scalp and hair shafts. **Tinea capitis** presents with scalp scaling and alopecia. The diffuse, patchy, or discrete alopecia may be associated with scalp pruritus and occipital adenopathy. The scalp sometimes develops a boggy sterile inflammatory mass called kerion.
- **Tinea corporis** (ringworm) typically appears as a single or multiple red, scaly, annular patch with central clearing, commonly on the trunk, legs, arms, and neck. The lesion can be slightly elevated with sharp margination. The borders may contain pustules or follicular papules with variable itching.
- **Tinea pedis (athlete's foot)** can occur in the interdigital form, which is characterized by itching, fissuring, maceration, and scaling in the interdigital spaces. Alternatively, the plantar skin becomes chronically scaly and thickened, with hyperkeratosis and erythema of soles, heels, and sides of feet.[3]
- **Tinea unguium (onychomycosis)** is a dermatophyte infection of the nail plate and bed. It occurs mostly in the big toe and leads to opaque, thickened, cracked, and hyperkeratotic nails. A white chalky patch pain and ulceration of the underlying nail bed are also common.

- **Tinea versicolor (pityriasis versicolor)** is caused by the lipophilic yeast flora Malassezia furfur. It is characterized by chronic hypopigmented, well-demarcated macules with fine scale on neck, chest, back, but less often on face. It is more common in adolescents and adults than in children.

Diagnosis

Skin fungal infections can readily be diagnosed based on history, physical examination, and potassium hydroxide (KOH) microscopy. Fungal presence is identified as hyphae or spores on KOH microscopy. Some cases may require Wood's lamp examination, and if the diagnosis is not conclusive or if it is not responding to treatment, fungal cultures or histologic investigations may be undertaken.[12]

CLINICAL PEARL: A key distinguishing feature for dermatophyte lesions is an inflammatory pattern at the edge of the lesion, usually accompanied by scaling, redness, and occasionally blistering. Recently, Wood's lamp examination has become less useful in diagnosing dermatophyte infections because a significant proportion of these infections is caused by Trichophyton species, which do not fluoresce in contrast to Microsporum species, which produce a bright blue–green fluorescence.

Tinea (pityriasis) versicolor produces pale yellow to white fluoresce, whereas tinea cruris or cutaneous candidiasis do not fluoresce.[12,13]

The most sensitive diagnostic method for tinea unguium (onychomycosis) is periodic acid–Schiff staining with histologic examination of the clipped, distal free edge of the nail and subungual debris.[14]

Management

Topical antifungal therapy is usually the initial management of skin fungal infection. For tinea capitis, tinea barbae, and onychomycosis, oral therapy is preferred.

- To treat **cutaneous candidiasis,** address the predisposing conditions, use topical nystatin cream/powder, ketoconazole, or clotrimazole two to four times per day.
- **Oral candidiasis** (thrush gray–white plaques with red base) can be treated with nystatin suspension (100,000 U/mL), wich is swished in the mouth and then spit out.
- **Disseminated or systemic candidiasis** should be treated with oral antifungals such as fluconazole, itraconazole, ketoconazole, or amphotericin B for severe disease.
- **Tinea capitis** is treated with oral griseofulvin. Provide 20 to 25 mg/kg/d in a single daily dose with fatty food. Treat for 6 to 12 weeks.
- Adjunctive use of selenium sulfide, ketoconazole, or ciclopirox shampoo decreases fungal shedding. Patient should wash fomites like combs, bedding, and hats.
- **Tinea corporis** treatment involves measures to decrease excessive moisture. Treat with topical antifungals twice daily for 2 to 4 weeks. These treatments can be clotrimazole, ketoconazole, miconazole, or econazole.

Second-line topical treatment may involve terbinafine, naftifine, butenafine, or ciclopirox.

- **Tinea pedis** (athlete's foot) is treated by applying antifungal cream to the foot web.
- **Tinea unguium (onychomycosis)** is treated with oral therapy (terbinafine, itraconazole, fluconazole). Topical ciclopirox nail gel is less efficacious. Tinea unguium is very difficult to eradicate and should be treated for a prolonged time (minimum 6 weeks for fingernail infections and minimum 12 weeks for toenail infections). Patients should debride dystrophic nails weekly and apply secondary prophylaxis with powder, antifungal creams lotions, or antiseptic gels.
- **Tinea versicolor (pityriasis versicolor)** is treated with topical selenium sulfide lotion or shampoo 2.5%; apply for 20 minutes and rinse, once daily for 7 days, then once weekly for 4 weeks. Systemic therapy with ketoconazole or fluconazole may also be useful.

CLINICAL PEARL: Topical treatment is not effective for tinea capitis and tinea unguium (onychomycosis). Systemic prolonged therapy is required to penetrate the hair follicles and nail system. Prolonged therapy is expensive and carries a risk for hepatotoxicity. Liver function should be monitored during treatment.

▧ SKIN INFECTIONS: VIRAL

Etiology

Common viral skin infections include warts, caused by human papillomavirus, molluscum contagiosum, HSV, varicella zoster, and viral exanthems. Most of these infections are asymptomatic, self-limited, or latent. In immunocompromised individuals, these infections may become persistent and extensive. Transmission can be via airborne droplets, skin-to-skin contact, in utero, intrapartum, through sexual intercourse, and/or via exposure to blood or other body secretions.

Epidemiology

The highest incidence for human papilloma virus (HPV) is in the 10- to 19-year-old age group. Molluscum contagiosum is more common in children, sexually active adults, and immunocompromised individuals, such as those with HIV/AIDS. Overall, the epidemiology of viral skin infection is evolving due to immunizations.

Clinical Presentation

- **Warts/HPV** include more than 150 subtypes, such as common warts (verruca vulgaris), plantar warts (verruca plantaris), and external genital warts. They present as firm, grainy papules, and hyperkeratotic vegetations. Warts can appear as red to brown dots with thrombosed dermal capillary loops. The skin distribution varies. They can occur as isolated lesions, as crops of verrucous papules, in confluent patterns, or in a cauliflower-like appearance.

- **Molluscum contagious lesions** are white, pink, or flesh-colored small raised lesions with a dimple in the center. They are usually smooth, firm, 2 to 3 mm in diameter, and can occur anywhere on the body.
- **HSV** lesions can present as a cluster of grouped pustules or vesicles arising from an erythematous base. Lymphadenopathy may be present. After a primary infection, HSV persists in sensory ganglia for the life of the patient. Healthy individuals can be symptomatic, but the disease may recur with lessening immunity.
- **Varicella zoster virus (VZV) disease** is characterized by disseminated multiple pruritic vesicles on an erythematous base. Primary infection (chicken pox) is always symptomatic and establishes lifelong infection in sensory ganglion. A potential complication of VZV occurs when there is reactivation of the virus causing **herpes zoster**. This eruption presents as grouped vesicles along a dermatome (shingles). See Figure 2.6 for an example of herpes zoster.

CLINICAL PEARL: Administer the varicella zoster vaccine to all adults ≥60 years of age to prevent or attenuate herpes zoster infection.

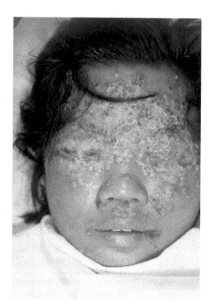

FIGURE 2.6 Example of herpes zoster infection.
Source: Lyons F, Ousley L. *Dermatology for the Advanced Practice Nurse.* New York, NY: Springer Publishing Company; 2014.

Other systemic viral infections with exanthems often present with characteristic mucocutaneous rashes accompanied by fever and/or other nonspecific symptoms such as coryza, sore throat, nausea, vomiting, abdominal pain, and headache (see Table 2.16). The most common presentation is a morbilliform, maculopapular blanchable rash on the trunk and face. The most common etiologies are enteroviruses in summer and respiratory viruses in winter. Viral exanthems are generally benign and are treated based on symptoms. They can be differentiated by history and rash appearance (Table 2.16).

Diagnosis

The diagnosis of viral skin infections is made clinically and can be confirmed by serology and viral cultures. Biopsy may be indicated to rule out viral-induced squamous cell carcinoma (SCC). Viral cultures can be used in the diagnosis of HSV. In infected specimens, acantholytic keratinocytes or multinucleated giant keratinocytes are detected. Polymerase chain reaction has emerged as a more rapid, sensitive, and specific method to confirm viral skin infections such as herpes simplex.

TABLE 2.16 Clinical Features of Viral Exanthems

Viral Exanthems Agent	Etiology	Characteristic Features
Measles	Paramyxovirus	An erythematous maculopapular rash and Koplik spots (small, irregular red spots with central gray or bluish-white specks that appear on the buccal mucosa) Incubation period is 8–12 days after initial exposure to the virus High fever, malaise, cough, coryza, conjunctivitis
Rubella	Rubella virus	Pink macules and papules, petechiae on the soft palate, mild fever, generalized lymphadenopathy, and transient joint pain The rash generally starts on the forehead, spreads inferiorly to face, trunk, and extremities during the first day The rash rarely last >5 days
Hand, foot, and mouth disease	Coxsackie A	Maculopapular vesicular rash on the hands and feet Ulcers on the tongue and oral mucosa
Erythema infectiosum	Parvovirus B19	Marked erythema of the cheeks (slapped cheek appearance) Erythematous, pruritic, reticular rash starting from the arms spreading to the trunk and legs.
Roseola infantum	Herpesvirus 6	Morbilliform rash appears after a high fever The rash starts on the trunk and spreads to the periphery

CLINICAL PEARL: The use of HPV-DNA testing is not recommended because test results do not alter clinical management.

Management

- **Molluscum lesions:** Conservative monitoring for spontaneous resolution, or if more extensive, curettage, cryotherapy, electrodessication, and imiquimod 5% cream.
- **Common warts**: Spontaneously resolve within months to a few years. Topical salicylic acid and lactic acid can be used for small lesions. Also, imiquimod 5% cream can be applied to sites that are not extensively keratinized. Cryotherapy with liquid nitrogen (multiple treatments) is effective in freezing the wart but has no effect on HPV. Warts can also be removed by occlusion therapy where patients are instructed to place and leave a piece of wart removal tape or duct tape on the wart for about 6 days.[15] Other therapies include immunotherapy, as well as electro and laser surgery.
- **HSV** can be managed with antiviral therapy (acyclovir, famciclovir, valacyclovir), which shortens the duration of symptoms and signs.
  - Oral Acyclovir: 400 mg, three times daily, or 200 mg five times daily for 7 to 10 days
  - Famciclovir: 250 mg, three times daily for 5 to 10 days
  - Valacyclovir: 1 g twice daily for 5 to 10 days
- Patients with severe, recurrent HSV should be managed by chronic suppressive therapy with daily antiviral therapy such as valacyclovir 500 mg daily.
- Pain and itching associated with viral skin diseases can be managed with acetaminophin and antihistamines. The use of NSAIDS is associated with an elevated risk of severe skin and soft-tissue complications of varicella zoster virus infection, mostly in children with varicella.[16]
- Aspirin should be avoided in a setting of viral exanthems due to increased risk of Reyes syndrome.

CLINICAL PEARL: Selection of treatment regimen depends on wart size, number, anatomic site morphology, patient preference, cost, adverse effects, and provider experience. Imiquimod should not be used during pregnancy.

REFERENCES

1. Wolff K, Johnson RA. *Fitzpatrick's Color Atlas and Synopsis of Clinical Dermatology.* New York, NY: McGraw Hill; 2009.
2. Hafner C, Vogt T. Seborrheic keratosis. *J Dtsch Dermatol Ges.* 2008;6:664. doi:10.1111/j.1610-0387.2008.06788.x
3. Rydholm A, Berg NO. Size, site and clinical incidence of lipoma. Factors in the differential diagnosis of lipoma and sarcoma. *Acta Orthop Scand.* 1983;54:929–934. doi:10.3109/17453678308992936

4. Plunkett A, Merlin K, Gill D, et al. The frequency of common nonmalignant skin conditions in adults in central Victoria, Australia. *Int J Dermatol*. 1999;38:901–908. doi:10.1046/j.1365-4362.1999.00856.x

5. Friedman RJ, Rigel DS, Kopf AW. Early detection of malignant melanoma: the role of physician examination and self-examination of the skin. *CA: Cancer J Clin*. 1985;35(3):130–151. doi:10.3322/canjclin.35.3.130

6. Islami F, Goding Sauer A, Miller KD, et al. Proportion and number of cancer cases and deaths attributable to potentially modifiable risk factors in the United States. *CA: Cancer J Clin*. 2018;68(1):31–54. doi:10.3322/caac.21440

7. Arora A, Attwood J. Common skin cancers and their precursors. *Surg Clin*. 2009;89(3):703–712. doi:10.1016/j.suc.2009.03.007

8. Breslow A. Thickness, cross-sectional areas and depth of invasion in the prognosis of cutaneous melanoma. *Ann Surg*. 1970;172(5):902. doi:10.1097/00000658-197011000-00017

9. Balch CM, Buzaid AC, Soong SJ, et al. Final version of the American Joint Committee on Cancer staging system for cutaneous melanoma. *J Clin Oncol*. 2001;19(16):3635–3648. doi:10.1200/JCO.2001.19.16.3635

10. Hersh AL, Chambers HF, Maselli JH, et al. National trends in ambulatory visits and antibiotic prescribing for skin and soft-tissue infections. *Arch Intern Med*. 2008;168(14):1585–1591. doi:10.1001/archinte.168.14.1585

11. Esposito S, Noviello S, Leone S. Epidemiology and microbiology of skin and soft tissue infections. *Curr Opin Infect Dis*. 2016;29(2):109–115. doi:10.1097/QCO.0000000000000239

12. Hainer BL. Dermatophyte infections. *Am Fam Physician*. 2003;67(1):101–110.

13. Aly R. Ecology, epidemiology and diagnosis of tinea capitis. *Pediatr Infect Dis J*. 1999;18(2):180–185. doi:10.1097/00006454-199902000-00025

14. Mehregan DR, Gee SL. The cost effectiveness of testing for onychomycosis versus empiric treatment of onychodystrophies with oral antifungal agents. *Cutis*. 1999;64(6):407–410.

15. Focht DR 3rd, Spicer C, Fairchok MP. The efficacy of duct tape vs cryotherapy in the treatment of verruca vulgaris (the common wart). *Arch Pediatr Adolesc Med*. 2002;156:971–974. doi:10.1001/archpedi.156.10.971

16. Mikaeloff Y, Kezouh A, Suissa S. Nonsteroidal anti-inflammatory drug use and the risk of severe skin and soft tissue complications in patients with varicella or zoster disease. *Br J Clin Pharmacol*. 2008;65(2):203–209. doi:10.1111/j.1365-2125.2007.02997.x

PSORIASIS/PSORIASIFORM DERMATOSES

Etiology

Psoriasis is a chronic inflammatory skin condition with several clinical manifestations. The etiology includes both genetic and environmental factors. About 30% of patients with psoriasis have a first-degree relative with the disease.[1] Psoriasis can be triggered by physiological stress, environmental factors, physical trauma, and Streptococcal throat infections. Certain drugs such as steroids, lithium, antimalarials, interferon, beta-blockers, alcohol ingestion, and smoking can also increase the risk and severity of psoriatic flares.[2]

Epidemiology

Psoriasis affects about 2% of the U.S. adult population and is often associated with systemic manifestations such as psoriatic arthritis (10%–25% of the patients).[3] It occurs in all ages, but early onset predicts a more serious and long-lasting disease. The prevalence is about equal between men and women. The disease has a low incidence in North and South American Indians, West Africans, and Japanese.

Clinical Presentation

- Psoriasis typically presents with chronic, recurring erythematous scaly patches, papules, and plaques. Clinical presentation varies according to the form of the disease:
  - ○ Psoriasis vulgaris (plaque, inverse, guttate, palmoplantar)
  - ○ Psoriatic erythroderma
  - ○ Pustular psoriasis
- Plaque psoriasis (the most common form) is characterized by well-defined round or oval plaques of varying sizes that often coalesce. These lesions are commonly found on the extensor surfaces of the arms, legs, scalp, buttocks, and trunk.[4]
- Inverse psoriasis is less scaly compared to plaque psoriasis. Lesions appear with brightly red erythematous glistening base and occur mostly in skin folds such as submammary, axillary, perineal, inguinal, and intergluteal regions.
- Guttate psoriasis appears as salmon-pink papules with fine silvery-white scales. In a chronic form, the papules coalesce into plaques to form large geographical regions. Lesions are usually on the trunk and buttocks and may appear several weeks after group A Streptococcal (GAS) pharyngitis.
- Unlike guttate psoriasis with scattered erythematous papules, psoriatic erythroderma is characterized by widespread generalized erythema and often accompanied with systemic symptoms.
- Pustular psoriasis presents in two forms: a chronic relapsing and localized form and a generalized acute psoriasis form. The localized form generally consists of pustules on the palms and soles, without plaque formation. The generalized acute form presents as burning, creamy-white coalescing pustules on a fiery-red erythematous base. It is also associated with fever and leukocytosis.

Diagnosis

A diagnosis of psoriasis is made clinically based on history and physical examination findings, particularly the presence of erythematous scaly patches, papules, and plaques. Patients with psoriasis are at increased risk for various comorbidities such as psoriatic arthritis, Crohn's disease, ulcerative colitis, malignancy, and depression. These conditions should be considered in the workup of these patients.

Management

The management of psoriasis is determined by a number of factors: age, type of psoriasis, site and extent of involvement, severity, previous treatments, and associated comorbidities such as arthritis or HIV/AIDS (see Figure 2.7).[2] The goal is to improve the skin, nails, and joint lesions, as well as to enhance the quality of life.

- For localized and mild cases, treat with topical therapies such as corticosteroids, vitamin D analogs, calcineurin inhibitors (tacrolimus or pimecrolimus), and retinoids such as tazarotene.

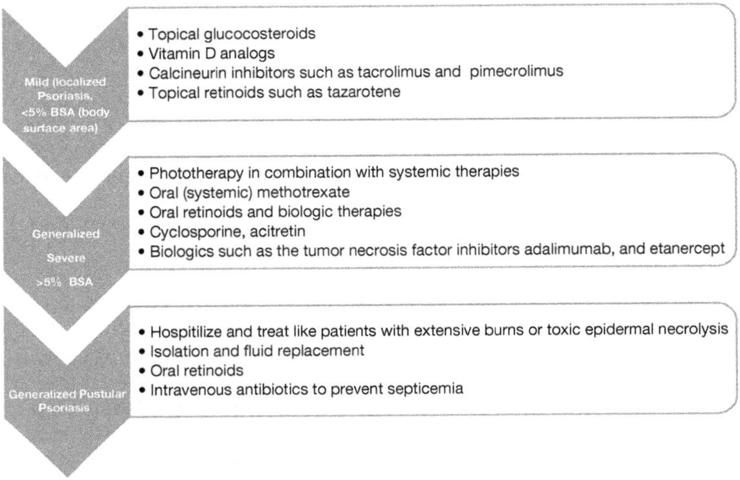

- Mild (localized Psoriasis, <5% BSA (body surface area)
  - Topical glucocosteroids
  - Vitamin D analogs
  - Calcineurin inhibitors such as tacrolimus and pimecrolimus
  - Topical retinoids such as tazarotene

- Generalized Severe >5% BSA
  - Phototherapy in combination with systemic therapies
  - Oral (systemic) methotrexate
  - Oral retinoids and biologic therapies
  - Cyclosporine, acitretin
  - Biologics such as the tumor necrosis factor inhibitors adalimumab, and etanercept

- Generalized Pustular Psoriasis
  - Hospitilize and treat like patients with extensive burns or toxic epidermal necrolysis
  - Isolation and fluid replacement
  - Oral retinoids
  - Intravenous antibiotics to prevent septicemia

FIGURE 2.7 Management of psoriasis.

- Psoriasis localized to the scalp often requires tar or ketoconazole shampoo followed by betamethasone. For psoriasis localized to the nails, topical treatment alone is not sufficient; add systemic therapy with methotrexate and corticosteroids.
- Patients with generalized and severe psoriasis require phototherapy in combination with systemic therapies.
- Biologicals such as tumor necrosis factor inhibitors are also effective for severe psoriasis or psoriatic arthritis.

CLINICAL PEARL: Most treatment options for psoriasis have significant side effects; monitor patients regularly and individualize treatment plans.

REFERENCES

1. Capon F, Trembath RC, Barker JN. An update on the genetics of psoriasis. *Dermatol Clin.* 2004;22(4):339–347. doi:10.1016/S0733-8635(03)00125-6
2. Menter A, Gottlieb A, Feldman SR, et al. Guidelines of care for the management of psoriasis and psoriatic arthritis: section 1. Overview of psoriasis and guidelines of care for the treatment of psoriasis with biologics. *J Am Acad Dermatol.* 2008;58(5):826–850. doi:10.1016/j.jaad.2008.02.039
3. Wolff K, Johnson RA. *Fitzpatrick's Color Atlas and Synopsis of Clinical Dermatology.* McGraw Hill; 2009.
4. Griffiths CE, Barker JN. Pathogenesis and clinical features of psoriasis. *Lancet.* 2007;370(9583):263–271. doi:10.1016/S0140-6736(07)61128-3

ENDOCRINE SYSTEM

ADRENAL DISORDERS: ADRENAL INSUFFICIENCY

Etiology

The main diseases of the adrenal glands are adrenal insufficiency (Addison's disease) and hypercortisolism (Cushing's disease and syndrome). Adrenal insufficiency occurs when there is impaired synthesis and release of adreno-cortical hormones. Hypercortisolism occurs when there are excessive levels of cortisol.

The most common cause of primary adrenal insufficiency in the industrialized world is autoimmune inflammation of the adrenal cortex.[1] The most common cause of adrenal insufficiency worldwide is tuberculosis. Other causes include infectious diseases, particularly fungal diseases, metastatic disease (from lung or breast cancer), and iatrogenic causes such as bilateral adrenalectomy.

Secondary adrenal insufficiency may result from long-term steroid therapy. Chronic suppression of corticotrophin-releasing hormone (CRH) and adrenocorticotropic hormone (ACTH) by exogenous steroids prevents the adrenal from releasing appropriate amount of cortisol. Secondary adrenal insufficiency may also be caused by other endocrine disorders such as hypothalamic diseases or hypopituitarism.[2] Adrenal crisis (acute and severe symptoms) can be precipitated by stress such as trauma, surgery, or infection and can be fatal if not managed effectively.

Epidemiology

In Western countries, the prevalence of Addison's disease is about 35 to 60 individuals per million.[3,4] Women are more often affected than men.[2]

Clinical Presentation

The most common signs and symptoms of Addison's disease include weakness, fatigue, anorexia, and weight loss. Most patients have hyperpigmentation, hypotension, and GI disturbances. Some patients crave salt may have postural symptoms, hypoglycemia, hyponatremia, and hyperkalemia. Patients with adrenal crisis present with acute and severe symptoms including severe hypotension and cardiac complications, abdominal pain, acute kidney injury, and death. Skin hyperpigmentation and hyperkalemia are found predominantly in primary adrenal insufficiency when ACTH is elevated (not in secondary disease when ACTH levels are low).

Diagnosis

Primary adrenal insufficiency is suspected when there is low plasma cortisol (<5 mcg/dL) at 8:00 a.m. accompanied by elevated ACTH.[5] If both the serum cortisol and the plasma ACTH concentrations are low, this implies a secondary adrenal insufficiency (Table 2.17).

TABLE **2.17** Differentiating Primary Versus Secondary Adrenal Insufficiency

Clinical Finding	Primary	Secondary
Cortisol	Low	Low
ACTH	High	Low
Glucose	Low (hypoglycemia)	Low (hypoglycemia)
Sodium	Low (hyponatremia)	Low (hyponatremia)
Potassium	High (hyperkalemia)	Normal
Blood pressure	Low (hypotension)	Low (hypotension)

ACTH, adrenocorticotropic hormone.

A definitive diagnosis of adrenal insufficiency is established by measuring the adrenal response to ACTH through the cosyntropin stimulation test. A patient with suspected adrenal insufficiency is given an IV infusion of synthetic ACTH, and plasma cortisol is then measured. In primary adrenal insufficiency, plasma cortisol does NOT increase sufficiently 30 to 60 minutes after infusion of synthetic ACTH. In secondary adrenal insufficiency, cortisol levels fail to respond to ACTH infusion.

Patients with suspected adrenal insufficiency should also be screened for antiadrenal antibodies, which are markers of autoimmune adrenalitis. Perform adrenal CT imaging if these tests are negative. Brain imaging by MRI should be performed if secondary adrenal insufficiency is diagnosed (Figure 2.8).

Management

Patients with primary adrenal insufficiency should be treated with daily oral hydrocortisone or prednisone and daily fludrocortisone. The management is outlined in Figure 2.8.

REFERENCES

1. Zelissen PM, Bast EJ, Croughs RJ. Associated autoimmunity in Addison's disease. *J Autoimmun.* 1995;8:121–130. doi:10.1006/jaut.1995.0009
2. Arlt W. Disorders of the adrenal cortex. In: Jameson J, Fauci AS, Kasper DL, et al., eds. *Harrison's Principles of Internal Medicine.* 20th ed. New York, NY: McGraw-Hill. http://accessmedicine.mhmedical.com/content.aspx?bookid=2129&sectionid=192 287137. Accessed September 20, 2018.
3. Willis AC, Vince FP. The prevalence of addison's disease in coventry, UK. *Postgrad Med J.* 1997;73:286. doi:10.1136/pgmj.73.859.286
4. Laureti S, Vecchi L, Santeusanio F, et al. Is the prevalence of Addison's disease underestimated? *J Clin Endocrinol Metab.* 1999;84:1762. doi:10.1210/jcem.84.5.5677-7
5. Hägg E, Asplund K, Lithner F. Value of basal plasma cortisol assays in the assessment of pituitary-adrenal insufficiency. *Clin Endocrinol (Oxf).* 1987;26:221. doi:10.1111/j.1365-2265.1987.tb00780.x

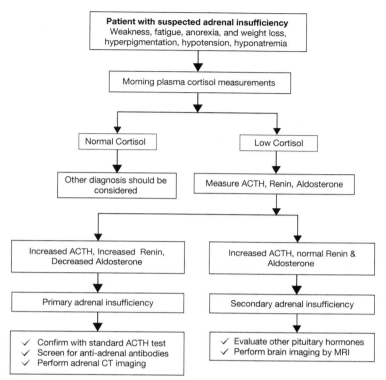

FIGURE 2.8   Approach to a patient with adrenal insufficiency.

ADRENAL DISORDERS—HYPERCORTISOLISM: CUSHING'S SYNDROME

Etiology

Cushing's syndrome or hypercortisolism occurs when there are excessive levels of glucocorticoids due to any cause. Cortisol is the principle glucocorticoid. Hypercortisolism can be exogenous or endogenous. The exogenous or iatrogenic form is usually caused by chronic use of prescribed glucocorticoids. Cushing's syndrome results from excessive secretion of ACTH by the pituitary. The chronic hypersecretion of ACTH results in adrenal hyperplasia, which leads to increased adrenocorticoid secretion of cortisol and androgens. Other causes of hypercortisolism include adrenal adenomas, carcinoma, and ectopic (nonpituitary) ACTH-producing tumors, which are frequently seen in patients with small-cell carcinoma of the lung.

Epidemiology

Cushing's syndrome is a relatively rare condition with an estimated annual incidence of two to three individuals per million. It is more prevalent in patients with poorly controlled diabetes and HTN compared to the general population. Cushing's disease is most common in premenopausal women.[1]

Clinical Presentation

The most common features of Cushing's sundrome include decreased libido, weight gain (central obesity), hirsutism, hypogonadism, menstrual changes in women, HTN, lethargy, depression, ecchymosis, and striae. Patients may have a moon face, "buffalo hump" on the upper back, acne, and easy bruising. Other common features ae proximal muscle wasting and weakness, osteoporosis, vertebral fractures, hypercalciuria, and kidney stones.

> **CLINICAL PEARL:** A number of clinical features associated with hypercortisolism are nonspecific, but pigmented striae, proximal muscle weakness, easy bruising, and virilization tend to be more specific.

Diagnosis

The initial step is to confirm that the patient has elevated cortisol levels. The second step is to determine the source of the excessive cortisol as from pituitary, adrenal, or other sources. Patients with Cushing's syndrome usually have an elevated 24-hour urine-free cortisol level (>100 mcg/24 h). A dexamethasone suppression test is performed to confirm the source of the elevated cortisol. A serum cortisol level >1.7 mcg/dL after the single-dose dexamethasone is considered a positive test for Cushing's disease (pituitary causes).[2,3]

MRI of the pituitary gland should be performed if a pituitary tumor is suspected. In ACTH-independent Cushing's syndrome, perform CT or MRI scanning for adrenocorticoid and other tumors.

Management

The goal of treatment is to remove the tumor that is producing excessive ACTH, correcting unregulated hypersecretion of adrenal hormones. Patients with Cushing's disease should be managed surgically with transsphenoidal resection and hydrocortisol replacement. Similarly, surgical removal of tumors is the treatment of choice for patients with Cushing's of nonpituitary causes. Alternative therapies include radiation and chemotherapy for patients with nonresectable tumors.

REFERENCES

1. Etxabe JVJA, Vazquez JA. Morbidity and mortality in Cushing's disease: an epidemiological approach. *Clin Endocrinol.* 1994;40(4):479–484. doi:10.1111/j.1365-2265.1994.tb02486.x
2. Nieman LK, Biller BM, Findling JW, et al. The diagnosis of Cushing's syndrome: an endocrine society clinical practice guideline. *J Clin Endocrinol Metab.* May 2008;93(5):1526–1540. doi:10.1210/jc.2008-0125
3. Yanovski JA, Cutler GB Jr, Chrousos GP, et al. Corticotropin-releasing hormone stimulation following low-dose dexamethasone administration, a new test to distinguish Cushing's syndrome from pseudo-Cushing's states. *JAMA.* May 5, 1993;269(17):2232–2238. doi:10.1001/jama.269.17.2232. PubMed 8386285.

DIABETES MELLITUS

Etiology

DM is a chronic metabolic disease caused by either absolute or relative insulin deficiency or varying degrees of insulin resistance leading to high blood glucose levels (hyperglycemia). Long-term complications are due to microvascular and macrovascular disease. If pancreatic beta cells do not produce enough insulin or the body does not respond to the insulin, then glucose builds up in the blood instead of being absorbed, leading to prediabetes or diabetes. Over time, high blood glucose damages nerves and blood vessels leading to complications.

Diabetes can be classified into the following general categories:

- Type 1 DM (due to beta-cell destruction leading to insulin deficiency)
- Type 2 DM (progressive loss of insulin secretion on the background of insulin resistance)
- Gestational DM (diagnosed in the second or third trimester)
- MODY (maturity onset diabetes of the young caused by mutations; most common forms are glucokinase, HNF alpha mutations)
- LADA (latent autoimmune DM in adults)

Epidemiology

Diabetes is one of the leading causes of death worldwide, with an age-adjusted prevalence over 10% in most places in North America.[1]

The risk factors for DM-2 include the following:

- Age 45 or older
- Overweight or obese
- Physically inactive
- Family history
- Family background that is African American, Alaska Native, American Indian, Asian American, Hispanic/Latino, or Pacific Islander American
- History of giving birth to a baby weighing more than 9 pounds
- History of gestational diabetes
- History of HTN
- HDL <35 mg/dL or triglyceride level above 250 mg/dL
- PCOS
- Prediabetes—A1C level of 5.7% to 6.4%; a fasting plasma glucose test result of 100 to 125 mg/dL; or a 2-hour oral glucose tolerance test result of 140 to 199
- History of CVD

Clinical Presentation

During history taking, review all systems and ask about symptoms of hypo- and hyperglycemia and assess for comorbidities, particularly cardiovascular diseases. Patients often present with frequent urination (polyuria), feeling very thirsty (polydipsia), feeling very hungry (polyphagia), extreme fatigue, blurry vision, cuts/bruises slow to heal, unintentional weight loss (type 1), tingling, pain, or numbness in the hands/feet (type 2).

> **CLINICAL PEARL:** Some people with type 2 diabetes have symptoms so mild that they go unnoticed.

It is important to perform a comprehensive physical examination, checking multiple organ manifestations of diabetes, such as dry skin, poor oral health, vision changes, peripheral vascular systems, and neural deficits. Vital signs may reveal increased weight and BMI. HTN should be noted if present as this further increases cardiovascular risk in patients with diabetes. Orthostatic BP may be noted in patients with autonomic dysfunction. Abnormal respiration patterns may be seen in conditions such as diabetic ketoacidosis.

One of the most important examinations to perform is the ophthalmologic evaluation. Retinopathy changes are common, in part due to the frequency of delayed recognition of diabetes. Findings include cotton wool spots, or yellow areas related to nerve infarction, as well as flame hemorrhages which occur secondary to microaneurysm. A complete cardiovascular examination should be performed. Note the presence of murmurs, S3, S4, and an irregular rhythm, a combination of which can be seen in HTN and HF. Listen for carotid bruits, and palpate all peripheral pulses. As diabetes predisposes to infection, poor wound healing, and peripheral neuropathy, a complete foot examination should include skin integrity and sensory evaluation.

Diagnosis

Use a motivational interviewing technique, perform a comprehensive medical history (including risk factors, lifestyle, diet and exercise, employment, and social support) and physical exam. Ask about exercise type, timing, and duration. Also inquire about meal types, amount, timing, who prepares them, and how they are prepared. Identify social factors such as stress that may raise blood sugar. Define illnesses and medications taken. Learn about family history. Assess for potential barriers to care, such as lack of understanding of the disease, drug cost, stigma, work issues, and living conditions.

Type 2 diabetes testing should be done in all adults who are overweight or obese (BMI ≥25 or ≥23 in Asian Americans) who have one or more diabetes risk factors, such as those listed earlier.[2]

Criteria for the diagnosis of diabetes includes any of the following:[3]

- Fasting plasma glucose ≥126 mg/dL (7.0 mmol/L). Fasting is defined as no caloric intake for at least 8 hours.
- 2-hour postprandial glucose ≥200 mg/dL (11.1 mmol/L) during an oral glucose tolerance test. The test should be performed using a glucose load containing the equivalent of 75 g anhydrous glucose dissolved in water.
- A1C ≥6.5% (48 mmol/mol). The test should be performed in a laboratory using a method that is National Glycohemoglobin Standardization Program (NGSP) certified and standardized to the Diabetes Control and Complications Trial (DCCT) assay.

- In a patient with classic symptoms of hyperglycemia or hyperglycemic crisis, a random plasma glucose ≥200 mg/dL (11.1 mmol/L).

CLINICAL PEARL: The American Diabetes Association (ADA) recommends that testing to detect prediabetes and type 2 diabetes be considered in adults who are overweight or obese and have one or more additional risk factors for diabetes. In adults without these risk factors, testing should begin at age 45.

Management

Management of diabetes requires an integrated and team-based approach, following chronic disease models. It is essential to use a patient-centered approach where care is respectful and responsive to individual patient preferences, needs, and values. Treatment goals should be individualized and focused on shared decision-making with the patient. Patients must be educated about diabetes and what they need to do to control blood glucose and prevent complications.

Testing for A1C should be performed at least *two times each year* in individuals who are meeting treatment targets and have stable glycemic control. The frequency of A1C testing can be increased to *quarterly* in individuals whose therapy has changed or who are not meeting glycemic targets.

Additional laboratory investigation should include fasting lipid panel, comprehensive metabolic panel, specifically evaluating renal function, and evaluation for microalbuminuria. Measuring the albumin-to-creatinine ratio in a urine sample provides an estimate of daily albumin excretion. A result >30 mg/g indicates albuminuria, which can accelerate renal damage and macrovascular disease.

For ongoing (chronic) management:

- Asses for glycemic control targets using A1C, initiate lifestyle modifications and pharmacological therapy
- Monitor for diabetic complications
- Educate patient about self-management
- Discuss diet and exercise as the cornerstone of DM management and discuss goals
- Arrange follow-up and referrals
- Provide resources and diabetes tool kit (glucometer, test strips, lancets, logbook, calorie, and carbohydrate counter books)
- Offer encouragement
- Routinely check urine for ketones and kidney function
- Offer appropriate immunizations (such as influenza and pneumonia vaccines)
- Monitor for complications with annual dilated eye exam, regular foot exams and monofilament assessment, BP and lipid level control monitoring, and check for albuminuria to monitor kidney function

> **CLINICAL PEARL:** Early glucose control has been shown to prevent microvascular complications such as nephropathy, neuropathy, retinopathy, and macrovascular complications such as stroke and MI (DCCT/Epidemiology of Diabetes Interventions and Complications).[2,4,5]

PHARMACOLOGICAL THERAPY FOR TYPE 2 DIABETES

The choice of pharmacologic therapy should be patient-based and consider efficacy, cost, resources, and the patient's comorbidities. Evaluate the potential side effects, including cardiovascular risk, possibilities of hypoglycemia, and effects on weight.

In general, more stringent glucose control should be considered in newly diagnosed individuals, those with low risk of hypoglycemia without comorbidities or vascular complications, those with long life expectancy, highly motivated patients, and those with readily available resources and support systems.

In the United States, the most popular noninsulin therapeutic options for type 2 diabetes are the following:

- Metformin, SGLT-2 inhibitors, glucagon-like peptide-1 (GLP-1) receptor agonists, DPP-4 inhibitors, thiazolidinediones, and sulfonylureas. Treatment considerations can be found in Table 2.18.

Insulin is eventually needed for many patients due to the progressive nature of type 2 diabetes. It is desirable to start insulin early and it may be the first-line drug if the patient is acutely symptomatic and has marked elevations in Hgb A1C. When adding insulin to the patient's regimen, be sure to educate the patient about insulin action and the potential for hypoglycemia, and monitor weight changes and hypoglycemia episodes. An overview of insulin preparation options can be found in Appendix B, Insulin Use in Primary Care.

TABLE 2.18 Medications for Hyperglycemia in Type 2 Diabetes Mellitus

At diagnosis, initiate lifestyle modifications, set A1C targets, initiate pharmacological therapy	
If A1C <9%, consider monotherapy **If A1C >9% consider dual therapy** **If A1C >10% + symptoms, consider combination injectable.**	
Metformin	Preferred initial therapy, if tolerated and not contraindicated, when lifestyle changes alone have not achieved or maintained glycemic goals
Consider insulin therapy with or without other agents	Initially in newly diagnosed patients with markedly symptomatic and/or elevated blood glucose levels or A1C
Add second oral agent, GLP-1 receptor agonist, or insulin	If noninsulin monotherapy at maximal tolerated dose does not achieve or maintain A1C target over 3 months

GLP-1, glucagon-like peptide.

> **CLINICAL PEARL:** To efficiently manage blood sugar to desired targets, teach the patient how to keep a log of carbohydrate intake, activity levels, medication dosing and frequency, hypo- and hyperglycemic episodes, as well as illness and stress conditions.

BARIATRIC SURGERY IN TYPE 2 DIABETES

Bariatric surgery can achieve near or complete normalization of glycemia 2 years after surgery. It should be considered for adults with BMI >35 kg/m^2, particularly if diabetes or associated comorbidities are difficult to control with lifestyle and pharmacologic therapy. It is important for patients to know that lifelong lifestyle support and medical monitoring are necessary postsurgery. Patients should also know that bariatric surgery is expensive, invasive, has variable outcomes depending on procedure, may predispose to long-term vitamin/mineral deficiencies, osteoporosis, and can cause severe hypoglycemia.

SELF-MANAGEMENT EDUCATION AND SUPPORT

In accordance with the national standards for diabetes self-management education (DSME) and support (DSMS), all DM patients should participate in self-management education to facilitate the knowledge, skills, and ability necessary for diabetes self-care both at diagnosis and as needed thereafter.[3] Key outcomes of DSME and DSMS should be measured and monitored as part of care.

REFERENCES

1. Fan W. Epidemiology in diabetes mellitus and cardiovascular disease. *Cardiovas Endocrinol Metab.* 2017;6(1):8–16. doi:10.1097/XCE.0000000000000116
2. American Diabetes Association. Standards of medical care in diabetes—2018. *Diabetes Care.* 2018;41:S1–S2. doi:10.2337/dc18-Sint01
3. Patel P, Macerollo A. Diabetes mellitus: diagnosis and screening. *Diabetes.* 2010;100:13.
4. Gæde P, Lund-Andersen H, Parving H, et al. Effect of a multifactorial intervention on mortality in type 2 diabetes. *N Eng J Med.* 2008;358:580–591. doi:10.1056/NEJMoa0706245
5. Turner R. Effect of intensive blood-glucose control with metformin on complications in overweight patients with type 2 diabetes (UKPDS 34). *Lancet.* 1998;352:854–865. doi:10.1016/S0140-6736(98)07037-8

PITUITARY DISORDERS

Etiology

The main diseases of the pituitary gland are pituitary adenomas which cause excessive or diminished hormones of the hypothalamic–pituitary axis.[1,2] The hormones produced by the anterior pituitary include adrenocorticotrophic hormone (ACTH), growth hormone (GH), luteinizing hormone (LH), follicle-stimulating hormone (FSH), prolactin, and TSH. The hormones produced by the posterior pituitary include antidiuretic hormone (ADH) and oxytocin.

Hypersecretion of these hormones causes hyperprolactinemia, acromegaly or gigantism, hyperthyroidism, and Cushing's disease. Diminished or inappropriate hormone secretion can cause dwarfism and diabetes insipidus. There are many forms of dwarfism of which achondroplasia is the most common.

Epidemiology

The average annual incidence of acromegaly is around three to four per million per year with prevalence of about 60 individuals per million.[3] It is more prevalent in families with a hereditary multiple endocrine neoplasia type 1 (MEN-1) or Wermer's syndrome. Achondroplasia (the most common form of dwarfism) is a genetic condition that affects about 1 in 15,000 to 1 in 40,000 people.[4]

Clinical Presentation

Pituitary tumors may cause headaches in some patients and can suppress normal function, leading to hormone deficiencies. If the pituitary mass compresses the optic chiasm, this can lead to vision changes. Patients may also develop seizures and cranial nerve defects when pituitary tumors invade the surrounding brain tissue.

- **Acromegaly and gigantism** are associated with excessive growth of hands, feet, and internal organs resulting in height that is above normal for age. The main difference between acromegaly and gigantism is that acromegaly occurs in adults, typically between the ages of 30 and 50. Patients will not have closure of their growth plates, which continue to grow into adult hood. Other features include moist handshake due to excessive perspiration, skin tags, cystic acne, thickened skin, arthritis, deep coarse voice, obstructive sleep apnea, insulin resistance, colon polyps, headaches, decreased libido, and menstrual abnormalities.
- **Dwarfism** or short stature is generally defined as an adult height of 4 feet 10 inches (147 cm) or less.[4] Patients are characterized by short limbs, long narrow trunks, and large heads with midface hypoplasia and prominent brows.
- **Diabetes insipidus** results from a deficiency (inadequate production) or resistance to ADH (vasopressin). Patients may have intense thirst and large-volume polyuria. Other features include dehydration, hypernatremia, and unremitting enuresis.
- **Hyperprolactinemia** refers to a condition of elevated serum prolactin. Prolactin is produced by the anterior pituitary gland and plays a vital role in the development of the breasts during pregnancy. Prolactin levels may be elevated for several reasons, such as a pituitary tumor (prolactinoma which directly secretes excessive prolactin while decreasing the levels of other sex hormones). Other causes of hyperprolactinemia include diseases that affect the hypothalamus, hypothyroidism, chronic liver or kidney diseases, and medications. Symptoms include infertility, gallactoria, infrequent or irregular periods, amenorrhea, loss of libido, breast pain, and painful intercourse due to vaginal dryness.

Diagnosis

- Acromegaly is diagnosed by combining the clinical features and results of biochemical assays. Measurement of excess serum IGF-1 (insulin-like growth factor) is a preferred screening test as levels do not fluctuate greatly during the day. Excess serum GH is confirmed with an oral glucose tolerance test. Glucose normally suppresses GH to <1 mcg/L so GH levels >1 mcg/L are diagnostic.
- MRI is preferred over CT for assessing pituitary adenomas.
- To diagnose diabetes insipidus, clinicians should assess serum glucose, BUN, calcium, uric acid, potassium, and sodium. Urine collection for 24 hours is essential to assess volume, glucose, and creatinine levels.
- The diagnosis of central diabetes insipidus is confirmed with vasopressin challenge test.

Management

The treatment of choice for acromegaly is transsphenoidal microsurgery to remove the pituitary adenoma. Medical therapy includes the following:

- Dopamine agonists for patients who fail surgical interventions
- Somatostatin analogs to inhibit GH secretion
- The treatment of choice for diabetes insipidus is desmopressin acetate

Stereotactic radiosurgery (gamma knife) may be offered to patients who are not responding to other treatment options.

REFERENCES

1. Famini P, Maya MM, Melmed S. Pituitary magnetic resonance imaging for sellar and parasellar masses: ten-year experience in 2598 patients. *J Clin Endocrinol Metab.* 2011;96(6):1633–1641. doi:10.1210/jc.2011-0168
2. Lake MG, Krook LS, Cruz SV. Pituitary adenomas: an overview. *Am Fam Physician.* 2013;88(5):319–327.
3. Holdaway IM, Rajasoorya C. Epidemiology of acromegaly. *Pituitary.* 1999;2(1):29–41. doi:10.1023/A:1009965803750
4. Dwarfism. Mayo Clinic website. https://www.mayoclinic.org/diseases-conditions/dwarfism/symptoms-causes/syc-20371969

THYROID DISORDERS

Etiology

Thyroid disorders commonly encountered in family medicine are hyperthyroidism, hypothyroidism, thyroiditis, thyroid storm, thyroid nodules, and thyroid cancer.[1] Autoimmune challenges to the thyroid gland can cause glandular destruction and hormone deficiency, as occurs with hypothyroidism, or can incite overproduction of thyroid hormone, leading to thyrotoxicosis. Graves' disease (diffuse toxic goiter) is the most common cause of hyperthyroidism. It is an autoimmune disorder in which antibodies bind to the TSH receptors (on surface of the thyroid cells) and trigger the synthesis of excess thyroid hormone. Other causes of hyperthyroidism include multinodular toxic goiter, toxic thyroid adenoma, Hashimoto's thyroiditis, postpartum thyroiditis, iodine-induced hyperthyroidism, and iatrogenic excessive doses of levothyroxine.

Epidemiology

Hyperthyroidism (Graves' disease) occurs more frequently in women (2%) than in men.[2] Similarly, hypothyroidism is about 10 times more common in women than in men and it is more prevalent in areas with iodine deficiency. Prevalence of both hyperthyroidism and hypothyroidism increases with age.[3]

HYPERTHYROIDISM

Clinical Presentation

Patients with hyperthyroidism may have nervousness, insomnia, irritability, tremors, excessive sweating, heat intolerance, weight loss, palpitations, and muscle weakness. In Graves' disease, the thyroid gland may be diffusely enlarged and a bruit may be present. Extrathyroidal features include proptosis, arrhythmias, pretibial myxedema, and brisk deep tendon reflexes.

> **CLINICAL PEARL:** Typical characteristics that are specific to Graves' disease are exophthalmos, pretibial myxedema, and a thyroid bruit.

Diagnosis

- Primary hyperthyroidism presents with low TSH levels, elevated free thyroid hormones T_4, T_3, and elevated thyroid resin uptake.
- In Graves' disease, the TSH receptor antibody and antithyroglobulin antibodies levels are elevated. Thyroid radioactive iodine uptake and scan show high uptake. MRI is the image of choice when evaluating ophthalmopathy associated with Graves' disease.

Management

Treatment goals for hyperthyroidism are to inhibit the production of thyroid hormones and to block the effects of the hormones on other systems in the body. Commonly used treatment modalities include pharmacologic, radioiodine, and surgical options.

Pharmacological interventions include the following:

- Methimazole and propylthiouracil (PTU), which inhibit thyroid hormone synthesis
- Beta-blockers that alleviate acute symptoms such as tachycardia, palpitations, anxiety, tremors, and sweating

Radioiodine interventions:

- This is the most commonly used therapy for Graves' disease
- When administered to a patient, radioactive iodine selectively destroys only thyroid cells (follicular) because these are the only cells in the body that absorb iodine.
- Contraindications include pregnancy and breastfeeding

Surgical interventions: This can either include full or partial removal of the thyroid gland.

● Risks of surgery include damage to the nerves that control vocal cords and damage to the parathyroid gland that controls the body's calcium. Patients should be monitored for hypocalcemia.

> **CLINICAL PEARL:** Agranulocytosis is a major side effect of drugs used for treating hyperthyroidism. Monitor leukocyte count on a regular basis.

HYPOTHYROIDISM

Clinical Presentation

Clinical manifestations of hypothyroidism can be subtle, vague, and nonspecific, but the most common symptoms are weakness, lethargy, cold intolerance, decreased sweating, forgetfulness, and constipation. Common signs are dry and pallor skin (coarse skin and hair), slow speech, eyelid and facial edema, cold skin to touch, and thick tongue.[4]

Diagnosis

● In hypothyroidism, TSH levels will be elevated whereas total and free T_4 may be low. T_3 may be normal.
● Occurrence of thyroid autoantibodies such as antithyroperoxidase in the serum confirms autoimmune causes.
● Patients will have increased antimicrosomal antibodies in Hashimoto's thyroiditis (most common cause of primary hypothyroidisms).
● If a structural abnormality is suspected, a thyroid ultrasound or radionuclide scanning may be indicated.

Management

Treatment of primary hypothyroidism is hormone supplementation with levothyroxine. Monitor treatment success by serial TSH levels and clinical manifestations. Levothyroxine doses should be titrated by 25 to 50 mcg every 2 months until normal TSH levels are achieved. Treatment is continued indefinitely.

> **CLINICAL PEARL:** Levothyroxine has a narrow therapeutic range and high potential for malabsorption due to drug-to-drug interactions. Pregnancy increases thyroid hormone requirements and should be accounted for when treating hypothyroidism in this population.

REFERENCES

1. Gardner DG, Shoback DM. *Greenspan's basic & clinical endocrinology.* New York, NY: McGraw-Hill Medical; 2011.
2. Vanderpump MP. The epidemiology of thyroid disease. *Br Med Bull.* 2011;99(1): 39–51. doi:10.1093/bmb/ldr030

3. Devdhar M, Ousman YH, Burman KD. Hypothyroidism. *Endocrinol Metab Clin North Am.* 2007;36:595. doi:10.1016/j.ecl.2007.04.008. PubMed: 17673121
4. Melmed S, Polonsky KS, Larsen PR, Kronenberg HM, eds. *Williams Textbook of Endocrinology.* 13th ed. Philadelphia, PA: Elsevier Health Sciences; 2016.

EYES, EARS, NOSE, AND THROAT

ALLERGIC RHINITIS

Etiology

Allergic rhinitis is inflammation of the nasal mucosa due to an IgE-mediated reaction to allergens. Dust mites, animals, pollen, and mold are common triggers. It is often noted concomitantly with asthma. Allergic rhinitis is a condition associated with atopy.

Epidemiology

In the United States, 15% to 30% of patients in adult and pediatric populations have allergic rhinitis.[1] It is a significant contributor to missed school and work, as well as sleep problems. It can occur seasonally or perennially. In episodic rhinitis, symptoms occur only when the patient is directly exposed to an allergen.

Clinical Presentation

The most common symptoms include nasal congestion, nasal pruritus, sneezing, clear rhinorrhea, and postnasal drip. Ocular symptoms such as itching, redness, and tearing may also be present. On examination, you may note clear rhinorrhea and pale nasal mucosa. Always perform a thorough examination of the eyes, ears, nose, and throat, as well as a pulmonary and skin exam to rule out other causes of symptoms or to detect other signs of atopy.

Diagnosis

The diagnosis of allergic rhinitis is made clinically. The American Academy of Otolaryngology criteria for diagnosis requires an allergic cause with at least one of the following symptoms:

- Nasal congestion, runny nose, itchy nose, or sneezing[2]

Response to empiric treatment can help confirm the diagnosis. Other conditions can cause chronic rhinitis symptoms. These include vasomotor rhinitis and nonallergic rhinitis. Routine diagnostic testing is not recommended. Because allergic rhinitis can occur with other atopic conditions or sleep-disordered breathing, these conditions should be considered in the evaluation of the patient.

Management

Patients should be advised to avoid known allergens and/or reduce exposure to allergens. This advice may include patient using home air-filtration systems, removing pets from the home, using allergen-reducing mattress covers and pillow cases, and keeping windows closed.

TABLE **2.19** Overview of Pharmacologic Management of Allergic Rhinitis

Drug Class	Drug Names	Additional Information
Intranasal corticosteroids	Budesonide, fluticasone, triamcinolone	Safe and effective; can be used for seasonal and perennial symptoms; may also benefit eye symptoms
Oral antihistamines *(second generation)*	Loratadine, fexofenadine, cetirizine	Mostly nonsedating; helps with sneezing and itching; not as effective as intranasal corticosteroids; low cost; helpful for intermittent symptoms
Intranasal antihistamines	Azelastine, olopadadine	For seasonal, perennial, or episodic symptoms; consider if oral antihistamines are not effective
Decongestants *(oral or intranasal)*	Phenylephrine, oxymetazoline, pseudoephedrine	Causes vasoconstriction that reduces inflammation in the nasal mucosa; short-term treatment recommended to avoid rebound congestion; caution with oral agents in patients with cardiovascular conditions, glaucoma, or who are at risk for urinary retention
Leukotriene receptor antagonists	Montelukast	Similar efficacy to oral antihistamines; not as effective as corticosteroids; beneficial for asthma symptoms

Source: Sur DKC, Plesa ML. Treatment of allergic rhinitis. *Am Fam Physician.* 2015;92:985–992.

For episodic symptoms, an oral or nasal antihistamine with or without an oral decongestant is recommended. For seasonal or perennial symptoms intranasal glucocorticoids are recommended as first-line treatment. When seasonal or perennial symptoms persist or are severe, additional agents such as antihistamines, decongestants, leukotriene receptor antagonists, or intranasal cromolyn can be added. An overview of pharmacologic options are detailed in Table 2.19.

If the initial treatment for allergic rhinitis is not effective, the patient should be referred for IgE allergy testing and consideration of immunotherapy. Patients who experience adverse effects from traditional therapy or those who do not wish to be on medications chronically should also consider immunotherapy. Patients are generally treated for 3 to 5 years, and the effects can last for up to 12 years after treatment.[2]

REFERENCES

1. Wheatley LM, Togias A. Allergic Rhinitis. *N Eng J Med.* 2015;372:456–463. doi:10.1056/NEJMcp1412282
2. Seidman MD, Gurgel RK, Lin SY, et al. Clinical practice guideline: allergic rhinitis. *Otolaryngol Head Neck Surg.* 2015;152:S1–S43. doi:10.1177/0194599814561600

CONJUNCTIVITIS

Etiology

Conjunctivitis is an inflammation of the conjunctiva of the eye and is a common presentation in family medicine. Although generally benign and easily treatable, you must rule out more serious causes of the patient's symptoms, particularly those that can threaten sight. Conjunctivitis can be viral, bacterial, or allergic in origin. Adenoviruses are the most likely pathogens in viral conjunctivitis. *S. aureus* and other staphylococcal pathogens are the most common causes of bacterial conjunctivitis, as well as *Streptococcus pneumoniae, Haemophilus influenzae,* and *Moraxella catarrhalis.*

Epidemiology

In total, cases of infectious conjunctivitis are most commonly due to viral causes, but children are more likely to present with bacterial conjunctivitis. Viral conjunctivitis is most common in summer, while bacterial conjunctivitis is prevalent in winter and early spring.[1] Allergic conjunctivitis is most commonly seen in spring and summer.[1]

Clinical Presentation

- Viral conjunctivitis commonly presents with conjunctival injection, clear, watery discharge, and may present as part of a viral upper respiratory infection (URI) syndrome or as conjunctivitis alone. Symptoms may begin unilaterally and progress to bilateral involvement over a few days and may be associated with mild itching. Adenovirus is a common cause and may cause associated preauricular adenopathy in addition to the general URI syndrome.
- Bacterial conjunctivitis generally presents with purulent or mucopurulent discharge, and the patient may report matting of the eyes upon waking in the morning.
- Allergic conjunctivitis tends to present with predominant symptoms of redness, itching, and tearing of the eyes. It is painless and may have watery discharge, although some patients report a gritty sensation.

> **CLINICAL PEARL:** Visual acuity should always be measured in a patient with an ocular complaint regardless of the practice setting.

Diagnosis

The diagnosis of conjunctivitis is made clinically, through history and physical examination. Although certain characteristics of the different types of conjunctivitis (such as descriptions of discharge) may help lead to the diagnosis, they are not always accurate and all aspects of the patient's presentation should be considered.

> **CLINICAL PEARL:** Cultures are generally only indicated for conjunctivitis in neonates, when suspecting gonococcal or chlamydial causes, or in cases in which there is lack of treatment response.[1]

Management

Viral conjunctivitis

- Symptomatic care; cold compresses, saline drops/artificial tears if needed
- Topical antibiotic drops do not prevent against a secondary bacterial infection
- Highly communicable; counsel on importance of handwashing, avoid sharing face cloths and other personal care items
- Those who encounter the public may return to work when there is no longer discharge from the eyes
- Should resolve in 7 to 10 days

Allergic conjunctivitis

- Avoid known allergens if possible
- Antihistamine eye drops, available over the counter (OTC)
- Saline or artificial tears may also help symptomatically
- The use of steroid drops should be reserved for ophthalmology

Bacterial conjunctivitis

- Most often treated with topical antibiotics, especially in children; can be self-limited in adults
- Use of antibiotic drops shortens duration of illness and decreases communicability
- Highly communicable; counsel on importance of handwashing, avoid sharing face cloths and other personal care items
- Generally, all antibiotic drops are effective; consider the patient's allergies, local resistance patterns, and cost when choosing an agent. The most common agents are outlined in Table 2.20
- Avoid topical steroids as they may worsen the condition

> **CLINICAL PEARL:** Hyperacute bacterial conjunctivitis presents with severe, copious purulent discharge; decreased vision; ocular pain; and eyelid swelling. This presentation is most commonly caused by Neisseria gonorrhoeae and requires emergent ophthalmologic evaluation.

TABLE 2.20 Commonly Prescribed Topical Antibiotics for Bacterial Conjunctivitis

Drug Name	Common Dose
Ciprofloxacin	1–2 drops into affected eye(s) QID × 7 days
Erythromycin ophthalmic ointment	½ inch to affected eye(s) QID × 7 days
Gentamicin ophthalmic ointment	½ inch to affected eye(s) QID × 7 days
Gentamicin ophthalmic solution	1–2 drops into affected eye(s) QID × 7 days
Sulfacetamide 10% solution	1–2 drops into affected eye(s) every 2–3 hours × 7 days
Tobramycin solution	1–2 drops into affected eye(s) QID × 7 days
Trimethoprim/polymyxin B	1–2 drops into affected eye(s) QID × 7 days

QID, four times a day.

TABLE **2.21** Bacterial Conjunctivitis Indications for Prompt Referral to Ophthalmology

	Immediate Referral	
Moderate or severe pain	Visual changes or loss	Involvement of the cornea
Conjunctival scarring	History of herpes simplex virus disease of the eye	Copious purulent discharge
	Consider Referral	
Contact lens wearers	Photophobia	Patients requiring steroids

Source: American Academy of Ophthalmology; Cornea/External Disease Panel. *Preferred Practice Pattern Guidelines: Conjunctivitis-Limited Revision.* San Francisco, CA: Author; 2011.

Table 2.21 outlines signs and symptoms for which you should immediately refer to ophthalmology and other presentations for which you should consider referral to ophthalmology.

> **CLINICAL PEARL:** Children with bacterial conjunctivitis who attend day care or school should not return until they have been treated with antibiotic drops for at least 24 hours.

REFERENCES

1. Azari A, Barney N. Conjunctivitis a systemic review of diagnosis and treatment. *JAMA.* 2013;310(16):1721–1729. doi:10.1001/jama.2013.280318

OTITIS EXTERNA

Etiology

Otitis externa is an inflammation of the auditory canal. Acute otitis externa is most commonly bacterial in origin, generally as a result of *Pseudomonas aeruginosa* or *S. aureus*, although it can be caused by other pathogens and can be polymicrobial.[1] Water exposure (generally through swimming) or improper cleaning of the ear canals are the primary causes. These mechanisms contribute to the removal of cerumen as a protective barrier, which can result in damage to the epithelium of the ear canal, leading to inflammation and infection. Otitis externa can also be more chronic; in these cases it generally has a fungal cause, such as *Candida*, or is seen in patients with inflammatory skin disorders and/or atopy.[1]

Epidemiology

Each year in the United States, there over two million visits to healthcare providers for otitis externa.[2] It is common in school-aged children and young adults. This condition is more commonly diagnosed in the summer months, and is seen more frequently in warmer regions, such as the southern United States, but can occur during any time of the year in any location.

Clinical Presentation

Patients will generally present with complaints of otalgia. The onset of symptoms is typically sudden, occurring over hours or 1 to 2 days. Pain can range from mild to severe. Itching and edema of the ear canal may also be reported. Be sure to inquire about a history of recent water exposure, instrumentation of the ear canal or atopy, as well as whether or not the patient has been previously diagnosed with otitis externa. Low-grade fever may be present but is not common. High fever is not expected with this condition, and if it occurs, you should suspect the infection has spread beyond the ear canal.

On examination, you may note edema and/or erythema of the ear canal. Manipulating the ear canal by way of palpation of the auricle and tragus will cause pain. In severe cases the canal will be entirely occluded due to edema. It is important to perform a thorough ear, nose, and throat (ENT) exam, as well as inspect the skin for a spreading cellulitis, and palpate the pre- and postauricular lymph nodes. When caused by a fungus, pruritus is often the predominant symptom. Otoscopy typically reveals thick debris in the canal.

Diagnosis

The diagnosis of otitis externa is made clinically through history and physical examination. It is important to rule out other causes of symptoms such as otitis media with a ruptured tympanic membrane, eczema, or seborrhea.

> **CLINICAL PEARL:** The term "malignant otitis externa" is often used to describe a severe case of otitis externa most commonly found in older patients, particularly those who have diabetes or are immunocompromised. This condition is a medical emergency. It involves infection of the mastoid process, and potentially underlying structures, and can be fatal.

Management

The American Academy of Otolaryngology set forth the following recommendations for the general treatment of otitis externa:[2]

- Topical therapy is appropriate for the initial treatment of uncomplicated otitis externa, which is localized to the ear canal.
- Patients should be educated on the proper administration of topical drops.
- If the ear canal is obstructed by debris or edema, an aural toilet and/or wick should be placed to allow adequate delivery of topical therapy.
- The patient's pain level should be assessed and appropriately managed.
- Patients who do not improve within 48 to 72 hours of initial therapy should be reassessed.
- Be sure to evaluate patients for risk factors such as nonintact tympanic membranes; tympanostomy tubes; diabetes; prior radiotherapy of the affected area; or immunocompromise. These patients are at risk for otomycosis and necrotizing otitis externa. They are more likely to require systemic treatment and will need closer monitoring.

TABLE 2.22 Topical Medications Used to Treat Otitis Externa

Drug Name	Common Dose
Acetic acid (otic) 2% solution	3–5 drops into affected ear(s) 3–4 times per day
Ciprofloxacin 0.2%, hydrocortisone 1%	3 drops into affected ear(s) twice daily
Ciprofloxacin 0.2%, dexamethasone 0.1%	4 drops into affected ear(s) twice daily
Neomycin, polymyxin B, hydrocortisone	4 drops into affected ear(s) every 6–8 hours
Ofloxacin 0.3%	10 drops into affected ear(s) once daily

Source: Centers for Disease Control and Prevention. Estimated burden of acute otitis externa—United States, 2003–2007. *MMWR Morb Mortal Wkly Rep.* 2011;60:605–609.

Topical preparations used to treat otitis externa have similar efficacy rates and are outlined in Table 2.22. Consider cost and the convenience of dosing schedules when prescribing. General length of treatment is 7 days. Some preparations also have a combination antimicrobial/glucocorticoid option.

REFERENCES

1. Schaefer P, Reginald F. Otitis externa: an update. *Am Fam Physician.* 2012; 86(11):1055–1061.
2. Centers for Disease Control and Prevention. Estimated burden of acute otitis externa—United States, 2003–2007. *MMWR Morb Mortal Wkly Rep.* 2011;60:605–609.

OTITIS MEDIA: ACUTE

Etiology

Acute otitis media (AOM) is an infection and inflammation of the middle ear. Obstruction or inflammation of the eustachian tube is often the inciting factor that leads to poor eustachian tube function and the development of an effusion in the middle ear space. Although it is most often bacterial in origin, some cases are viral. The most common bacterial pathogens are *S. pneumoniae*, *M. catarrhalis*, and *H. influenzae*.

Epidemiology

Although it is seen in children and adults, AOM is more common in children, and as such, is the most common reason antibiotics are prescribed in this population. Approximately two million cases of AOM are diagnosed in the United States annually. Most children will have at least one case of AOM before they enter school. Young children who attend day care are more likely to develop AOM due to more frequent exposure to respiratory pathogens and infections. Exposure to secondhand smoke can increase a child's risk of developing AOM, and breastfeeding can be mildly protective.

Clinical Presentation

Otalgia is the most common symptom of AOM and can range from mild to severe. Although older children and adults may be able to verbalize this pain, younger children often cannot. Common signs of ear pain in younger children include pulling, tugging, or rubbing the ear; fussiness; or a change in sleep habits. Fever is a common symptom. AOM can occur during, after, or independent of an upper respiratory infection.

> **CLINICAL PEARL:** Infants and toddlers who have frequent cases of AOM with resulting persisting middle ear effusions are at risk for speech and language delay. You should be particularly attentive to these areas during developmental screening and surveillance.

Diagnosis

Examination of the tympanic membrane is necessary to accurately diagnose AOM. At times, examination may be difficult in children due to lack of compliance with the exam, crying, excessive cerumen in the ear canal, or other factors. The American Academy of Pediatrics (AAP) recommends diagnosing AOM in children when the following criteria are present: recent onset of otalgia (<48 hours); moderate or severe bulging of the tympanic membrane; or intense erythema of the tympanic membrane.[1] The presence of a bulging tympanic membrane is highly correlated with a bacterial cause of AOM. The use of pneumatic otoscopy is essential in aiding the diagnosis.

Be sure to examine the eyes, nose, and throat of a patient with a complaint of otalgia to look for alternative causes of pain. Cardiac, pulmonary, lymphatic, and skin exams are also indicated. In cases of high fever or excessive fussiness maintain a high index of suspicion for more dangerous conditions in the differential diagnosis, such as meningitis, pneumonia, or bacteremia.

> **CLINICAL PEARL:** It is important to distinguish the difference between a normal tympanic membrane, a middle ear effusion, and AOM to reduce the unnecessary use of antibiotics. Making the correct diagnosis can be difficult for clinicians in training.

Management

Antibiotics are the mainstay of treatment for AOM and can reduce the duration of illness, as well as aid in the reduction of pain. Observation, without antibiotic therapy, may be appropriate. This recommendation should be the result of shared decision-making between the clinician and the parent/caregiver. In these instances, close follow-up is necessary. Follow-up within 48 to 72 hours from the onset of symptoms must be possible, on the part of the child/family and clinician, if the child's condition worsens or does not improve so antibiotics can be prescribed. Observation and treatment options are outlined in Tables 2.23 and 2.24. The AAP defines severe signs and symptoms of AOM as moderate or severe otalgia for at least 48 hours or temperature of 102.2°F.[1]

The AAP recommends amoxicillin as initial empiric treatment for AOM in children as long as the child has not received antibiotics in the last 30 days and does not have concurrent purulent conjunctivitis. If either of these qualifiers exists, prescribe an antibiotic with beta-lactamase coverage, such as amoxicillin-clavulanate. For those children who have a history of recurrent AOM that has not been responsive to amoxicillin in the past, a beta-lactam

TABLE 2.23 American Academy of Pediatrics Recommendations Regarding Observation for AOM

Age	Presentation	Recommended Treatment
Children ≤6 months	Bilateral or unilateral AOM plus severe signs and symptoms	Antibiotic therapy
Children 6–23 months	Bilateral AOM plus nonsevere signs and symptoms	Antibiotic therapy
Children 6–23 months	Unilateral AOM plus nonsevere signs and symptoms	Antibiotic therapy or observation
Children ≥24 months	Bilateral or unilateral plus nonsevere signs and symptoms	Antibiotic therapy or observation

AOM, acute otitis media.
Source: Harmes, K. M., Blackwood, R. A., Burrows, H. L., et al. (2013). Otitis media: diagnosis and treatment. *American Family Physician,* 88:435–440.

TABLE 2.24 Antibiotic Options for Acute Otitis Media

	Recommended First Line	Dose	Duration	Alternatives
Initial empiric treatment for AOM in children[2]	Amoxicillin	80–90 mg/kg/d, two divided doses	Severe symptoms, any age: 10 days to <2 years old, mild to moderate symptoms: 10 days	Cefdinir, cefuroxime, cefpodoxime, ceftriaxone, azithromycin
	Amoxicillin-clavulanate	90 mg/kg/d, two divided doses; high dose (amoxicillin to clavulanate ratio 14:1)	2–5 years old, mild to moderate symptoms, 7 days; 6 years or older, mild to moderate symptoms, 5–7 days	

AOM, acute otitis media.

is recommended as initial therapy. Amoxicillin should be avoided in children with a penicillin allergy.

Regardless of whether you choose to treat with antibiotics or observe, pain management is necessary. The AAP recommends assessing the child's pain, and if present, recommending treatment to reduce pain. Oral acetaminophen or ibuprofen at standard recommended doses are most effective and should be continued as long as necessary. Pain is often most severe in the first few days of the illness but can persist.

All children with AOM should be reassessed in 48 to 72 hours if they fail to improve, or sooner if their condition worsens. Refer to an ENT specialist for tympanostomy tubes if a child has three episodes of AOM in 6 months, or four episodes in 1 year, with one episode in the preceding 6 months.[2]

REFERENCES

1. Lieberthal AS, Carroll AE, Chonmaitree T, et al. The diagnosis and management of acute otitis media. *Pediatrics*. 2013;131:e964–e999. doi:10.1542/peds.2012-3488
2. Randel A. AAO-HNSF releases guideline on tympanostomy tubes in children. *Am Fam Physician*. 2014;89:754–761.

PHARYNGITIS

Etiology

Pharyngitis is an inflammation and infection of the throat. Most cases of pharyngitis are viral in origin and can be caused by various pathogens, including rhinovirus, adenovirus, and coronavirus.[1] Bacteria, such as Group A *streptococcus*, can also be the causative agent in cases of pharyngitis. If untreated, bacterial pharyngitis can result in local complications, such as abscess, and can lead to significant cardiovascular and renal sequelae. The appropriate treatment for pharyngitis is based upon the specific etiology.

Epidemiology

In the United States, there are approximately 15 million primary care visits per year for pharyngitis.[2] Of these visits, 20% to 30% of children, and fewer adults, will have GAS pharyngitis. Among bacterial causes of pharyngitis, Group A *streptococcus* is the most common pathogen, accounting for 5% to 15% of cases in adults, and 20% to 30% in children.[2] GAS pharyngitis is most common in late winter and early spring.[3]

Clinical Presentation

Patients most commonly present with a chief complaint of a sore throat which may be an isolated complaint or may occur in addition to other upper respiratory symptoms. Additional symptoms can include fever, painful lymph nodes, cough, coryza, malaise, headache, and/or rash. Physical examination will confirm these symptoms and can help rule out other causes such as otitis media and sinusitis. An examination of the pharynx may reveal erythema with or without exudate amd tender and enlarged cervical lymph nodes.

CLINICAL PEARL: Be vigilant when examining the pharynx to be sure there is no evidence of peritonsillar or parapharyngeal abscess.

Diagnosis

Because the presentations of streptococcal and nonstreptococcal pharyngitis are similar, a purely clinical diagnosis is unreliable. Generally, a sore throat that is accompanied by other symptoms such as cough, rhinorrhea, hoarseness, and oral ulcers is more likely to be viral in origin.[2] For patients with symptoms more suggestive of GAS pharyngitis, a rapid antigen detection test (RADT) or culture from a throat swab is the most accurate way to diagnose streptococcal pharyngitis and to distinguish it from nonstreptococcal causes.[2] RADT can be performed quickly and easily in an office setting. If negative, you should order a confirmatory throat culture in pediatric patients, but this is not necessary in adult patients[3] because significant complications of an untreated group A streptococcal (GAS) infection, such as glomerulonephritis, are less common in adults. A positive RADT does not need to be confirmed with a throat culture.[2]

The modified Centor score can be helpful in determining the best diagnostic course of action. Patients are assigned a score according to the following criteria: age 4 to 14 years (1 point), 15 to 44 years (0 points), ≥45 years (−1 point); tonsillar swelling or exudate (1 point); absence of cough (1 point); temperature >100.4°F (1 point); tender anterior cervical lymph nodes (1 point).[4] Patients with a score of 0 to 1 are low risk and do not require testing or antibiotic treatment; patients with a score of 2 to 3 should be tested with RADT or throat culture; patients with a score of 4 or more are considered high risk and can be treated empirically for GAS pharyngitis.[4]

Management

For GAS pharyngitis, antibiotic treatment is recommended. Penicillin or amoxicillin is the first-line treatment in children and adults.[2] For those with a penicillin allergy, cephalexin, azithromycin, or clindamycin are appropriate alternatives.[3] Nonpharmacologic treatment is indicated for streptococcal and nonstreptococcal pharyngitis to minimize symptoms and discomfort. Analgesics such as acetaminophen or NSAIDS can reduce pain and fever. Patients may also experience relief from lozenges and saltwater gargles. Improvement is expected within 2 to 3 days, and patients should be advised to return to clinic if not improving in that time or seek care sooner if their symptoms worsen.

> **CLINICAL PEARL:** Although evidence varies on whether or not tonsillectomy prevents further cases of streptococcal pharyngitis, patients with recurrent GAS pharyngitis, those who have multiple antibiotic allergies or are otherwise difficult to treat, or those who have had complications from throat infections should be referred to otolaryngology for consultation regarding tonsillectomy.

REFERENCES

1. Gore J. Quick recertification series; acute pharyngitis. *JAAPA*. 2013;26(2):57–58. doi:10.1097/01720610-201302000-00012
2. Shulman S, Bisno AL, Clegg HW, et al. Clinical practice guideline for the diagnosis and management of group A streptococcal pharyngitis: 2012 update by the infectious diseases society of America. *Clin Infect Dis*. 2012;55(10):e86–e102. doi:10.1093/cid/cis629
3. Karla M, Higgins K, Perez E. Common questions about streptococcal pharyngitis. *Am Fam Physician*. 2016;94(1):24–31.
4. McIsaac WJ, White D, Tannenbaum D, et al. A clinical score to reduce unnecessary antibiotic use in patients with sore throat. *CMAJ*. 1998;158:75–83.

SINUSITIS

Etiology

Sinusitis, technically known as rhinosinusitis, is a condition in which the mucosa of the nasal cavity and paranasal sinuses are inflamed. Most cases of sinusitis are viral. The most common bacterial pathogens are *S. pneumoniae*, *M. catarrhalis*, and *H. influenza*.[1] Bacterial sinusitis can occur as the sequelae of a viral URI, due to obstruction of the sinuses from a deviated septum or nasal polyps, from decreased ciliary motility seen in patients who smoke, or even from dental infections or procedures.

When the infection from sinusitis is limited to the nasal cavity and sinuses, it is considered uncomplicated sinusitis, but extension of the infection to other areas of the body (i.e., skin/soft tissues, central nervous system) is more serious and is termed complicated sinusitis.

Epidemiology

Sinusitis is a common condition seen in adults and children in the family medicine setting. It is diagnosed more than 30 million times per year in the United States Sinusitis is also one of the most common reasons for which providers prescribe antibiotics.[1]

Clinical Presentation

Chiefly, patients will report nasal congestion, rhinorrhea, or sinus congestion/pressure/pain. Additionally, they may report fatigue, fever, cough, postnasal drip, headache, halitosis, pressure in the ears, or anosmia. Early sinusitis presents similarly to a viral URI.[1]

Physical examination may reveal tenderness upon palpation or percussion of the frontal and/or maxillary sinuses and red, inflamed nasal mucosa with discharge ranging from clear or mucoid to purulent. Be sure to examine the ears, pharynx, dentition/gingiva, and lungs to exclude other sites of infection. It is important to rule out complicated sinusitis by examining the skin of the preseptal and periorbital areas to rule out cellulitis, An examination of the neck and basic neurologic exam to evaluate for central nervous system infection should also be included in the evaluation.

> **CLINICAL PEARL:** Complicated sinusitis can result in meningitis, intracranial abscess, facial cellulitis, cavernous sinus thrombosis, or osteomyelitis. These conditions require emergent intervention.

Diagnosis

The diagnosis of sinusitis is most commonly made clinically through history and physical examination. It is important to distinguish between viral and bacterial sinusitis (see Table 2.25).

Management

The appropriate treatment for sinusitis is based on making an accurate diagnosis. Symptomatic and supportive care can benefit patients with viral or bacterial sinusitis. Some common supportive care measures include the following:

- OTC analgesics such as acetaminophen and ibuprofen, as needed, at standard dosages
- Nasal saline irrigation; this can also be purchased in a sterile form OTC
- Oral decongestants such as pseudoephedrine or phenylephrine; available OTC

TABLE 2.25 Distinguishing Bacterial Sinusitis From Viral Sinusitis

Findings Consistent With Bacterial Sinusitis	Findings Consistent With Viral Sinusitis
Symptoms persist for ≥10 days	Symptoms last <10 days
Illness begins with severe symptoms: high fever, facial pain, purulent nasal discharge	Illness begins with mild, general upper respiratory symptoms
Symptoms specific to sinusitis worsen over the course of the illness after an initial improvement after 5–6 days, i.e., "double sickening"	Symptoms gradually improve over the course of the illness or do not worsen

Source: Adapted from Chow AW, Benninger MS, Brook I, et al. IDSA clinical practice guideline for acute bacterial rhinosinusitis in children and adults. *Clin Infect Dis. 2012;*54(8):e72–e112. doi:10.1093/cid/cis370

- Topical decongestants such as oxymetazoline; available OTC
- Oral mucolytics, such as guaifenesin, may also be helpful; available OTC
- Intranasal corticosteroids such as fluticasone, triamcinolone; available OTC

CLINICAL PEARL: Patients should be encouraged to utilize these supportive therapies, whether or not an antibiotic is prescribed, because these therapies will improve their symptoms and overall comfort.

Antibiotic therapy is recommended for patients with suspected bacterial sinusitis. Table 2.26 lists common antibiotics. Generally, adults should be treated for 5 to 7 days and children for 10 to 14 days.[2] If there is worsening after 48 to 72 hours, or no improvement after 3 to 5 days on antibiotics, a different class of antibiotic should be prescribed.[2] Patients who do not improve or worsen after changing antibiotics should be referred to otolaryngology.

Patients at risk for antibiotic resistance[2] include:

- Those in a region with high resistance rates
- Extremes of age (<2 years or >65 years)
- Day-care attendance
- Received antibiotics within the last month
- Have been hospitalized within the past 5 days
- With comorbidities
- Immunocompromised

CLINICAL PEARL: Because sinusitis is a common reason for antibiotic prescriptions, use your best judgment to determine when antibiotics are needed in order to reduce inappropriate use and decrease the potential for antibiotic resistance.

Patients should be referred to an otolaryngologist if:[2]

- Condition worsens or does not improve after appropriate antibiotic treatment

TABLE 2.26 Recommended Antibiotics for Bacterial Sinusitis

Drug Name	Indications
Amoxicillin/clavulanate	Preferred first-line empiric treatment for adults and children Use high dose for adults (2 g PO BID) and children (90 mg/kg/d PO) at risk of resistance
Azithromycin	Generally not recommended as empiric therapy due to risk of resistance
Doxycycline	Acceptable alternative first-line treatment, or if penicillin allergic Not appropriate for children
Levofloxacin	Second-line treatment, or if penicillin allergic
Moxifloxacin	Second-line treatment, or if penicillin allergic
Clindamycin *plus* cefixime *or* clindamycin *plus* cefpodoxime	Second-line treatment, or if nontype I penicillin allergy
Trimethoprim-sulfamethoxazole	Generally not recommended as empiric therapy due to risk of resistance

BID, twice a day; PO, by mouth.

Source: Adapted from Chow AW, Benninger MS, Brook I, et al. IDSA clinical practice guideline for acute bacterial rhinosinusitis in children and adults. *Clin Infect Dis.* 2012;54(8):e72–e112. doi:10.1093/cid/cis370

- They are seriously ill and immunocompromised
- They have recurrent cases of sinusitis

REFERENCES

1. Aring AM, Chan MM. Current concepts in adult acute rhinosinusitis. *Am Fam Physician.* 2016;94(2):97–105.
2. Chow AW, Benninger MS, Brook I, et al. IDSA clinical practice guideline for acute bacterial rhinosinusitis in children and adults. *Clin Infect Dis.* 2012;54(8):e72–e112. doi:10.1093/cid/cis370

GI System

Alcoholic Liver Disease

Etiology

Liver disease occurs secondary to acute or chronic liver cell injury from a variety of causes. Known causes of acute and chronic liver disease include viruses, alcohol, steatosis (nonalcoholic fatty liver disease [NAFLD], steatohepatitis). These types of liver disease can occur secondary to obesity, drugs, cholestasis, metabolic diseases, autoimmune disorders, parasites, and venous obstruction (Budd-Chiari). If the cause of the injury is not accurately diagnosed and treated, ongoing inflammation will result in fibrosis and cirrhosis. Alcoholic liver disease, steatosis, and steatohepatitis remain the top underlying causes of chronic liver disease.

Alcohol misuse is defined as alcohol ingestion that exceeds 20 g (two alcoholic drinks) in women or 30 g (three drinks) in men a day. The standard drink is any drink that contains about 14 g of pure alcohol. Alcohol causes direct hepatocellular injury. It acts as a direct oxidative stressor and endotoxin that activates Kupffer cells in the liver. Acetaldehyde, the toxic metabolite of alcohol, targets an enzyme—methionine synthase. This enzyme is needed to form methionine, which is the essential amino acid required for the processing and the elimination of fats. Failure to process fat ultimately results in steatosis, which may result in steatohepatitis. Those patients who have a history of alcohol use disorder will all have some degree of fatty liver disease. Approximately 10% to 15% advance to alcoholic hepatitis, fibrosis, and cirrhosis.[1]

CLINICAL PEARL: Individuals who develop cirrhosis have a greater risk of developing hepatocellular carcinoma (HCC).

Epidemiology

Approximately 10% of individuals in the United States admit to excessive drinking (2+ drinks per day; 24 ounces beer or 12 ounces wine). Alcohol is the third leading cause of preventable death and second most common cause for liver transplant. Alcoholic hepatitis occurs in approximately 1/3 of patients with chronic use and is associated with a mortality rate of up to 48%.[2] Women are more susceptible than men to the toxic effects of alcohol on the liver.[1]

Clinical Presentation

Appropriate historical questions to ask all patients whom you suspect have underlying liver disease include possible parenteral exposures, transfusions, IV and intranasal drug use, tattoos, sexual activity, needle-stick injury, recent travel, exposure to individuals with jaundice, exposure to contaminated foods, occupational exposure to hepatotoxins, and alcohol consumption. Review all medications, including prescription, OTC, and supplements.

In general, patients may report weakness, fatigue, appetite loss, and fluid retention. They may also experience skin rashes, diffuse itching, easy bruising, or jaundice. GI complaints include nausea, vomiting, abdominal pain and bloating, increased abdominal girth, light stools, and hematemesis. Urine may appear dark in color. They can have arthralgias and myalgias. Neurological complaints can range from subtle confusion, memory loss, disorientation, lethargy to difficulty to arouse.

On physical exam the patient may be febrile. The skin can be jaundiced, along with spider nevi and palmar erythema. Head, eyes, ears, nose, and throat (HEENT) exam findings may include parotid gland enlargement, scleral icterus, and conjunctival pallor. The exam can be positive for left supraclavicular/periumbilical adenopathy and gynecomastia. The patient may have ascites, RUQ tenderness, abdominal mass, hepatomegaly, splenomegaly, or caput medusae on abdominal exam. Testicular atrophy can be present. Bilateral lower extremity edema is associated with hepatic congestion. Neurological findings include mental status changes, asterixis, muscle wasting in the temporal areas and proximal muscle groups, and the presence of Dupuyten's contractures.

Diagnosis

Primary diagnosis can be determined noninvasively in the majority of cases. The initial diagnostic evaluation for alcohol-related liver disease should begin with a hepatic panel. Abnormal patterns in transaminases, alkaline phosphatase, bilirubin, and protein values can guide the provider to the underlying pathology, as seen in Tables 2.27 and 2.28.

TABLE 2.27 Type of Injury and Associated Aminotransferase Elevation in Alcohol-Related Liver Disease

Direct Hepatocellular Injury	Cholestasis	Synthetic Liver Function
Serum ALT	Serum bilirubin	Bili
Serum AST	Serum ALP	Albumin
Serum ALP		Prothrombin time
Serum GGT		

ALP, alkaline phosphatase; ALT, alanine aminotransferase; AST, aspartate aminotransferase; GGT, gamma glutamyltransferase.

TABLE 2.28 Specific Disease Patterns and Labs in Alcohol-Related Liver Disease

Condition	Labs
NAFLD	AST/ALT ratio <1 Minor elevation AST/ALT (<100 IU/L)
ETOH	Elevated GGTP AST/ALT ratio >2:1 (<100–300 IU/L)
Chronic hepatitis C, B	Minor to moderate elevation AST/ALT (<100–300 IU/L)
Acute viral hepatitis	Major AST/ALT elevation (>1,000 IU/L)
Cholestasis	ALP 3–5 X ULN Mild elevation transaminases (<100 IU/L)
Wilson's disease	Moderate elevation AST/ALT (100–300 IU/L) Decreased ceruloplasmin
Autoimmune hepatitis	Moderate elevation AST/ALT (100–300 IU/L) Serum protein electrophoresis
PBC	AMA
PSC	ASMA, pANCA
Hemochromatosis	Iron C282Y, HFEH63D, trans sat >45%
Hereditary alpha-1 antitrypsin deficiency	Alpha-1 antitrypsin levels
Drug toxicity, especially acetaminophen	Major AST/ALT elevation (>1,000 IU/L)
Ischemic liver	Major AST/ALT elevation (>1,000 IU/L)

ALP, alkaline phosphatase; ALT, alanine aminotransferase; AMA, antimitochondrial antibody; ASMA, antismooth muscle antibody; AST, aspartate aminotransferase; NAFLD, nonalcoholic fatty liver disease; pANCA, perinuclear antineutrophil cytoplasmic antibody; PBC, primary biliary cirrhosis; PSC, primary sclerosing cholangitis; ULN, upper limit of normal.

The typical enzyme patterns seen with alcohol-induced liver disease are the following:

- Aspartate aminotransferase (AST): alanine aminotransferase (ALT) ratio ≥2:1
- Rare for the AST >8× normal
- Less common for the ALT >5× normal
- Gamma-glutamyl transpeptidase (GGTP): twofold elevation in a patient with an AST: ALT ratio >2:1

> **CLINICAL PEARL:** Minor elevation in AST and ALT (<2× normal) may not be clinically important (if certain conditions have been excluded) or may not even be abnormal as 5% of the results obtained from normal persons fall outside the defined normal range.

Additional blood work can include the following:

- CBC: Anemia, thrombocytopenia
- Prothrombin time (PT) and partial thromboplastin time (PTT): Prolonged
- Electrolytes: Hyponatremia, hyperkalemia, hypoglycemia
- Renal function: Reduced GFR, elevated BUN, Cr seen with the hepatorenal syndrome
- If the diagnosis is uncertain, additional testing may include ceruloplasmin, serum protein electrophoresis, antimitochondrial antibody (AMA), anti-smooth muscle antibody (ASMA), perinuclear antineutrophil cytoplasmic antibody (pANCA), iron C282Y, HFEH63D, iron studies, alpha-1 antitrypsin levels, and alpha feta protein (AFP) when there is a suspicion of HCC

Options for imaging the liver include the following:

- Ultrasound: Shows evidence of fat infiltration, presence of gallstones
- Triphasic CT or MRI: Identifies cirrhotic changes, portal HTN, and liver masses
- FibroScan: Used to indirectly measure/estimate the degree of scarring/fibrosis within the liver and to assess the degree of fibrosis
- Liver biopsy: The gold standard for determining the degree of fibrosis, cirrhosis; may be indicated to exclude inflammatory and or fibrotic changes
- Trichrome staining: Can show bridging fibrosis, steatosis, and the presence of steatohepatitis

Management

- Alcohol cessation program
- Weight loss
- Avoid hepatotoxins
- Immunize against hepatitis A, hepatitis B
- Monitoring:
  - Laboratory studies: hepatic panel, electrolytes, renal function
  - Imaging: U/S, blood work—alpha feta protein levels (tumor marker AFP) every 6 months to identify early changes that may reflect HCC in patients with cirrhosis

○ Endoscopic screening to document the presence/absence of esophageal varices[2]

REFERENCES

1. Singal AK, Anand BS. Recent trends in the epidemiology of alcoholic liver disease. *Clin Liver Dis.* April 2013;2(2):53–56. doi:10.1002/cld.168
2. Singal AK, Bataller R, Ahn J, et al. ACG clinical guideline: alcoholic liver disease. *Am J Gastroenterol.* 2018;113:175. doi:10.1038/ajg.2017.469

CHOLECYSTITIS

Etiology

Acute cholecystitis occurs when there is cystic duct obstruction resulting in gallbladder (GB) inflammation. Inflammation results from the increase in ductal pressures, bile inflammation due to stasis, and bacterial colonization. Complications can result from cystic duct obstruction leading to a secondary bacterial infection or ascending cholangitis.

Epidemiology

Calculous cholecystitis is the most common cause of acute cholecystitis. Acalculus cholecystitis is responsible for the remaining 10% of cases.[1] Acalculous cholecystitis is associated with a higher morbidity and mortality. Known risk factors include CAD, diabetes, infections, sepsis, mechanical ventilation, multiple transfusions, total parenteral nutrition, and medications such as opiates and sunitinib. The definitive treatment is a cholecystectomy.

Clinical Presentation

Patients will have a similar presentation to those with choledocholithiasis. This presentation can include biliary colic radiating to the right interscapular or back region, with diaphoresis, nausea, and vomiting. Jaundice may be present if there is ductal obstruction. The pain can continue for 24 hours and is accompanied by fever, and or chills.

On examination, the patient will be febrile and tachycardic. Abdominal examination reveals RUQ tenderness, positive Murphy's sign, and guarding. Bowel sounds may be diminished or absent when complicated by the presence of an ileus.

Diagnosis

Leukocytosis with a preponderance of neutrophils and circulating immature bands. Hepatic panel abnormalities represent a "cholestatic" picture, with an elevated alkaline phosphatase and total (+ conjugated) bilirubin within a range of 1.8 to 4 mg/dL. Mild transaminase elevations may be present. Amylase and lipase can be elevated with secondary pancreatic inflammation.

Ultrasound abnormalities include thick-walled, edematous GB, adjacent fluid, presence of a common bile duct (CBD) stone, and dilated (>6 mm) CBD. Air can be seen in the biliary tree with fistula formation. Hepatobiliary iminodiacetic acid (HIDA) scan supplies functional information about GB emptying and can be used to evaluate for biliary dyskinesia (dysfunction) and inflammation. Normal GB ejection fraction is >40%. IV isotope technetium-99 m hepatolite is injected into the patient and taken up by hepatocytes, excreted into bile, then concentrated in the GB. The patient is given a cholecystokinin (CCK) injection causing the GB to contract and empty. Patients with dyskinesia, obstruction, or inflammation may experience nausea, vomiting, pain, or delayed emptying. Reduced tracer can be seen in the GB and is consistent with blockage or obstruction. No radioactive tracer seen in the GB indicates acute inflammation (acute cholecystitis).

Management

Surgical consultation is recommended for cholecystectomy during admission for an acute attack once the infection and fever is controlled. If not, increased risk of gangrene, empyema, perforation, and cholecystenteric fistula (to duodenum, colon, stomach) can develop. Readmission rates in older patients may be as high as 38%.[2] Endoscopic retrograde cholangiopancreatography (ERCP) with biliary decompression, sphincterotomy, and stone extraction is an option if the patient is not considered a surgical candidate.

Antibiotic regimens should be initiated according to microbial sensitivities. Common regimens include the following:

- Monotherapy with ampicillin and sulbactam
- Pipercillin and tazobactam
- Ceftriaxone plus metronidazole
- Fluoroquinolone plus metronidazole

REFERENCES

1. Ganpathi IS, Diddapur RK, Eugene H, et al. Acute acalculous cholecystitis: challenging the myths. *HPB (Oxford)*. 2007;9(2):131–134. doi:10.1080/13651820701315307
2. Riall TS, Zhang D, Townsend CM, et al. Failure to perform cholecystectomy for acute cholecystitis in elderly patients is associated with increased morbidity, mortality, and cost. *J Am Coll Surg*. 2010;210(5):668–677. doi:10.1016/j.jamcollsurg.2009.12.031
3. Giljaca V, Gurusamy KS, Takwoingi Y, et al. Endoscopic ultrasound versus magnetic resonance cholangiopancreatography for common bile duct stones. *Cochrane Database Syst Rev*. 2015:CD011549. doi:10.1002/14651858.CD011549

CHOLEDOCHOLITHIASIS

Etiology

The two major categories of bile duct dilation are obstructive, including strictures and stones, and nonobstructive. Choledocholithiasis, "calculi in the bile ducts," is the most common cause of biliary obstruction. Cholesterol or cholesterol predominant (mixed) stones account for majority of cases. The cholesterol saturated bile promotes a decrease in GB motility resulting in stasis. Less common causes of stone formation include the black-pigmented stones that can be seen in patients with hemolytic diseases such as sickle cell anemia, hereditary spherocytosis, thalassemia, and cirrhosis. Brown-pigmented stones are the result of stasis complicated by infection with common organisms such as the *Escherichia coli* and Klebsiella spp. seen within the biliary tract system.

Epidemiology

The risk factors associated with cholelithiasis include obesity, diabetes, age >40, female (women have twice the risk), pregnancy, parenteral nutrition, prolonged fasting, and hemolysis. Factors thought to reduce the risk of developing gallbladder disease are statins, ascorbic acid, coffee, and vegetable proteins.

Clinical Presentation

Patients may present with any of the following findings: biliary colic; obstructive jaundice; inflammation of bile ducts (cholangitis), GB, or pancreas; or "gallstone ileus." Two-thirds of patients are asymptomatic. Symptoms will develop when the stones cause inflammation or obstruct the cystic or CBD. Biliary colic is described as a dull, steady ache in the RUQ or epigastric, or substernal area. The pain may radiate into the right interscapular or back region. This discomfort is due to GB distension and can be triggered by a fatty meal. The pain may last for up to 30 minutes, slowly subsiding over several hours, with the entire attack lasting <6 hours. Associated symptoms include diaphoresis, nausea, and vomiting. Stool may be lighter in color. When the bilirubin levels are elevated, the patient will become jaundiced, signifying ductal obstruction. Most of these attacks can be treated at home with analgesia and antiemetics. A patient who develops symptoms such as pain >24 hours, and/or a fever, should be evaluated for cholecystitis. Disorders of the liver, peptic ulcer disease (PUD), pancreatitis, or esophageal spasm have a similar clinical presentation.

The physical examination can be normal. Jaundice may be present if there is ductal obstruction. Positive findings on abdominal exam include RUQ tenderness, abdominal distension, and a positive Murphy's sign. Bowel sounds may be diminished or absent when complicated by the presence of an ileus.

Diagnosis

Initial blood work should include CBC, urinalysis, a hepatic panel, amylase, and lipase.

- The hepatic panel may reveal an elevated bilirubin, primarily direct; however, both fractions may be elevated. There may also be a normal to slight elevation in aminotransferases, but rarely greater than 500 IU. Alkaline phosphatase often can be elevated to >4 times the upper limit of normal (ULN).
- Lipase and amylase can also become elevated if there is an obstruction of the pancreatic ducts. Lipid values can be elevated.
- There may be a normocytic normochromic anemia on the CBC. The peripheral smear may reveal fragmented red blood cells (RBCs), spherocytes, or sickle cells, all consistent with a hemolysis as the cause of stone formation.
- Urine is often positive for bilirubinuria.

Diagnostic imaging:
- Ultrasonography (US) is highly sensitive in detecting stones over 4 mm. Positive findings on US include visualization of the stones, GB wall thickening, edema, free fluid, and "shadowing appearing as gray-black on images, which refers to the absence of echoes posterior to the calculi.
- CT will show GB wall thickening, pericholecystic stranding that is seen with inflammation and GB, and ductal distension.
- Endoscopic ultrasound (EUS) will identify similar abnormalities; however, study quality is better due to closer proximity. EUS can also serve as a therapeutic tool to obtain biopsies or drain cysts.[1,2]

- Magnetic resonance cholangiopancreatography (MRCP) is commonly used to evaluate for obstruction and dilation of the bile or pancreatic ducts, stones within the ducts or GB, or congenital anomalies. MRCP is also used when CT is inconclusive but clinical suspicion is high.
- ERCP will show dilated intra- and extrahepatic biliary system and multiple filling defects due to stone formation. This test is primarily utilized in the diagnosis and management of pancreatic-biliary disorders. CBD stones that are <1 cm in diameter can be removed through a biliary endoscopic sphincterotomy and extraction procedure.

Management

Lifestyle modification:

- Low-fat diet
- Weight loss

ERCP with division of sphincter of Oddi (sphincterotomy):

- Stones <1 cm diameter
- <4 stones
- Functioning GB
- Patent cystic duct
- Mild symptoms

Surgical referral:

Monitor patients for signs of cholangitis, cholecystitis, pancreatitis, and ileus.

REFERENCES

1. Ganpathi IS, Diddapur RK, Eugene H, et al. Acute acalculous cholecystitis: challenging the myths. *HPB (Oxford)*. 2007;9(2):131–134. doi:10.1080/13651820701315307
2. Tse F, Liu L, Barkun AN, et al. EUS: a meta-analysis of test performance in suspected choledocholithiasis. *Gastrointest Endosc*. 2008;67:235. doi:10.1016/j.gie.2007.09.047

DIVERTICULITIS

Etiology

Diverticulitis is defined as an inflammation of a diverticulum. It is more common in patients with a history of diverticulosis. Nonsteroidal use, obesity, sedentary lifestyle, and increased age are several risk factors associated with diverticulitis.

Epidemiology

Patients diagnosed with diverticulosis have a lifetime risk of developing diverticulitis of approximately 25%. Studies have shown the rate of recurrence varies from 9% to 36%.[1] There is an increased incidence of admissions for acute diverticulitis during the summer months.

Clinical Presentation

The patient may complain of a fever and chills and may develop sudden left lower quadrant (LLQ) abdominal pain that can become continuous. Pain is often associated with anorexia, nausea, constipation, or diarrhea. There may be associated rectal bleeding, hematochezia, as well as dysuria.

Positive physical examination findings include a fever, tachycardia, and hypotension, depending upon severity. There is often LLQ tenderness on abdominal exam, with or without associated rebound. A palpable mass may be felt in the LLQ. Distension may also be present and is suggestive of peritonitis. Rectal exam may reveal tenderness, mass, and the stool sample may be positive for occult blood.

> **CLINICAL PEARL:**   Differential diagnosis should include inflammatory bowel disease, irritable bowel syndrome (IBS), gastroenteritis, nephrolithiasis, UTI, CRC ectopic pregnancy, and tubo-ovarian abscess.

Diagnosis

- Leukocytosis is found in over 50% of cases. Additional blood work should include a metabolic panel for electrolytes and renal function. C–reactive protein can be elevated; values can be greater than 50 mg/L. Urinalysis should be obtained to rule out infection and HCG to rule out pregnancy when indicated.
- Plain films of the abdomen can show free air consistent with perforation.
- CT scan is the imaging test of choice to rule out secondary complications of acute diverticulitis. Findings include bowel wall thickening, fat stranding, abscess formation, phlegmon, intramural air, sinus tracts, or free air.
- Ultrasound is less able to identify the extent of larger abscesses or the presence of free air within the abdominal cavity. MRI is also accurate in diagnosing diverticulitis; however, the length of time required to complete the test may be inappropriate for the critically ill patient.
- Colonoscopy is contraindicated in acute diverticulitis because of the concern for perforation and bleeding risks; however, it is recommended 4 to 6 weeks after the acute episode has resolved.[2]

> **CLINICAL PEARL:**   The presence of LLQ tenderness, no vomiting, and CRP result >50 mg/L represents a significant likelihood of acute diverticulitis.[3]

Management

Management is guided by a diagnosis of complicated versus uncomplicated diverticulitis. Diverticulitis is considered complicated if it is associated with an abscess, phlegmon, fistula, obstruction, bleeding, or perforation. All other cases are uncomplicated.

Uncomplicated mild disease: outpatient management:[4]

- Current evidence recommends that patients with mild, stable, improving symptoms do not require antibiotic therapy
- Diet: Clear liquids
- Follow up in 48 to 72 hours
- If symptoms are persistent or worsening, oral antibiotics are warranted

Complicated–moderate–severe: inpatient management:

- Diet: Nothing by mouth (NPO), IV therapy with lactated Ringer's, 0.9% saline
- Antibiotic therapy as outlined in Table 2.29

Other considerations in management:

- Diverticulitis may be associated with secondary peritonitis, which always warrants close evaluation. Risk factors for peritonitis include[5,6] the following:
  - Age >50, female sex, organ failure, malignancy, preoperative peritonitis, sepsis, diffuse peritonitis, and exudates
- Statistically significant predictors for death include organ failure and fecal exudates

TABLE 2.29 Antibiotic Therapy Choices for Diverticulitis

Medication	Dose
Mild with persistent symptoms outpatient: primary regimen	
Trimethoprim/sulfamethoxazole DS, 160/800 mg	Every 12 hours
Ciprofloxacin 750 mg	Every 12 hours
Levofloxacin 750 mg	Every 24 hours
Plus	
Metronidazole 500 mg	Every 6 hours
Mild with persistent symptoms outpatient: alternative regimen	
Amoxicillin/clavulanate extended release 1,000/62.5 mg	Two tablets every 12 hours
Moxifloxacin 400 mg	Every 24 hours
Moderate/severe inpatient therapy: primary regimen	
Piperacillin/tazobactam 3.375 g IV	Every 6 hours
Ticarcillin/clavulanate 3.1 g IV	Every 6 hours
Ertapenem 1 g IV	Every 24 hours
Moxifloxacin 400 mg IV	Every 24 hours
Moderate/severe inpatient therapy: alternative regimen	
Ciprofloxacin 400 mg	Every 12 hours
Levofloxacin 750 mg	Every 24 hours
Plus	
Metronidazole 500 mg	Every 6 hours
Tigecycline 100 mg, 50 mg	100 mg first dose, followed by 50 mg IV every 12 hours
Moxifloxacin 400 mg	Every 24 hours
Severe (life threatening): primary regimen	
Imipenem/cilastatin, 500 mg IV	Every 6 hours
Meropenem 1 g IV	Every 8 hours
Doripenem 500 mg	Every 8 hours
Severe (life threatening): alternative regimen	
Ampicillin, 2 g IV plus	Every 6 hours
Metronidazole 500 mg plus	Every 6 hours
Ciprofloxacin, 400 mg or Levofloxacin	Cipro every 12 hours, levofloxacin evert 24 hours

- Thirty percent of patients who develop acute diverticulitis experience a complication that will require surgical intervention[1]

Patient education to prevent recurrence:

- Maintain a diet high in fiber. Current evidence reveals that avoiding nuts, corn, or popcorn has no effect in decreasing the risk of diverticulosis or diverticular complication.
- Lifestyle changes should include exercise, weight loss, and counseling for smoking cessation.

REFERENCES

1. Wilkins T, Embry K, George R. Diagnosis and management of acute diverticulitis. *Am Fam Physician.* 2013;87(9):612–620.
2. Laméris W, van Randen A, van Gulik TM, et al. A clinical decision rule to establish the diagnosis of acute diverticulitis at the emergency department. *Dis Colon Rectum.* 2010;53(6):896–904. doi:10.1007/DCR.0b013e3181d98d86
3. Etzioni DA, Chiu VY, Cannom RR, et al. Outpatient treatment of acute diverticulitis: rates and predictors of failure. *Dis Colon Rectum.* 2010;53(6):861–865. doi:10.1007/DCR.0b013e3181cdb243
4. Muralidhar VA, Madhu CP, Sudhir S, et al. Efficacy of Mannheim Peritonitis Index (MPI) score in patients with secondary peritonitis. *J Clin Diagn Res.* December 2014;8(12):NC01–NC03.
5. Wacha H, Linder MM, Feldman U, et al. Mannheim peritonitis index – prediction of risk of death from peritonitis: construction of a statistical and validation of an empirically based index. *Theoretical Surg.* 1987;1:169–177.
6. Rafferty J, Shellito P, Hyman NH, et al. Practice parameters for sigmoid diverticulitis. *Dis Colon Rectum.* 2006;49(7):939–944. doi:10.1007/s10350-006-0578-2

DIVERTICULOSIS

Etiology

Diverticuli are out pouchings of the mucosa through the muscularis. Diverticuli occur most commonly in the descending and sigmoid colon. They may be associated with an increase in intracolonic pressure and slow motility resulting in constipation. An association with a diet low in fiber is controversial.

Epidemiology

Diverticulosis occurs in up to 10% of individuals >45 years of age and in approximately 80% of individuals over the age of 85. Additional risks may include smoking and obesity.[1] There is a genetic predisposition.[2]

Clinical Presentation

Most patients are asymptomatic. Diagnosis commonly occurs as an incidental finding at the time of colonoscopy, during routine screening, or when evaluating the patient for some other condition. Patients may complain of intermittent LLQ discomfort, pain, bloating, or a change in bowel habits. Bleeding can occur with vessel rupture. Bleeding is described as red or maroon colored. Patients may have a history of constipation and a diet high in fats, low in fiber.

Most often, patients will have a normal exam; however, when examining the abdomen, there may be mild distension, along with mild-moderate LLQ tenderness to palpation. On rectal exam the stool may be heme positive.

> **CLINICAL PEARL:** Individuals who present at an older age, have a family history of diverticular disease, have persistent anorectal bleeding despite treatment, or have weight loss or iron deficiency anemia should be referred for colonoscopy.

Diagnosis

Colonoscopy is the test of choice; it enables the provider direct visualization of any out pouchings in the mucosa. CT scan with oral contrast obtains cross-sectional images identifying the diverticuli along with any findings suggestive of inflammatory or infectious complications. Nuclear medicine bleeding scans can localize site of bleed if undetectable by a scope.

Management

A diet high in fiber is recommended to prevent constipation. Bulking agents and stool softeners may be needed. Avoidance of fruits, nuts, corn, and seeds is not necessary.

REFERENCES

1. Turunen P, Wikström H, Carpelan-Holmström M, et al. Smoking increases the incidence of complicated diverticular disease of the sigmoid colon. *Scand J Surg.* 2010;99(1):14–17. doi:10.1177/145749691009900104
2. Wilkins T, Embry K, George R. Diagnosis and management of acute diverticulitis. *Am Fam Physician.* 2013;87(9):612–620.

DUMPING SYNDROME

Etiology

The dumping syndrome is defined as the rapid emptying of gastric contents into the small bowel due to the rapid transit of a large and hyperosmolar concentration chyme from the stomach to the duodenum. This condition is associated with gastric surgery, vagotomy, GB surgery, DM, previous history of gastroenteritis, anxiety, depression, or idiopathic. Postoperative changes can result in reduced stomach volume, inhibition of stomach's receptive relaxation properties (e.g., fundoplication), or the disruption of neural mechanisms retarding gastric emptying (vagotomy). The dumping syndrome can also be related to hormonal and neuronal changes of VIP, serotonin, norepinephrine, GLP-1, GIP, and insulin. Shifts in fluid from circulation to the intestinal lumen result in increased contractility and/or distention of the small bowel. Clinical findings are due to the autonomic responses to intestinal distension.

Epidemiology

Symptoms of dumping syndrome can be found in up to approximately 50% of patients who have had gastric surgery. In approximately 5% of patients, symptoms can become severe. The rates of early dumping syndrome are higher than those of late dumping syndrome.[1] Women are affected more than men.

Clinical Presentation

With early dumping, patients will note symptoms within 10 to 30 minutes after meals, which can include abdominal distension, nausea, bloating, abdominal cramps, explosive diarrhea, and palpitations. Stools are watery or soft, with no evidence of bleeding. Late dumping presents 1 to 3 hours after a meal, following insulin release. Carbohydrates are most likely to trigger symptoms. Pertinent negatives include lack of fever, vomiting, and bleeding with bowel movements (BMs). Systemic symptoms include flushing, diaphoresis, dizziness, palpitations, and an intense desire to lie down due to a reactive hypoglycemia. Lying down helps to minimize symptoms.

The patient is afebrile on exam, ruling out an infectious process. The patient may show signs of dehydration, tachycardia, dry mucous membranes, orthostasis, and postural hypotension. Examination of the abdomen may reveal evidence of previous surgery, and hyperactive bowel sounds may be present. Patients often have a history of anxiety and depression.[1]

Diagnosis

A complete blood cell count should be obtained to look for anemia or leukocytosis. Serum electrolytes and renal function testing will detect nutrient losses. Gastric emptying study when performed will reveal a rapid emptying time of <1 hour.[1]

Management

Dietary:

- Avoid liquids for at least 30 minutes after a solid meal
- Eat smaller more frequent (at least six) meals a day
- Reduce carbohydrates; eat complex, rather than simple sugars
- Avoid milk and dairy products
- Increase protein and fat intake to meet daily needs
- Dietary fibers, bran, and methycellulose fibers, can be used to manage hypoglycemia

Medications: antimotility drugs; dicyclomine, octreotide

REFERENCE

1. Berg P, McCallum RW, Hall M, Sarosiek I. Dumping syndrome: updated perspectives on etiologies and diagnosis. *Pract Gastroenterol.* 2014;38(10):30–38.

GASTROESOPHAGEAL REFLUX DISEASE

Etiology

Reflux disease is associated with the transient relaxation or incompetence of the lower esophageal sphincter (LES) that results in mucosal damage from the chronic exposure to gastric acids, pepsin, and bile salts. Saliva acts as a protective mechanism by triggering peristalsis and neutralizing the acids present in the esophagus. Lower esophageal tone can be affected by a variety of hormonal, neural, and dietary factors, as outlined in Table 2.30. Gastric motor dysfunction (gastroparesis) and visceral hypersensitivity can also affect reflux.

TABLE 2.30 Mediators of Lower Esophageal Sphincter Tone

	Increases Resting Tone	**Decreases Resting Tone**
Hormonal mediators	Gastrin	Estrogen, progesterone, glucagon, secretin, cholecystokinin
Neural mediators	Vagus nerve	
Medications	Bethanechol, metoclopramide, histamine, antacids	Theophylline, meperidine, calcium channel blockers

Epidemiology

Gastroesophageal reflux disease (GERD) constitutes a large proportion of primary care practice, with a prevalence of 10% to 20% in the United States.[1] Patient risk factors include obesity and diets that are high in fat and carbohydrates. Exercise after meals is also known to cause reflux in patients with no underlying pathology. Tobacco and alcohol cessation have resulted in no significant change in patient symptoms or changes in esophageal pH. The presence of a hiatal hernia may worsen lower esophageal tone and can function as a reservoir for refluxed gastric contents; however, recent evidence has found that it is of less importance than previously thought.

Clinical Presentation

Common presenting symptoms include retrosternal aching or burning, "heartburn," that occurs 30 to 60 minutes following a meal and chest pain or heaviness that radiates to the neck, jaw, and shoulder region. Dysphagia or odynophagia represents chronic reflux causing inflammation and strictures. The symptoms of GERD can be similar to angina in patients with CAD. Regurgitation of stomach contents may awaken patients from sleep with a cough. Aspiration of stomach contents may result in chronic cough, pneumonia, or bronchospasm. Sore throat, hoarseness, laryngitis, and erosion of tooth enamel can also occur. Barrett's esophagus (BE) may represent the tissue repair from longstanding reflux. Patients can also present with an iron deficiency anemia secondary to gradual blood loss from chronic inflammation (esophagitis). Medications such as NSAIDs, potassium chloride tablets, tetracyclines, and bisphosphonates can also result in esophageal injury.

The physical exam is often normal. There may be dental erosions, pharyngeal erythema, and hoarseness on the HEENT portion of the exam. Wheezing may be heard in the chest. Epigastric tenderness or mass may be present. Rectal exam may reveal dark, heme positive stools.

CLINICAL PEARL: Differential diagnosis for GERD may include any of the following: myocardial ischemia, esophageal spasm (scleroderma), cholelithiasis, PUD, cancer, gastroparesis, and infections of the esophagus (cytomegalovirus [CMV], herpes, candida) in an immunocompromised host.

Diagnosis

- The CBC can reveal a microcytic anemia secondary to an erosive esophagitis, gastritis.
- Endoscopy is recommended in the presence of alarm symptoms, such as dysphagia, odynophagia, unexplained weight loss, or iron deficiency anemia. Also consider endoscopy for those at high risk for complications, such as patients with a >5-year history of severe symptoms, Caucasian males, and those >65 years. Endoscopy with biopsy identifies the presence and degree of inflammation, strictures, and ability to obtain biopsies ruling out dysplastic changes, BE.
- 24-hour ambulatory esophageal pH monitoring can be ordered when the diagnosis is in question, refractory symptoms exist, or before consideration of endoscopic or surgical therapy.
- Ambulatory reflux monitoring is the only test that is available to assess actual reflux with symptom association.
- Esophageal manometry is also recommended for preoperative evaluation when surgery is considered.

Management

Patient education:

- Elevate head of bed on 6-inch blocks
- Avoid late high-fat content meals (nothing 2 hours before bedtime)
- Weight loss when indicated
- Cessation of chocolate, caffeine, spices, citrus, carbonated beverages is not always necessary but can be considered on an individual patient basis if known to precipitate symptoms
- Avoid lying down after meals
- Complications such as erosive esophagitis, bleeding, anemia, Barrett's esophagus, and esophageal malignancy should be discussed with the patient

Pharmacologic therapy: Empiric trial of proton pump inhibitors (PPIs) is recommended for those patients with typical symptoms of heartburn and regurgitation and no warning signs. There is no major difference in efficacy between the various PPIs.

- PPI administered 30 to 60 minutes before the first meal of the day for an 8-week course
- Twice daily dosing can be considered for nighttime symptoms, variable schedules, and/or sleep disturbance
- Maintenance PPI therapy can be continued in patients with ongoing symptoms and those patients diagnosed with erosive esophagitis and Barrett's esophagus
- Because of onset and mechanism of action, histamine-2 blockers such as ranitidine 150 mg or famotidine 20 mg, prescribed at bedtime, may offer a greater benefit with nighttime reflux
- In patients who have a partial response, consider increasing the dose to twice daily or switching to a different PPI

> **CLINICAL PEARL:** PPIs can decrease calcium absorption.

> **CLINICAL PEARL:** PPIs are safe in pregnant patients when clinically indicated.

Surgery may be indicated if earlier methods have failed; endoscopic procedures or laparoscopic fundoplication can be considered as an option in select patients. Referral to an ENT, pulmonologist, or allergist should be considered in those patients who do not respond to PPI s or who present with atypical otolaryngologic symptoms.

SCREENING FOR AND MANAGEMENT OF BE

BE consists of a change in the normal squamous lining of the lower esophagus to columnar epithelium and remains one of the most common conditions seen in gastroenterology. BE is associated with GERD. Additional risk factors include male sex, central obesity, and age over >50 years.[2] Once low-grade dysplasia is confirmed, endoscopic eradication therapy is indicated.

Alcohol consumption does not increase risk of BE, and wine may even be a protective factor.[3] Patients diagnosed with BE should undergo endoscopic surveillance at routine intervals because of the small but higher risk than the general population of developing dysplastic changes and esophageal adenocarcinoma. Screening guidelines are outlined in Box 2.2.

Box 2.2 American College of Gastroenterology Current Guidelines for Patient Screening for Barrett's Esophagus

1. Considered in men with chronic GERD (>5 years)
2. Frequent (weekly or more) symptoms of gastroesophageal reflux (heartburn or acid regurgitation)

And two or more of the following risk factors

>50 years

Caucasian race

Waist circumference >102 cm or WHR >0.9

Current or past smoker

First-degree relative with a history of BE or esophageal adenocarcinoma

BE, Barrett's esophagus; GERD, gastroesophageal reflux disease; WHR, waist–hip ratio.
Source: Shaheen NJ, Falk GW, Iyer PG, Gerson L. ACG clinical guideline: diagnosis and management of Barrett's esophagus. *Am J Gastroenterol. 2016;*111:30–50. doi:10.1038/ajg.2015.322

> **CLINICAL PEARL:** The majority (>90%) of patients diagnosed with BE will die of causes other than esophageal cancer.[3]

The management of Barrett's esophagus has two goals:
1. Identify and appropriately manage the esophagitis
2. Early detection/prevention of cancer.

> **CLINICAL PEARL:** Screening for BE in females is not routinely recommended due to the low risk of esophageal cancer, but may be considered if multiple risk factors are present.

Surveillance intervals:
- Endoscopy at 3- to 5-year intervals in patients with BE without dysplasia
- Endoscopy annually in patients with BE uncertain if dysplasia is present

Medication:
- Once-daily PPI therapy
- Avoid routine use of aspirin and NSAIDs

Surgical options:
- Endoscopic ablative therapies, photodynamic therapy, radiofrequency ablation, cryotherapy
- Esophagectomy
- Antireflux surgery

REFERENCES

1. Cohen E, Bolus R, Khanna D, et al. GERD symptoms in the general population: prevalence and severity versus care-seeking patients. *Dig Dis Sci.* October 2014;59(10):2488–2496. doi:10.1007/s10620-014-3181-8
2. Wang KK, Sampliner RE. Updated guidelines 2008 for the diagnosis, surveillance and therapy of Barrett's esophagus. *Am J Gastroenterol.* 2008;103:788–797. doi:10.1111/j.1572-0241.2008.01835.x
3. Shaheen NJ, Falk GW, Iyer PG, Gerson L. ACG clinical guideline: diagnosis and management of Barrett's esophagus. *Am J Gastroenterol.* 2016;111:30–50. doi:10.1038/ajg.2015.322. http://gi.org/wp-content/uploads/2015/11/ACG-2015-Barretts-Esophagus-Guideline.pdf. Accessed May 5, 2018

GASTROPARESIS

Etiology

Gastroparesis is defined as a delay in the emptying of gastric contents resulting from poor antro-pyloro-duodeno synchronization. Abnormal vagal innervation leads to fewer antral contractions, decreased gastric tone, antral hypomotility, and pylorospasm. Gastroparesis is considered a diagnosis of exclusion after a mechanical obstruction of the stomach, pylorus, or small bowel has been ruled out. The etiology is idiopathic in the majority (50%–60%) of cases. The remaining cases are secondary to diabetes (29%), postgastric/esophageal surgeries (13%), postinfectious episodes (21%), collagen vascular diseases (5%), Parkinson's disease (8%), and certain medications (narcotics, anticholinergics, GLP-1, and amylin analogs).[1]

Epidemiology

Gastroparesis affects approximately 10 million people in the United States. Caucasian women are affected more often than males, the mean age of onset is 44 years, and most patients are high school or college educated.[2] Depression, physical abuse, and sexual abuse have been found to exist in up to 62% of women diagnosed with idiopathic gastroparesis.[1]

Clinical Presentation

Patients commonly present with signs and symptoms associated with a delay in stomach emptying and include nausea, vomiting, postprandial fullness, early satiety, epigastric/upper abdominal pressure, fullness, distension, and dehydration. Delayed gastric emptying is also known to exacerbate GERD symptoms. Symptoms prompting evaluation often include vomiting for diabetic gastroparesis and abdominal pain for idiopathic gastroparesis. Medications known to aggravate the symptoms include narcotics, anticholinergics, GLP-1 and amylin analogs, calcium channel blockers, and cannabinoids. Patients may also have a past medical history significant for diabetes, gastric/esophageal surgeries, collagen vascular diseases, and Parkinson's disease.

General exam findings occur secondary to dehydration and can include tachycardia, hypotension, orthostatic changes, mucosal dryness, and diminished skin turgor. The abdominal exam may be positive for distension and epigastric and/or upper abdominal tenderness.

Diagnosis

Blood testing should include electrolytes, hepatic panel, and renal function to determine that the patient is receiving adequate intake and is not intravascularly volume depleted. Blood glucose and A1C should be checked to rule out DM as a potential etiology. Obtain thyroid studies to rule out hypothyroidism.

Gastric emptying study (scintigraphy) confirms delayed emptying after 4 hours if >10% of the isotope remains in the stomach.[1] Wireless motility capsule can visualize any obstructions. Breath testing can be performed using C-octanoate or spirulina, and results are similar to those of gastric emptying scintigraphy.[1,3] Endoscopy may be required both for diagnostic and therapeutic indications.

Management

Patients may require restoration of fluids and electrolytes if symptoms are severe enough.

Lifestyle modifications include the following:

- Dietary counseling: Low in fats and soluble fiber, smaller more frequent meals (4–5 a day), greater liquid nutrients, enteral (jejunal) feedings
- Glucose control
- Avoid alcohol and tobacco

Pharmacologic therapy:

- Prokinetic agents:[3]
  - ○ Metoclopramide 5 to 10 mg three times a day before meals and at night (limiting tolerance due to parkinsonian effects)
  - ○ Domperidone 10 mg three to four times daily (caution prolonged QT syndrome) under a physician licensed to prescribe this medication
  - ○ Erythromycin 250 to 500 mg before a meal three times daily
- Antiemetics:
  - ○ Scopolamine 1.5 mg patch every 72 hours for nausea
  - ○ Ondansetron dissolvable pill (ODT; 4 mg, 8 mg) as needed
  - ○ Tricyclic antidepressants (TCAs) may be considered with refractory nausea and vomiting
  - ○ Pyloric botulinum toxin injections

Surgical: Gastric electrical stimulation, pyloroplasty, jejunostomy tube placement, gastrectomy

Cognitive behavioral therapy: Address pain and psychological aspects when indicated

Acupuncture: May be considered as an alternative therapy (evidence of effectiveness is controversial, lacking)

REFERENCES

1. Avalos DJ, Nail P, McCallum RW. Understanding the etiology and spectrum of idiopathic gastroparesis. *Pract Gastroenterol*. April 2017;41(4):38–50.
2. Jung HK, Choung RS, Locke GR III, et al. The incidence, prevalence, and outcomes of patients with gastroparesis in Olmsted County, Minnesota, from 1996 to 2006. *Gastroenterology*. 2009;136:1225–1233. doi:10.1053/j.gastro.2008.12.047
3. Camilleri M, Parkman HP, Shafi MA, et al. Clinical guideline: management of gastroparesis. The *Am J Gastroenterol*. 2013;108:18–37. doi:10.1038/ajg.2012.373

HEMORRHOIDS

Etiology

Hemorrhoidal disease involves the enlargement of AV vessels of the anorectal region. Hemorrhoids can be caused by an increase in venous pressure associated with standing upright and straining with BM, AV communications within the local tissues, and laxed tissue secondary to loss of support. Clinical conditions that are associated with them include constipation, portal HTN, and pregnancy. Depending upon the anatomic site of origin, hemorrhoids are categorized as internal (above the dentate line) or external (below the dentate line).

Epidemiology

Hemorrhoids are the most common anorectal condition, affecting approximately 50% of patients older than 50 years old, and can affect up to 80% of the primary care population.[1] Hemorrhoids are one of the most common causes of lower GI bleeding. They are associated with an elevated BMI[2] and diets that are high in fats and low in fiber.

TABLE 2.31 Hemorrhoid Grading

Grade I	Grade II	Grade III	Grade IV
Small, no prolapse	Medium sized, prolapsed but reduced spontaneously	Large, prolapsed but can be manually reduced	Largest, cannot be reduced

Clinical Presentation

Patients most commonly present with painless bleeding with BM, typically seen on the toilet tissue. Rectal pain is associated with external hemorrhoids. Internal hemorrhoids are not associated with pain because they do not have somatic sensory innervation. The patient may have a history of constipation, straining with BMs, pruritus, rectal bleeding with BMs, intermittent-reducible protrusion (prolapse), aching following BMs, and rectal discharge. External hemorrhoids that have thrombosed present as a painful rectal bluish lump or mass. A skin tag represents previous, thrombosed hemorrhoids. Internal hemorrhoids are assigned a functional grade based upon patient history, as outlined in Table 2.31

Digital rectal exam: Perform a perianal inspection to evaluate for the presence of skin tags. Assess rectal tone by having the patient squeeze/contract sphincter and perform Valsalva maneuver. There should be a decrease in anal canal pressure around the examiner's finger. A contraction around the finger suggests defecatory disorder. A tender, swollen blue lump at the anal verge is reflective of a thrombosed external hemorrhoid.

Diagnosis

- Anorectal manometry: Assesses sphincter tone and confirms elevated anal sphincter resting pressures
- Anoscopy: To visualize the canal and mucosa
- Colonoscopy: Assesses for lesions or an anatomic, structural abnormality in the large bowel, and is indicated in patients who are ≥50 years old

CLINICAL PEARL: Individuals with CRC have an increased incidence of hemorrhoidal disease.

Management

The mainstay of managing hemorrhoidal disease is with local therapies such as suppositories and topical agents as well as a routine bowel regimen that includes dietary modifications to regulate bowel habits. There is a small subset of these patients who fail this primary treatment regimen and will require more definitive therapy. The two most common forms of therapy include band ligation and infrared photocoagulation (IRC), with response rates up to 80% to 90%.[3]

Noninvasive therapies center around patient education:

- Avoiding straining
- Limiting time spent on the commode
- Increasing fiber in diet, bulking agents

- Liberalizing fluids
- Taking stool softeners
- Using suppositories
- Applying topical therapies: Astringents, analgesics, cold packs, and anti-inflammatories (1% hydrocortisone) for Grade I hemorrhoids
- Applying cold packs during the first few hours for pain
- Taking sitz baths twice a day for 20 to 30 minutes

Invasive therapies: (antibiotic prophylaxis is not indicated for hemorrhoidal procedures)

- Infrared coagulator* (Grades I, II)
- Rubber band ligation* (Grades II, III)
- Sclerotherapy* (Grades I, II)
- Stapled hemorrhoidopexy (Grades III, IV)
- Surgical excision (Grades III, IV), thrombosed external hemorrhoid if presents within <72 hours. Excision is also associated with higher remission rates.

*Office-based procedures.

REFERENCES

1. Fargo MV, Latimer KM. Evaluation and management of common anorectal conditions. *Am Fam Physician.* 2012;85(6):624–630.
2. Riss S, Weiser FA, Schwameis K, et al. The prevalence of hemorrhoids in adults. *Int J Colorectal Dis.* 2012;27:215–220. doi:10.1007/s00384-011-1316-3
3. Wald A, Bharucha AE, Cosman BC, Whitehead WE. ACG clinical guideline: management of benign anorectal disorders. *Am J Gastroenterol.* 2015;109:1141–1157. doi:10.1038/ajg.2014.190. https://www.nature.com/articles/ajg2014190

HEPATITIS A

Etiology

There are several known viruses that can affect the liver; however, the most common are hepatitis A (HAV), B (HBV), and C (HCV). They each differ according to virus type, source, method of prevention/transmission, infection risk, response to treatment, and whether or not they progress to diseases resulting in greater morbidity (fibrosis) and mortality (cirrhosis and HCC). Refer to Table 2.33 at the end of section for comparisons. HAV is a RNA Picornaviridae virus. It has an incubation period of 14 to 28 days. It does not lead to chronic infection.

Epidemiology

HAV is associated with poor hygiene and sanitation and lack of clean water for drinking. HAV is found in feces and transmitted via the fecal–oral route. The HAV can survive in the environment for long periods and is commonly associated with local outbreaks. Up to 50% of cases of HAV reported in the United States have no identifiable risk factors. HAV is successfully prevented by vaccination and ensuring safe food and drinking water. Acute HAV infection has been associated with a high morbidity/low mortality secondary to acute liver failure. More severe complications are possible in patients with chronic liver disease. The two most frequent causes of HAV are international travel and food-related infection.[1]

Clinical Presentation

Symptoms are age related. Most children under the age of 6 are asymptomatic, while the majority of older children and adults are symptomatic. When present, symptoms appear 15 to 50 days (average of 28 days) after exposure. The illness generally lasts ≤2 months, but can persist for up to 6 months.[1] Most commonly, patients will complain of fatigue and malaise. Coryza, photophobia, and headaches can be present. Patients may relay a history of sudden onset of nausea and vomiting, anorexia, RUQ pain, diarrhea, and pale-colored stools. The urine can be darker in color. They may have a recent history of myalgias and change in sense of smell or taste. They may report sick contacts as well.

Patients may be febrile. They may have jaundice (profound with HAV and can last for several months). There also may be a maculopapular rash. The abdominal exam will be positive for RUQ tenderness, hepatomegaly, and splenomegaly. Generalized lymphadenopathy may also be present in a small percentage of patients.

Diagnosis

Blood work should include the following:

- CBC may reveal leukocytosis.
- PT and PTT can be elevated with impaired function of the liver.
- Hepatic panel pattern of elevated aminotransferases can be >25 times ULN, low albumin levels.
- Basic metabolic panel can reveal hyponatremia, hypoglycemia. BUN, Cr may be elevated, along with a reduction in GFR.
- Measurement of serum IgG and IgM ab can help to determine how long the patient has had the virus, how recent was the exposure.
- Measurement of the viral load in the blood. Anti-HAV is detectable 2 weeks before the onset of symptoms to 6 months afterward. False-negative tests can occur in the severely immunosuppressed host (HIV, solid organ transplants, hypogammaglobulinemia, hemodialysis patients).

Imaging studies may include the following:

- Ultrasound: Evidence of a fatty liver, cirrhosis
- Triphasic CT: Fibrosis, cirrhosis, mass
- MRI: Fibrosis, cirrhosis, mass

A liver biopsy may also be indicated to rule out inflammatory and/or fibrotic changes, prior to therapy, as well as to determine patient response to treatment. Trichrome staining can show bridging fibrosis steatosis, or the presence of steatohepatitis.

Management

- Conservative, supportive therapy
- Notify contacts of possible exposure
- Document immunization status; HCV and HBV antibody and vaccinate for HBV if Ab are not present
- Monitor for acute liver failure
- Avoid hepatotoxic substances: NSAIDS, acetaminophen, alcohol
- Repeat serological testing in 3 months

> **CLINICAL PEARL:** Viral hepatitis is a reportable disease.

REFERENCE

1. Nelson NP, Murphy TV. Hepatitis a: the changing epidemiology of hepatitis A. *Clin Liver Dis.* July 2013;2(6):227–230. doi:10.1002/cld.230

HEPATITIS B VIRUS

Etiology

Hepatitis B is a DNA virus from the Hepadnaviridae family. It has a mean incubation period of 80 days, with a range of 28 to 160. There are several genotypes of HBV; however, A, B, and C are most prevalent in the United States. Genotypes A and B respond better to antiviral therapy. Genotype B is associated with sustained remission after treatment, less active hepatic necroinflammation, slower rate of progression to cirrhosis, and a lower rate of HCC development compared to genotype C. Genotype C carries with it a greater risk of progression to cirrhosis. Genotype D infection has the greatest risk of developing into acute hepatic failure.

Epidemiology

HBV is found in blood and body fluid and can be transmitted through percutaneous/permucosal routes. HBV can lead to chronic infection and cirrhosis, and is associated with a 15% risk of developing HCC. HBV can be prevented by pre-/postexposure immunization and modifying behaviors that can increase risk. Approximately 50% of acute infections in adults are asymptomatic. About 1% to 2% of acute infections progress to fulminant hepatitis, and this is associated with a significant mortality rate. About 10% of patients remain positive for hepatitis B surface antigen, and 20% develop fibrosis, which can lead to cirrhosis. Patients with the greatest risk of progressing to chronic hepatitis B are those who are diagnosed at a younger age, which is most commonly acquired in the perinatal period. Not all patients with acute HBV require therapy as they may have the ability to clear the virus on their own. HBV is a vaccine preventable disease.[1] Additional risk factors are outlined in Box 2.3.

Clinical Presentation

In general, patients will complain of fatigue and malaise. Coryza, photophobia, and headaches can be present. Patients may relay a history of sudden onset of nausea and vomiting, anorexia, RUQ pain, diarrhea, and pale-colored stools. The urine can be darker in color. They may have a recent history of myalgias and change in sense of smell or taste. Patients with both HBV and HCV can develop a "serum sickness" consisting of immune complex deposition, rash, arthralgias, and a positive rheumatoid factor.[2]

On examination, patients may be febrile or jaundiced. Jaundice occurs in approximately one-third of patients with the acute infection.[3] There also may be a maculopapular rash. The abdominal exam will be positive for RUQ tenderness, hepatomegaly, and splenomegaly. Generalized lymphadenopathy may also be present in a small percentage of patients.

> **Box 2.3   Risk factors for the development of viral infections of the liver**
>
> Hepatitis Screening
>
> 1. Individuals born in areas of high or intermediate prevalence rates
> 2. U.S.-born persons not vaccinated as infants whose parents were born in regions with high HBV rate of infection
> 3. Household and sexual contacts of HBsAg-positive persons
> 4. Persons who have ever injected drugs
> 5. Persons with multiple sexual partners or history of sexually transmitted disease
> 6. Men who have sex with men
> 7. Inmates of correctional facilities
> 8. Individuals with chronically elevated ALT or AST
> 9. Individuals infected with HCV or HIV
> 10. Patients undergoing renal dialysis
> 11. All pregnant women
> 12. Persons needing immunosuppressive therapy
>
> ALT, aminotransferase; AST, aspartate aminotransferase; HBsAg, hepatitis B virus surface antigen; HBV, hepatitis B virus; HCV, hepatitis C virus.

Diagnosis

Blood work will include the following:

- CBC may reveal leukocytosis
- PT and PTT can be elevated with impaired function of the liver
- Hepatic panel pattern of elevated aminotransferases that can reach levels >25′ ULN, low albumin levels
- Basic metabolic panel: hyponatremia, hypoglycemia. BUN, Cr may be elevated, along with a reduction in GFR
- Serum IgG and IgM ab can help to determine how long the patient has had the virus and how recent the exposure was
- Hepatitis B surface antigen, hepatitis B surface antibody, hepatitis B core antibody, hepatitis B e antigen, hepatitis B e antibody, and hepatitis B virus DNA
- False-negative tests can occur in severely immunosuppressed host (HIV, solid organ transplants, hypogammaglobulinemia, hemodialysis patients)

Interpretation of results is outlined in Table 2.32.

    a. Hepatitis B surface antibody (HBsAb+) hepatitis B core antibody (HBcAb+) = presence of immunity

    b. Hepatitis B virus surface antigen (HBsAg+) HBcAb+ = presence of infection

    c. B e antigen+ = active viral replication

    d. HBsAb+ = vaccination

Definitions:

- Chronic (replicative) HBV infection: HBsAg seropositive status at 6 months or beyond, HBeAg+ indicating active viral replication—infectious

TABLE **2.32** Diagnostic Criteria of Acute versus Chronic Hepatitis B Virus Infection

Marker	Acute (Early Phase)	Acute (Window Phase)	Acute (Recovery Phase)	Chronic (Replicative)	Chronic (Non replicative)	Chronic (Flare)
HBsAg	+			+	+	+
HBeAg	+			+		+
IgM anti-HBc	+	+				+
IgG anti-HBc			+	+	+	+
Anti-HBs			+			
Anti-HBe			+		+	
HBV DNA	+	+	+	+	+	+

- Acute early phase is indicative of infection within the past 6 months
- Acute recovery phase represents the period representing a distant HBV infection cleared by the immune system or that may persist
- Chronic (replicative) HBV infection: HBsAg seropositive status at 6 months or beyond with active viral replication
- Chronic (nonreplicative) HBV infection: HBsAg seropositive status at 6 months or beyond
- Chronic (flare) in an acute exacerbation or flare of hepatitis in chronic HBV-infected patient is defined as intermittent elevations of serum aminotransferase level to more than five times the ULN and more than twice the baseline value

Imaging studies include the following:

- Ultrasound: Evidence of a fatty liver, cirrhosis
- Triphasic CT: Fibrosis, cirrhosis, mass
- MRI: Fibrosis, cirrhosis, mass
- A liver biopsy may also be indicted to rule out inflammatory and/or fibrotic changes, prior to therapy, as well as to determine patient response to treatment.
- Trichrome staining can show bridging fibrosis steatosis, presence of steatohepatitis.

Management

General management of acute episodes:

- Conservative supportive therapy
- Notify contacts
- Document immunization status; with concomitant acute HCV vaccinate for HAV, HBV if Ab are not present
- Monitor liver failure
- Avoid hepatotoxic substances
- Repeat serological testing in 3 months

Specific antiviral therapy:[4,5]

- Entecavir 0.5 mg daily
- Tenofovir 300 mg daily
- Lamivudine 100 mg daily

The course of therapy can be up to 48 weeks with the goal of reducing the risk of cirrhosis and HCC.

REFERENCES

1. Kim BH, Kim WR. Epidemiology of hepatitis B virus infection in the United States. *Clin Liver Dis.* July 2018;12(1):1–4. doi:10.1002/cld.732
2. Liang TJ. Hepatitis B: the virus and disease. *Hepatology.* May 2009;49(5 suppl):S13–S21. doi:10.1002/hep.22881. NIH Public Access.
3. Liaw YF, Tsai SL, Sheen IS, et al. Clinical and virological course of chronic hepatitis B virus infection with hepatitis C and D virus markers. *Am J Gastroenterol.* 1998;93:354. doi:10.1111/j.1572-0241.1998.00354.x
4. Lok AS, McMahon BJ, Brown RS Jr, et al. Antiviral therapy for chronic hepatitis B viral infection in adults: a systematic review and meta-analysis. *Hepatology.* 2016;63:284–306. doi:10.1002/hep.28280
5. Ahn J, Lee HM, Lim JK, et al. Entecavir safety and effectiveness in a national cohort of treatment-naïve chronic hepatitis B patients in the US - the ENUMERATE study. *Aliment Pharmacol Ther.* 2016;43:134–144. doi:10.1111/apt.13440

HEPATITIS C VIRUS

Etiology

Hepatitis C is an RNA virus from the Flaviviridae family. It has a mean incubation period of 80 days, with a range of 28 to 160. Six genotypes have been isolated worldwide. Current antiviral therapy significantly improves clinical outcomes and is considered to result in a sustained virologic response (SVR). Successful treatment early in the disease can significantly reduce the progression of liver disease. There is no vaccine available for HCV.

Epidemiology

There are an estimated four million Americans positive for antibodies to hepatitis C.[1,2] HCV is found in blood and body fluid and can be transmitted through percutaneous/permucosal routes. HCV can lead to chronic infection. Patients who are at greatest risk are those with a history of parenteral exposure (blood transfusions before 1992, IV drug use, occupational). HCV can be prevented by blood donor screening and avoiding behaviors that are associated with greater risk. Additional risk factors include cocaine use, tattoos, body piercing, high-risk sexual behavior, need of long-term hemodialysis, born to an HCV-infected mother, incarceration, and intranasal drug use.

In the United States, 97% of all HCV infections result from genotype 1, 2, or 3. Eighty percent of patients that go untreated will go on to develop persistent infection. Of that subset:

- 30% have stable disease
- 30% go on to develop severe liver disease
- 40% have variable progression[1,2]

Clinical Presentation

In general, patients may complain of weakness, fatigue, appetite loss, fluid retention. They may complain of a skin rash, diffuse itching, easy bruising, or become jaundiced. GI complaints include nausea, vomiting, abdominal pain and bloating, increased abdominal girth, light stools, and hematemesis. Their urine may appear dark in color. They can have arthralgias and myalgias. Neurological complaints can range from subtle confusion, memory loss, disorientation, lethargy to difficulty to arouse. Patients may also become more sensitive to medications. They may participate in at-risk behaviors. Patients may develop a "serum sickness" consisting of immune complex deposition, rash, arthralgia, and +rheumatoid factor.

On physical exam, patients may be febrile. The skin can be jaundiced, along with spider nevi and palmar erythema. HEENT exam findings may include parotid gland enlargement, scleral icterus, and conjunctival pallor. The exam can be positive for left supraclavicular/periumbilical adenopathy and gynecomastia. Patients may have ascites, RUQ tenderness, mass, hepatomegaly, splenomegaly, and caput medusae on abdominal exam. Testicular atrophy can be present. Bilateral lower extremity edema is associated with hepatic congestion. Neurological findings include mental status changes, asterixis, muscle wasting in the temporal areas and proximal muscle groups, and the presence of Dupuyten's contractures.

Diagnosis

Initial testing should include the following:

- Hepatitis C antibody enzyme immunoassay. Anti-HCV screening tests can detect antibodies 4 to 10 weeks after infection, and in the majority of patients will be detected by 6 months after exposure
- Serum HCV RNA by PCR to confirm viral load. False-negative tests can be seen in the severely immunosuppressed host (HIV, solid organ transplants, hypogammaglobulinemia, hemodialysis patients)
- One-time hepatitis C testing is recommended for persons born from 1945 through 1965 independent of risk factors[3]

Additional blood work will include the following:

- CBC that may reveal leukocytosis
- The PT and PTT can be elevated with impaired function of the liver
- Hepatic panel pattern of elevated aminotransferases, low albumin levels
- Basic metabolic panel may reveal hyponatremia, hypoglycemia. BUN, Cr may be elevated, along with a reduction in GFR
- Serum IgG and IgM ab can help to determine how long the patient has had the virus and how recent the exposure was

> **CLINICAL PEARL:** Coexistent HBV and HCV infection rates can be up to 10% to 15%.

Imaging studies include the following:

- Ultrasound: Evidence of a fatty liver, cirrhosis
- Triphasic CT: Fibrosis, cirrhosis, mass

- MRI: Fibrosis, cirrhosis, mass
- A liver biopsy may also be indicted to rule out inflammatory and/or fibrotic changes, prior to therapy, as well as to determine patient response to treatment. Trichrome staining can show bridging fibrosis steatosis, presence of steatohepatitis.

Management

General Management of acute episodes:

- Conservative supportive therapy
- Notify contacts
- Document immunization status; with acute HCV vaccinate for HAV, HBV if Ab are not present
- Monitor liver failure
- Avoid hepatotoxic substances
- Serological testing should be repeated in 3 months
  Specific antiviral therapy is complex and often managed by hepatologists.

CLINICAL PEARL: Complications of HCV if untreated include chronic liver disease, cirrhosis within 25 years, HCC, or decompensated liver disease. Eighty percent of all HCV + patients progress to chronic infection.

A summary of the different viral hepatitis infections is outlined in Table 2.33.

REFERENCES

1. Denniston MM, Jiles RB, Drobeniuc J, et al. Chronic hepatitis C virus infection in the United States National Health and Nutrition Examination Survey 2003 to 2010. *Ann Intern Med.* 2014;160:293. doi:10.7326/M13-1133
2. Edlin BR, Eckhardt BJ, Shu MA, et al. Toward a more accurate estimate of the prevalence of hepatitis C in the United States. *Hepatology.* 2015;62:1353. doi:10.1002/hep.27978
3. American Association for the Study of Liver Diseases, & Infectious Diseases Society of America. Recommendations for Testing, Managing, and Treating Hepatitis C. Joint panel from the American Association of the Study of Liver Diseases and the Infectious Diseases Society of America; 2014.

ELECTRONIC RESOURCES

Hepatitis C Virus Guidance: Recommendations for Testing, Managing, and Treating Hepatitis C

https://www.hcvguidelines.org/

IRRITABLE BOWEL SYNDROME

Etiology

IBS is classified as a functional bowel disorder of intestinal motility and visceral hypersensitivity, characterized by abdominal pain associated with changes in bowel habits. IBS has a strong association with emotional factors.[1] Patients who have a history of receiving multiple antibiotics for various reasons can develop a disruption in their normal gut flora that can be associated

TABLE 2.33 Differentiating the Common Viral Hepatitis Infections

Type	A	B	C	D	E
Virus	Picornaviridae	Hepadnaviridae	Flaviviridae	Deltaviridae	Calciviridae
Nucleic acid	RNA	DVA	RNA	RNA	RNA
Mean incubation period (days)	30 (15–50)	80 (28–160)	50 (14–160)	Variable	40 (15–45)
Source	Feces	Blood and body fluids	Blood and body fluids	Blood and body fluids	Feces
Transmission	Fecal–oral	Percutaneous, permucosal	Percutaneous, permucosal	Percutaneous, permucosal	Fecal–oral
Chronicity	No	Yes	Yes	Yes	No
Prevention	Pre/postexposure immunization; ensure safe food and drinking water	Pre/postexposure immunization; risk behavior modification	Blood donor screening; risk behavior modification	Pre/postexposure immunization against HBV; risk behavior modification	Ensure safe food and drinking water
Vaccine	Yes	Yes	No	No	No

HBV, hepatitis B virus.

with IBS (especially IBS-D). Past medical history may be positive for infections with Campylobacter, Salmonella, and Shigella that may be the initial trigger.

Epidemiology

IBS affects approximately 16% of people in the United States, the majority of which are women. Almost half of the patients with IBS experience their first symptoms before the age of 35.[1,2]

Clinical Presentation

The Rome IV criteria for IBS include recurrent abdominal pain for at least 1 day a week in the last 3 months that is associated with at least two of the following: pain associated with defecation, pain onset with a change in stool frequency or form. Symptoms must be present for 6 months. IBS is divided into three subgroups with the predominant complaint of abdominal pain (19%–49%), constipation (19%–44%), or diarrhea (15%–36%).[1-3] Generally, patients will give a history of hypersensitivity—hyperalgesia, hypervigilance to noxious stimulation. Patients will describe exaggerated pain referral patterns (perception of pain outside the normal anatomic sites normally activated in healthy individuals), sleep disturbances, repeated nocturnal awakening, arising in the morning feeling unrested.

GI complaints include nausea, reflux, abdominal pain relieved with defecation, bloating, distension, change in bowel habits, frequency, consistency, passage of mucous, difficulty passing stools, allodynia, exaggerated colorectal motor activity, changes in rectal tone, and increases in rectal hypersensitivity.

It is critical to review all medications the patient may be taking prescribed and OTC as many drugs are associated with GI side effects. Medical history is often positive for fibromyalgia, chronic migraines, interstitial cystitis, and temporomandibular joint (TMJ) syndrome.

The following signs and symptoms are not commonly associated with functional bowel disorder and suggest underlying pathology: unintended weight loss of >10 lb, fever or chills, high-volume diarrhea (>300 mL/d), nocturnal diarrhea, family history of GI malignancy/IBD/celiac disease, 50 years of age or older upon presentation, iron deficiency anemia, or rectal bleeding.

Physical examination is often normal with IBS and is performed to rule out organic disease. The abdomen may be distended and diffusely tender. Visceral hypersensitivity, presenting as tenderness to touch, on abdominal exam may be present. Stool may be palpated throughout the abdomen. Rectal exam will be normal.

Diagnosis

There is little consensus for a specific diagnostic workup except in those patients who present with alarm symptoms/findings; approach is patient dependent.

Laboratory studies that are routinely performed to rule out underlying pathology include the following:

- CBCs and a comprehensive metabolic panel to rule out a nutritional, malabsorptive process
- Thyroid function tests: Underlying over- or underactive thyroid
- C-reactive protein elevation may be reflective of an underlying inflammatory process such as inflammatory bowel disease

- HLA-DQ2/8 serology, tissue transglutaminase IgA, and total IgA levels to rule out celiac disease
- Stool studies: Fecal leukocytes, bacteria, ova, and parasites for infection
- Lactulose breath test: Enzyme deficiency[4]

Diagnostic imaging can include the following:

- Plain films of the abdomen to quantify stool content, especially if there is concern for "overflow" diarrhea
- Colon transit (marker) study performed to evaluate colonic inertia. If after 5 days, most markers are scattered about the colon, the patient most likely has hypomotility or colonic inertia. If most markers are gathered in the rectosigmoid, the patient may have functional outlet obstruction, internal rectal prolapse, or anismus.
- Screening colonoscopy is recommended for patients >50 years old (African Americans 45 years old) and anyone presenting with alarm features.

Management

Requires a multidisciplinary approach, including the following:

- Gastroenterologist
- Primary care provider
- Nutritionist
- Psychologist: Psychotherapy, behavioral therapies
- Nursing
- Dietary modifications:[5–7]
  - Alter intake of dairy, fructose, wheat products, corn, tea, citrus fruits, and caffeine
  - Small meals and higher fiber intake
  - Avoid fatty foods, milk products, carbohydrates, caffeine, alcohol, high-protein foods (meats)
  - Do not mix liquids and solids (with meals)
  - Follow diet low in carbohydrates such as fruit sugar (fructose) and milk sugar (lactose), and consume FODMAPs (fermentable oligo-, di-, monosaccharides, and polyols), which can help improve digestive symptoms

  Medications:[1,7]
- Antidepressants:
  - TCAs for abdominal pain and diarrhea
  - Selective serotonin reuptake inhibitors (SSRIs) for abdominal pain and constipation
  - Serotonin–norepinephrine reuptake inhibitors (SNRIs) for abdominal discomfort
- Antibiotics: Rifaximin 550 mg three times daily × 14 days for gas, bloating, diarrhea
- IBS-D
  - Antispasmodics: Hyoscamine, dicyclomine, chlordiazepoxide/clidinium bromide, peppermint oil (IBgard)
  - Loperamide
  - Eluxadoline: 75 to 100 mg twice daily binds to peripheral opioid receptors in the GI tract to slow motility and reduce secretions

- IBS-C[1]
  - Laxatives: Polyethylene glycol, bisacodyl
  - Linaclotide: Stimulates secretion of chloride and bicarbonate increases fluid within intestines
  - Lubiprostone: Activates chloride channels, increases fluid and motility
  - Fiber
  - Promotility agents: Metoclopramide, renzapride
- Probiotics most commonly used with chronic constipation, to reduce gas, bloating, and abdominal distension have received mixed responses:
  - Examples: Bifidobacterium infantis 35624, Lactobacillus species, *Saccharomyces* sp.

REFERENCES

1. Mearin F, Lacy BE, Chang L, et al. Bowel disorders. *Gastroenterology.* 2016;150:1393–1407. doi:10.1053/j.gastro.2016.02.031
2. Naik P, McCallum RW. Current treatment strategies for irritable bowel syndrome. *Pract Gastroenterol.* November 2016;40(11):50–59.
3. Ford AC, Bercik P, Morgan DG, et al. Validation of the Rome III criteria for the diagnosis of irritable bowel syndrome in secondary care. *Gastroenterology.* 2013;145:1262–1270. doi:10.1053/j.gastro.2013.08.048
4. Menees SB, Powell C, Kurlander J, et al. A meta-analysis of the utility of C-reactive protein, erythrocyte sedimentation rate, fecal calprotectin, and fecal lactoferrin to exclude inflammatory bowel disease in adults with IBS. *Am J Gastroenterol.* 2015;110:444–454. doi:10.1038/ajg.2015.6
5. Zhu Y, Zheng X, Cong Y, et al. Bloating and distention in irritable bowel syndrome: the role of gas production and visceral sensation after lactose ingestion in a population with lactase deficiency. *Am J Gastroenterol.* 2013;108:1516–1525. doi:10.1038/ajg.2013.198
6. American College of Gastroenterology Task Force on Irritable Bowel Syndrome, Brandt LJ, Chey WD, et al. An evidence-based position statement on the management of irritable bowel syndrome. *Am J Gastroenterol.* 2009;104(suppl 1):S1–S35. doi:10.1038/ajg.2009.134
7. Ford AC, Moayyedi P, Lacy BE, et al. American College of Gastroenterology monograph on the management of irritable bowel syndrome and chronic idiopathic constipation. *Am J Gastroenterol.* 2014;109(suppl 1):S2–S26. doi:10.1038/ajg.2014.187

NONALCOHOLIC FATTY LIVER DISEASE

Etiology

The natural history of NAFLD consists of two distinct pathophysiologic entities. Simple steatosis represents 80% to 90% of cases. It presents as excessive amounts of fat in the liver, mostly benign and nonprogressive. Approximately 10% of patients will progress to steatosis with inflammation, termed "steatohepatitis." Of these, approximately 60% progress to fibrosis and 30% will progress to cirrhosis. There is also a greater risk of HCC as hepatic fibrosis progresses.[1] NAFLD is also associated with increased rates of insulin resistance, DM, HTN, and dyslipidemia and is considered the hepatic component to the metabolic syndrome.

Epidemiology

NAFLD is the most common chronic liver disease in Western countries and occurs in 30% of the general adult population. Prevalence in the diabetic or obese patient is 69% to 90%. NAFLD affects men and women equally. It occurs in all age groups, but the highest is in the 40- to 49-year-old patient population. The known risk factors for NAFLD are obesity, diets high in fructose corn syrup and saturated fats, a sedentary lifestyle, and genetic predisposition. Fatty liver disease is now the third most common cause for liver transplant.[1-3]

Clinical Presentation

Most patients are asymptomatic with the only objective finding being an incidental finding of elevated transaminases on routine blood work. Nonspecific symptoms may include fatigue and vague RUQ discomfort. Physical exam can be essentially normal. Patients are often obese and hypertensive.[4]

Diagnosis

Laboratory studies should include a hepatic panel that reveals minor elevations in AST/ALT (<100 IU/L); AST/ALT ratio <1; and elevated ALT usually <4' ULN. Both the serum glucose and lipid profiles may be elevated. The two types of noninvasive tests used to diagnose liver fibrosis include serum markers and radiography. The fibrosure test includes the following group of markers: alpha-2 macroglobulin, alpha-2 globulin (haptoglobin), gamma globulin, apolipoprotein A1, GGTP, and total bilirubin. The results combined with the patient's age and sex are used to determine the degree of fibrosis, either mild, significant, or indeterminate.

Imaging of the liver includes an ultrasound that may show evidence of a fatty liver and/or the presence of gallstones. A FibroScan image can reveal inflammatory and/or fibrotic changes within the liver. Liver biopsy remains the gold standard and may be indicated to further identify the extent of damage and tor rule out inflammatory and/or fibrotic changes. Trichrome staining can show bridging fibrosis steatosis and presence of steatohepatitis. Because of the overlap in findings, liver scanning is becoming the go-to test to first identify fibrotic changes in the liver.[4,5]

Management

Steatosis "fatty liver":

- Avoid known hepatotoxins
- Vaccinations against HAV, HBV
- Weight loss:
  - 6 to 12 months (reduced intake + exercise)
  - Calorie restriction, diet <30% fat (1–2 lbs/wk)
  - 3% to 5% loss of body weight required to improve steatosis
  - 10% loss of body weight required to improve inflammation
- Medications:
  - Orlistat PO 120 mg three times daily
  - Metformin: Control blood sugars
- Monitor for extrahepatic complications: cardiovascular disease, coronary heart disease, stroke, HTN, DM-2, chronic kidney disease, CRC, obstructive sleep apnea, hypothyroidism, polycystic ovarian syndrome (PCOS), osteoporosis

Steatohepatitis "fatty liver with inflammation":

- Same as above

- Maximize treatment of associated conditions
- Avoid any hepatotoxins
- Immunize against hepatitis A, hepatitis B
- Vitamin E (α-tocopherol) at 800 IU/daily if biopsy-proven nonalcoholic steatohepatitis (NASH)

> **CLINICAL PEARL:** Once fibrosis has begun, no oral regimen to date has had statistically significant effect on decreasing/reversing the fibrotic changes.

REFERENCES

1. Oda K, Uto H, Mawatari S, et al. Clinical features of hepatocellular carcinoma associated with nonalcoholic fatty liver disease: a review of human studies. *Clin J Gastroenterol.* 2015;8:1–9. doi:10.1007/s12328-014-0548-5
2. Do A, Lim JK. Epidemiology of nonalcoholic fatty liver disease: a primer. *Clin Liver Dis.* May 2016;7(5):106–108. doi:10.1002/cld.547
3. Lazo M, Hernaez R, Eberhardt MS, et al. Prevalence of nonalcoholic fatty liver disease in the United States: the third national health and nutrition examination survey, 1988–1994. *Am J Epidemiol.* 2013;178:38. doi:10.1093/aje/kws448
4. Chalasani N, Younossi Z, Lavine JE, et al. The diagnosis and management of nonalcoholic fatty liver disease: practice guidance from the American Association for the Study of Liver Diseases. *Hepatology.* 2018;67:328. doi:10.1002/hep.29367
5. Williams CD, Stengel J, Asike MI, et al. Prevalence of nonalcoholic fatty liver disease and nonalcoholic steatohepatitis among a largely middle-aged population utilizing ultrasound and liver biopsy: a prospective study. *Gastroenterology.* 2011;140:124. doi:10.1053/j.gastro.2010.09.038

PANCREATITIS: ACUTE

Etiology

Acute pancreatitis is a generalized inflammation of pancreatic tissue, resulting in the retention of what are normally inactive proteolytic enzymes. Due to the obstruction and disruption of drainage, these enzymes become activated. Once activated within the pancreas, these enzymes can trigger a local inflammatory response, most often self-limiting. Occasionally, the patient will develop a fulminating course leading to pancreatic necrosis, sepsis, and multiorgan system failure.

Acute pancreatitis is characterized by two distinct phases: early (within 1 week), characterized by a SIRS and/ or organ failure, and late (> 1 week), characterized by local complications which include peripancreatic fluid collections, pancreatic and peripancreatic necrosis (sterile or infected), pseudocysts, and walled-off necrosis (sterile or infected).

Epidemiology

The two most common risk factors for acute pancreatitis are gallstones and alcohol use. Other less common causes include hypertriglyceridemia (levels >400 mg/dL), hypercalcemia, hyperparathyroidism, certain medications such as 6-mercaptopurine, azathioprine, thiazides, ACE inhibitors, estrogens, and steroids. Anatomic and physiologic anomalies causing acute pancreatitis include pancreas divisum, pancreatic masses (especially in patients >40 years), or sphincter of Oddi dysfunction. Genetic causes should be considered in the younger patients (<30 years) with a known family history of pancreatic disease. Autoimmune reactions, viral illness, and following certain procedures; ERCP (5%), cardiac/abdominal surgeries are also known to cause pancreatic inflammation. Acute pancreatitis is responsible for over 280,000 hospital admissions annually and can be associated with 15% mortality.[1]

Clinical Presentation

Patients often present with epigastric or left upper quadrant pain. They may describe the pain as constant with radiation to the back, chest, or flanks. Intensity is usually severe but can be variable and does not correlate with severity. Associated symptoms include nausea and vomiting.

General findings on examination include low-grade fever, tachycardia, and hypotension. Erythematous nodules due to subcutaneous fat necrosis may be seen on examination of the skin. Basilar rales, diminished breath sounds with left pleural effusion, are associated pulmonary findings. Exam of the abdomen can reveal diffuse tenderness, rigidity, and hypoactive bowel sounds. Retroperitoneal bleeding may appear as bruising of the flanks (Grey Turner sign) or periumbilical ecchymosis (Cullen sign), both of which are associated with severe acute pancreatitis and a high mortality. Findings on initial assessment that are associated with greater risk of severity include age >55 years, BMI >30 kg/m^2, altered mental status, and comorbidities.

Inquire about a previous history of pancreatitis, gallstones, alcohol use, current medications, and if there is a family history of pancreatic diseases. Other potential critical conditions to be ruled out by history and physical exam include biliary colic, bowel obstruction/perforation, MI, or abdominal aortic aneurysm.

Diagnosis

Routine blood work indicated to diagnose acute pancreatitis includes the following:

- Serum amylase: 3′ ULN. Generally rises within a few hours after the onset of symptoms and returns to normal values within 3 to 5 days. May be normal in alcohol-induced acute pancreatitis and hypertriglyceridemia
- Serum lipase: 3′ ULN. Lipase is preferred, as it is more specific for the pancreas and remains elevated longer than amylase after the disease presents. Lipase can also be elevated with renal disease, appendicitis, cholecystitis, perforated ulcer, and bowel infarction/obstruction
- CBC: Leukocytosis
- Hepatic panel: Transaminitis, with ALT level >150 U/L within 48 hours after onset of symptoms discriminates biliary pancreatitis[2]
- Comprehensive metabolic panel: Hypercalcemia, hypocalcemia, hyperglycemia
- Lipid panel: Hypertriglyceridemia with triglycerides >400 mg/dL
- Creactive protein: >150 mg/dL

> **CLINICAL PEARL:** No lab is consistently accurate in predicting severity of pancreatitis, nor is there any definite correlation between the severity of pancreatitis and the degree of serum lipase and amylase elevations.

Diagnostic imaging may include the following:

- Abdominal ultrasound is recommended in all patients with acute pancreatitis. Images show characteristics findings of edema, inflammation, fluid surrounding the gland.
- Contrast-enhanced computed tomographic (CECT) is recommended when the diagnosis is unclear, the patient fails to improve clinically within the first 48 to 72 hours after hospital admission, the patient has persistent pain, fever, nausea, or is unable to begin oral feeding, or to assess for possible local complications such as pancreatic necrosis.
- MRI can be performed in patients with contrast allergy or renal insufficiency.
- MRCP can be performed to better visualize ductal anatomy, stones, strictures, or other anatomic variants.
- EUS is technically better at direct visualization of the pancreas and can perform biopsies, drain peripancreatic fluid if present, obtain cultures/cytology, as well as perform celiac plexus block for pain.
- ERCP with biliary sphincterotomy is reserved for therapeutic interventions such as treatment of choledocholithiasis in biliary pancreatitis.

To establish the diagnosis of AP, the presence of two of the following three criteria should be met:[3]

1. Abdominal pain consistent with the disease
2. Serum amylase and/or lipase greater than three times the ULN
3. Characteristic findings on CECT or MRI

Management

There exists a variety of scoring systems, including Glasgow, Ranson, and APACHE II, to aid in determining the severity but are limited in their value. It is best to rely upon your own clinical assessment to determine the severity and direct patient management accordingly. Primary treatment goals include appropriate fluid resuscitation, antibiotic use when indicated, adequate nutritional support, and monitoring for, diagnosing, and treating any associated ductal disruption and necrosis. Patients with acute fulminant pancreatitis are commonly managed in the intensive care unit. Potential complications of pancreatitis are outlined in Table 2.34.

Initial management:[4–6] Hemodynamic status must quickly be determined and volume replacement initiated:

- Early aggressive IV hydration because of hypovolemia that occurs secondary to vomiting, reduced oral intake, third spacing of fluids, increased respiratory losses, and diaphoresis
- 250 to 500 mL per hour of isotonic crystalloid solution (lactated Ringer's as it provides both calcium and bicarbonate and is more pH balanced)

TABLE **2.34** Complications of Acute Pancreatitis

Local	Systemic
Enlargement of pancreas due to edema	Sepsis
Peripancreatic inflammation: linear strands in the peripancreatic fat	Acute lung injury
	Pleural effusions
Phlegmon	Ileus
Acute suppurative inflammation affecting the surrounding tissue	GI obstruction
	Acute renal failure
Necrosis	Multi organ system failure
Pseudocysts: liquefaction of necrotic pancreatic tissue	
Abscesses	
Hemorrhage	
Chronic pancreatitis	

GI, gastrointestinal.

- Routine use of antibiotics is not recommended, but is indicated in the presence of extrapancreatic infection and pancreatic necrosis

> **CLINICAL PEARL:** Early and adequate fluid resuscitation remains the cornerstone of initial acute pancreatitis management. Failure to administer appropriate fluids can be associated with pancreatic necrosis, prolonged hospital stays, and organ failure.[1]

Surgical indications:

- Presence of gallstones: Laparoscopic cholecystectomy with intraoperative cholangiography
- Pancreatic necrosis: Confirm by fine-needle aspirate, options include debridement via endoscopy, interventional radiology, or video-assisted retroperitoneal laparoscopy if not responsive to a 7 to 10 day course of antibiotics

REFERENCES

1. Wu BU, Banks PA. Clinical management of patients with acute pancreatitis. *Gastroenterology.* 2013;144:1272. doi:10.1053/j.gastro.2013.01.075
2. Working Group IAP/APA Acute Pancreatitis Guidelines. IAP/APA evidence-based guidelines for the management of acute pancreatitis. *Pancreatology.* 2013;13:e1 doi:10.1016/j.pan.2013.07.063
3. Tenner S, Baillie J, DeWitt J, et al. American College of Gastroenterology guideline: management of acute pancreatitis. *Am J Gastroenterol.* 2013;108:1400–1415. doi:10.1038/ajg.2013.218
4. de-Madaria E, Banks PA, Moya-Hoyo N, et al. Early factors associated with fluid sequestration and outcomes of patients with acute pancreatitis. *Clin Gastroenterol Hepatol.* 2014;12:997–1002. doi:10.1016/j.cgh.2013.10.017
5. Roberts KM, Conwell D. Acute pancreatitis: how soon should we feed patients? *Ann Intern Med.* 2017;166:903. doi:10.7326/M17-1123
6. Haydock MD, Mittal A, Wilms HR, et al. Fluid therapy in acute pancreatitis: anybody's guess. *Ann Surg.* 2013;257:182. doi:10.1097/SLA.0b013e31827773ff

PANCREATITIS: CHRONIC

Etiology

Chronic pancreatitis results from an ongoing inflammatory process in the pancreas that ultimately results in permanent damage to the gland. The end result is loss of both endocrine and exocrine function. Known causes of chronic pancreatitis are more likely related to alcohol use disorder, genetics, ductal obstruction/scarring, autoimmune, or systemic conditions.

Epidemiology

In the United States, alcohol has been found to account for approximately 45% of cases of chronic pancreatitis. It is the most common cause in men, and the least common cause in women. Cigarette smoking has also been associated with both acute and chronic pancreatitis.[1] In the younger patient population presenting in the first and second decades of life, hereditary causes are the most common. Hereditary causes of chronic pancreatitis carry greater risk of pancreatic adenocarcinoma.[2] Those cases of chronic pancreatitis that are not attributable to alcohol or hereditary causes are idiopathic.

Clinical Presentation

Chronic disease of the pancreas differs from the acute form in that the patient with chronic pancreatitis can be asymptomatic. Patients may present with the symptoms associated with pancreatic insufficiency, including a dull, achy, epigastric pain, nausea, vomiting, weight loss, steatorrhea, and glucose intolerance. These symptoms may not be apparent until over 90% of pancreatic function is lost.

Diagnosis

There is no specific lab test for chronic pancreatitis; however, hepatic panel, amylase test, and lipase test are commonly ordered and tend to be normal. Erythrocyte sedimentation rate (ESR), IgA, rheumatoid factor, ANA, antismooth muscle antibody may be abnormal in familial, autoimmune conditions. Fecal elastase is useful if steatorrhea is present.[3] Impaired glucose tolerance may be present. A secretin stimulation test is sensitive for exocrine deficiency. Diffuse calcifications across the midline, anterior to the L1 to L3 vertebral bodies, can be picked up on plain films of abdomen.

MRCP will show dilatation of the main pancreatic duct, with ectasia of the side branches. ERCP reveals classic findings of irregular dilatation of the pancreatic duct with or without strictures, intrapancreatic stones, cysts, and CBD strictures. Biopsy will confirm the presence of extensive fibrosis, chronic inflammation, obliteration of the ducts, and no acinar tissue.

Management

Multidisciplinary approach to treatment:

- Indicated to minimize the complications listed in Table 2.35
- Patient education to enhance behavior modifications: stop smoking, stop alcohol
- Pain control: Referral to a chronic pain center, celiac nerve block, radiotherapy[4]

TABLE **2.35** Complications Associated With Chronic Inflammation in the Pancreas

Local	Systemic
Fibrosis	Malnutrition
Fat necrosis	Hyperglycemia
Calcification	
Strictures in the main pancreatic duct	
Pseudocysts	
Chronic abdominal pain	
Splenic vein thrombosis	
Varices (gastric, esophageal)	
GI bleeding	
Carcinoma	

GI, gastrointestinal.

- Dietitian consult: General dietary recommendations include small meals with fluids, minimize fat intake
- Pancreatic enzyme supplements containing lipase, protease, amylase
- Control blood glucose levels
- Referral to psychologist for chronic disease management
- Surgery: Resection, islet cell transplant[5]

REFERENCES

1. Coté GA, Yadav D, Slivka A, et al. Alcohol and smoking as risk factors in an epidemiology study of patients with chronic pancreatitis. *Clin Gastroenterol Hepatol.* 2011;9:266. doi:10.1016/j.cgh.2010.10.015
2. Sossenheimer MJ, Aston CE, Preston RA, et al. Clinical characteristics of hereditary pancreatitis in a large family, based on high-risk haplotype. The Midwest Multicenter Pancreatic Study Group (MMPSG). *Am J Gastroenterol.* 1997;92:1113.
3. Keim V, Teich N, Moessner J. Clinical value of a new fecal elastase test for detection of chronic pancreatitis. *Clin Lab.* 2003;49:209.
4. Sutherland DE, Radosevich DM, Bellin MD, et al. Total pancreatectomy and islet autotransplantation for chronic pancreatitis. *J Am Coll Surg.* 2012;214:409. doi:10.1016/j.jamcollsurg.2011.12.040
5. Guarner L, Navalpotro B, Molero X, et al. Management of painful chronic pancreatitis with single-dose radiotherapy. *Am J Gastroenterol.* 2009;104:349. doi:10.1038/ajg.2008.128

PEPTIC ULCER DISEASE

Etiology

Peptic diseases refer to disorders of the upper GI tract related to the action of acid and pepsin or, in some instances, bacteria that exist within the GI tract. Ulcers are the erosions that can develop as a result in the gastric or duodenal mucosa, extending through the muscularis. The most common causes of PUD are Helicobacter pylori infection and the use of NSAIDs.[1] The extent of peptic disease ranges from undetectable mucosal injury to erythema, erosions, and ultimately ulcerations. Gastroduodenal mucosal injury results from the imbalance between mediators that damage mucosa and mediators known to protect it, as outlined in Table 2.36. Aspirin and NSAIDS can cause mucosal

TABLE 2.36 Factors Known to Influence Peptic Ulcer Disease

Aggravators	Protective Factors
Exogenous	Mucous
Ethanol	Bicarbonate
Aspirin	Phospholipid membrane surface of epithelial
NSAIDs	cell layers
Corticosteroids	Mucosal blood flow
Tobacco	Parietal cell secretion of bicarbonate
Endogenous	Epithelial regeneration
Acid	Prostaglandins
Pepsin	Epidermal growth factors
Bile acid	
Helicobacter pylori	

NSAIDs, nonsteroidal anti-inflammatory drugs.

injury from the esophagus through the duodenum by directly irritating the mucosa and inhibiting the protective prostaglandins.

> **CLINICAL PEARL:** Patients who are at an increased risk for NSAID GI toxicity include those with a history of previous ulcer, age >65 years, high-dose therapy, and concurrent use of aspirin, corticosteroids, or anticoagulants.

Epidemiology

H. pylori, a Gram-negative bacterium, is transmitted via fecal–oral route and is seen in 95% of duodenal ulcers and 70% of gastric ulcers. PUD has decreased over time; however, the incidence of gastritis and duodenitis is increasing.[1]

> **CLINICAL PEARL:** H. pylori infection increases the risk of NSAID-related GI complications. All patients with a history of ulcers who require NSAIDS should be tested for H. pylori, and if the infection is present, eradication therapy should be given.

Clinical Presentation

Patients can present to the office with signs and symptoms of acute ulcer disease, as well as complications associated with peptic ulcers. These include bleeding, perforation, gastric outlet obstruction, and gastric cancer. Common presenting complaints include epigastric pain and burning that may worsen on an empty stomach. The epigastric pain can radiate to the left upper abdomen, or to the back in the case of duodenal ulcerations. Associated symptoms may include nausea, vomiting that may be secondary to gastric outlet obstruction, anorexia, weight loss (mass), bleeding, hematemesis, coffee ground emesis, black tarry stools (melena), and anemia. Past medical history may be significant for drug use, alcohol use, smoking, previous ulcer, or family members with peptic diseases.

Physical examination can often be normal. On abdominal exam there may be epigastric, upper quadrant tenderness, or a palpable mass. Exam findings of guarding, rigidity, and quiet/absent bowel sounds can be suggestive of perforation. Rectal exam may be positive for black, tarry-colored stool, if bleeding is present. Because many of the signs and symptoms of disorders involving the GI tract can overlap, it is import that the history and physical examination be thorough enough to rule out other causes such as functional dyspepsia, gastritis, GERD, esophagitis, gastroenteritis, and cholelithiasis.

> **CLINICAL PEARL:** The severity of patient history or symptoms has not been proven to be associated with disease severity, functional causes, or organic disease.

Diagnosis

Blood work can include the following:

- CBC to identify any evidence of blood loss; microcytic, hypochromic red cell indices suggest iron loss
- Electrolytes to evaluate the possibility of a metabolic alkalosis secondary to loss of chloride ions from nausea and vomiting
- Depending upon the patient history and exam findings, amylase or lipase may be indicated to rule out a pancreatitis and a hepatic panel to rule out hepatitis or cholelithiasis
- Special studies: *H. pylori* testing in all patients with active PUD, history of PUD, dyspepsia, or gastric lymphoma; urea breath tests can be used for initial diagnosis, as well as follow-up 4 to 6 weeks after treatment is completed to confirm eradication of infection; stool studies for *H. pylori* can detect active infection, and serum gastrin levels will be elevated with gastrinoma (Zollinger Ellison) syndrome, antral G-cell hyperplasia, and gastric outlet obstruction
- Endoscopy affords the ability to confirm the diagnosis and treat abnormalities and obtain tissue for biopsy and cultures, including the presence of *H. pylori*.

> **CLINICAL PEARL:** Indications to perform an endoscopy include significant weight loss, nausea and repeated vomiting, evidence of bleeding, iron deficiency, progressive dysphagia, odynophagia and age >65 years.

Management

If PUD is suspected, consider a trial of empiric treatment for 2 weeks with PPI. If there is no improvement, consider endoscopy. Endoscopy is recommended in patients 55 years or older if symptoms persist despite trial of PPIs, or presence of alarm symptoms.

Eradication therapy for *H. Pylori*, depending upon patient allergy profile

- PPI (BID), clarithromycin (500 mg QD), and amoxicillin (1-g QD) or metronidazole (500 mg TID) for 14 days
- PPI (BID), bismuth (120–300 mg QID), tetracycline (500 mg QID), and metronidazole (250–500 mg QID) for 10 to 14 days is a recommended first-line treatment option
- PPI (BID), clarithromycin (500 mg QD), amoxicillin (1-g QD), and nitroimidazole (500 mg) for 10 to 14 days
- Patients should undergo testing to prove eradication 4 weeks after completing treatment and PPI with urea breath test, fecal antigen test, or biopsy

When prescribing anti-inflammatory agents:

- Consider either misoprostol at a dose of 800 mcg/d or proton pump inhibitors when prescribing NSAIDS to patients at risk for PUD
- Consider COX-2 inhibitors as opposed to NSAIDS in managing patients due to a lower incidence of gastric and duodenal ulcers when compared to traditional NSAIDS

Surgery: Secondary to the advancements in understanding the pathophysiology and treatments of ulcer disease, surgery is primarily indicated for management of ulcer complications: lesions that are refractory to treatment, bleeding, perforation, or obstruction.

REFERENCES

1. Fashner J, Gitu AC. Diagnosis and treatment of peptic ulcer disease and H. pylori Infection. *Am Fam Physician*. February 15, 2015;91(4):236–242.

ELECTRONIC RESOURCES

American College of Gastroenterology: Clinical Guidelines.

http://gi.org/clinical-guidelines/clinical-guidelines-sortable-list/

GENITOURINARY SYSTEM

BENIGN PROSTATIC HYPERPLASIA

Etiology

Benign prostatic hyperplasia (BPH) is an enlargement of the prostate gland due to a noncancerous cause, and it is generally seen in men over the age of 50 years. This condition occurs due to excessive proliferation of connective tissue, smooth muscle, and epithelium. The enlargement can lead to difficulty with urination due to obstruction of the urethra.

Epidemiology

Nearly all men, if they live long enough, will develop some degree of BPH. Not all patients will seek treatment for it. Symptomatic BPH affects approximately 15 million men in the United States, and the prevalence increases with age. Some sources suggest the prevalence is about 50% of men by age 50 years, and 80% to 90% among men 80 years of age or older.[1]

Risk factors for BPH:[1,2]

- Increasing age
- Genetic predisposition
- Obesity
- Sedentary lifestyle
- Metabolic syndrome
- Hispanic and Black race
- Smoking
- Diet high in meats and carbohydrates
- Excessive alcohol intake

Protective factors against BPH:[1,2]

- Increased physical activity
- Moderate or decreased alcohol intake
- Increased consumption of vegetables

Clinical Presentation

Symptoms associated with BPH include frequent urination, weak urine stream, nocturia, urine leakage/incontinence, difficulty initiating urine stream, straining to void, and incomplete bladder emptying. Ask about these symptoms and their onset, duration, and severity. The American Urological Association Symptom Index (AUASI) or the International Prostate Symptom Score (IPSS) are questionnaires that can be given to the patient to assess the severity of symptoms and their effect on the patient's life.

Be sure to ask additional questions to rule out urinary tract infection (fever, chills, dysuria), as well as review the patient's medication list to see if urinary difficulty may be a side effect of a current medication. An examination of the abdomen and assessing for bladder distention, as well as a neurologic assessment of the lower extremities is indicated. A digital rectal examination to assess prostate size, symmetry, and consistency can help confirm the diagnosis and can help screen for signs of malignancy.

Diagnosis

Often BPH can be diagnosed based on history and physical examination. The prostate-specific antigen (PSA) level may correlate with prostate size, but it is not required to diagnose BPH. A urinalysis should be ordered to rule out other causes of symptoms such as a urinary tract infection. Renal function (BUN/creatinine) should also be monitored in the setting of BPH to ensure there are no renal complications. If necessary, ultrasound can measure postvoid residual as well as the size and shape of the prostate gland.

Management

Treatment is guided by the severity of symptoms. For mild symptoms, observation and regular monitoring and surveillance are recommended. Supportive care includes reducing fluid intake in the evening to lessen symptoms of nocturia, reducing caffeine and alcohol, and avoiding antihistamines as they may lead to urinary retention. Men with moderate to severe symptoms without impaired renal function, urinary retention, or recurrent urinary infections may also elect observation. Medical and surgical options also exist for the treatment of BPH. Pharmacologic options are listed in Table 2.37.

TABLE 2.37 Pharmacologic Treatment of Benign Prostatic Hyperplasia

Drug Class	Drug Names	Adverse Effects	Comments
Nonselective alpha blockers	Doxazosin Terazosin	Orthostatic hypotension Avoid in older adults due to risk of orthostatic hypotension and syncope Risk of floppy iris syndrome; avoid if cataract surgery is planned	Cause smooth muscle cell relaxation in prostate and bladder; improves urinary flow Does not reduce prostate size May aid in hypertension treatment for patients with concurrent diseases Full effect in 2–4 weeks
Selective alpha blockers	Alfuzosin Silodosin Tamsulosin	Less dizziness and hypotension than nonselective alpha blockers Risk of floppy iris syndrome; avoid if cataract surgery is planned	Mechanism of action is similar, but affects receptors in urinary tract more selectively Does not reduce prostate size Full effect in 2–4 weeks
5-alpha reductase inhibitors	Dutasteride Finasteride	Decreased libido Erectile dysfunction	Reduces prostate size, slows progression of disease Can be combined with alpha-blockers Reduces PSA levels; consider this when using for cancer screening Full effect in 3–6 months
Anticholinergic agents	Oxybutynin Solifenacin Tolterodine	Dry mouth and eyes May worsen constipation and cognitive impairment—use with caution in older adults Increases risk of urinary retention; check postvoid residual before prescribing	Used as an addition to alpha-blockers when they are not effective Decreases bladder contractions Helpful with symptoms of frequency and urgency
Phosphodiesterase-5 enzyme inhibitor	Tadalafil	Headache Risk of priapism Do not coadminister with nitrates	Primary indication for erectile dysfunction; consider in men with concurrent disease Decreases prostatic hyperplasia Full effect in 4 weeks

Source: Pearson R, Williams PM. Common questions about the diagnosis and management of benign prostatic hyperplasia. *Am Fam Physician.* 2014;90:769–774B.

> **CLINICAL PEARL:** A urology consult is recommended for those patients with increasing PSA levels, urinary retention, concern for prostate cancer, inadequate response to treatment, or frequent UTIs.

Surgical management of BPH should be considered in patients with moderate to severe symptoms when a patient requests it, if medical treatment fails, or if there are complications of BPH such as recurrent urinary tract infections, renal insufficiency or renal failure, or refractory gross hematuria. Surgical options range from endoscopic transurethral procedures using loops, lasers, or microwaves to traditionally open surgical procedures. The determination of which procedure is most appropriate for a particular patient is best left to the urologist.

REFERENCES

1. Skinder D, Zacharia I, Studin J, et al. Benign prostatic hyperplasia: a clinical review. *JAAPA*. 2016;29:19–23. doi:10.1097/01.JAA.0000488689.58176.0a
2. Egan KB. The epidemiology of benign prostatic hyperplasia associated with lower urinary tract symptoms: prevalence and incident rates. *Urol Clin North Am*. 2016;43:289. doi:10.1016/j.ucl.2016.04.001

CYSTITIS: UNCOMPLICATED

Etiology

Uncomplicated cystitis is often referred to as a "bladder infection." Uncomplicated cystitis occurs in premenopausal, nonpregnant women who are healthy and who do not have any anomalies of the urinary tract.[1] Bacteria, generally fecal flora, enter the urinary tract at the urethra and travel upward into the bladder. The vast majority of cases of cystitis are caused by *E.coli*. Other common pathogens include *Klebsiella pneumoniae, Staphylococcus saprophyticus, Enterococcus faecalis*, and group B streptococcus.[2] Although generally uncomplicated in healthy women, cystitis can progress to pyelonephritis.

Epidemiology

Most women will have at least one episode of cystitis at some point in their lifetime. In the outpatient setting, more than eight million visits per year are due to cystitis. Risk factors for cystitis include recent sexual intercourse, use of spermicide, and a previous history of cystitis.

Clinical Presentation

Dysuria is the hallmark symptom of cystitis. Urinary frequency, urinary urgency, and suprapubic pain are often also present. Gross hematuria can occur. Fever, flank pain, nausea, and vaginal discharge are not typically seen with cystitis, and these symptoms suggest pyelonephritis or another more serious infection.

Be attentive to vital signs and date of last menstrual period, perform an abdominal exam, assess for costovertebral angle tenderness, and consider the need for a pelvic exam for women who present with cystitis symptoms.

> **CLINICAL PEARL:** Signs and symptoms of complicated cystitis include fever, flank pain, malaise, or other signs of systemic illness.

Diagnosis

The diagnosis of cystitis can be supported by an office dipstick urinalysis. Positive findings for leukocyte esterase and nitrites are the most accurate predictors of cystitis.[3] Interpretation of urine dipstick results is often difficult, or impossible, if the patient has taken a urinary analgesic (such as phenazopyridine) prior to giving the urine sample. A negative urine dipstick result does not necessarily rule out cystitis.

A urine culture and sensitivity can help confirm the diagnosis of cystitis when it is in question, and it should always be ordered if there is a concern for a complicated urinary tract infection. In cases of recurrent cystitis, a history of resistant pathogens, or in those patients who have taken antibiotics, a urine culture, is also recommended. It is not necessary to order a urine culture and sensitivity in obvious cases of cystitis in healthy women.[3]

> **CLINICAL PEARL:** The differential diagnosis for cystitis should include vaginitis and sexually transmitted infections.

Management

Antibiotics aid in the rapid resolution of uncomplicated cystitis. Although it is important to be aware of local resistance patterns, those patterns are most often based on complicated cystitis, and most cases of uncomplicated cystitis in the ambulatory care setting will respond to the general recommendations for empiric therapy. Empiric treatments are outlined in Table 2.38.

The Infectious Diseases Society of America (IDSA) recommends using the following criteria when choosing among first-line options: patient allergy,

TABLE 2.38 Empiric Treatments for Uncomplicated Cystitis in Women

Drug Name	Common Dose	Recommendation
Trimethoprim-sulfamethoxazole DS	160/800 mg BID × 3 days *Avoid if patient has taken it in the last 3 months for cystitis*	First-line option
Nitrofurantoin	100 mg BID × 5 days	First-line option
Fluoroquinolones	Ciprofloxacin 250 mg BID × 3 days Levofloxacin 250–500 mg QD × 3 days	Second-line option
Beta-lactams	Amoxicillin-clavulanate, cefdinir, cefaclor treat for 3–7 days	Second-line option

Sources: Gupta K, Hooton TM, Naber KG, et al. International clinical practice guidelines for the treatment of acute uncomplicated cystitis and pyelonephritis in women: A 2010 update by the Infectious Diseases Society of America and the European Society for Microbiology and Infectious Diseases. *Clin Infect Dis.* 2011;52:e103–e120. doi:10.1093/cid/ciq257; Hooton TM. Uncomplicated urinary tract infection. *N Eng J Med.* 2012;366:1028–1037. doi:10.1056/NEJMcp1104429

compliance history, availability, cost, local practice patterns, local community resistance. Fluoroquinolones, although commonly used, should be avoided as first-line therapy as they are frequently not necessary and contribute to overall antimicrobial resistance.[2] Additionally, the U.S. Food and Drug Administration (FDA) has recently strengthened its black box warning for fluoroquinolones, making these agents less desirable options. Due to lack of efficacy and high levels of resistance, amoxicillin is not recommended by the IDSA for empiric therapy.[2]

When treated appropriately, cystitis responds rapidly to antibiotics, with some patients experiencing relief of symptoms in as little as a few hours, but most commonly within 24 to 48 hours. OTC urinary analgesics such as phenazopyridine can be used to mitigate irritative voiding symptoms. This treatment should not be needed or used for longer than 2 to 3 days. If symptoms are persisting beyond that time frame, the patient should be reassessed. Routine urine cultures after treatment are not recommended if a patient is nonpregnant, symptoms resolve with treatment, and do not recur within 2 weeks.[3]

> **CLINICAL PEARL:** Although it has been widely recommended, postcoital urination does not seem to reduce the incidence of cystitis.

REFERENCES

1. Grigoryan L, Trautner BW, Gupta K. Diagnosis and management of urinary tract infections in the outpatient setting: a review. *JAMA*. 2014;312:1677–1684. doi:10.1001/jama.2014.12842
2. Gupta K, Hooton TM, Naber KG, et al. International clinical practice guidelines for the treatment of acute uncomplicated cystitis and pyelonephritis in women: a 2010 update by the Infectious Diseases Society of America and the European Society for Microbiology and Infectious Diseases. *Clin Infect Dis*. 2011;52:e103–e120. doi:10.1093/cid/ciq257
3. Hooton TM. Uncomplicated urinary tract infection. *N Eng J Med*. 2012;366:1028–1037. doi:10.1056/NEJMcp1104429

PROSTATITIS: ACUTE BACTERIAL

Etiology

Prostatitis is an infection or inflammation of the prostate gland. Prostatitis can be classified as acute bacterial, chronic bacterial, chronic prostatitis/pelvic pain syndrome, or asymptomatic.[1] *E. coli* is the most commonly isolated pathogen in acute bacterial prostatitis, but other Gram-negative bacteria such as *P. aeruginosa, Klebsiella*, and *Enterobacter* are also potential pathogens.[2] *N. gonorrhoeae* and *Chlamydia trachomatis* should be considered in young sexually active men or in any man who participates in high-risk sexual behaviors.[2]

Epidemiology

The incidence of acute bacterial prostatitis is highest in men between the ages of 20 and 40 years and in men older than 70 years of age.[2]

Clinical Presentation

Pelvic and/or perineal pain, urinary urgency, urinary frequency, and dysuria are all common symptoms of acute bacterial prostatitis. Patients may also experience urinary hesitancy, weak urine stream, and hematospermia. Patients may also have fever, chills, nausea, and malaise. Although these are not uncommon with prostatitis, they also can indicate a progression to sepsis and should be considered in the diagnostic evaluation.

Physical examination should include attention to vital signs, an abdominal exam, palpation of bladder to ensure it is not distended suggesting urinary retention, and assessment of costovertebral angle tenderness. A genital exam and gentle examination of the prostate is indicated. Prostatic massage should be avoided as it can result in bacteremia. On examination, the prostate will be tender and boggy.

Diagnosis

Although the diagnosis is often made through history and physical examination, additional testing is recommended. Pyuria will be noted on urinalysis. A urine culture should also be ordered. If acute bacterial prostatitis is suspected, empiric antibiotics should be prescribed at the time of the visit without waiting for the results of the urine culture.

.Other tests to consider based on the patient's presentation include a CBC with differential, electrolytes, and renal function. Blood cultures should be considered in febrile patients. Testing for sexually transmitted infections should be considered if risk factors exist. Generally, imaging is not helpful unless there is no or poor response to therapy.[2] In these cases, a transrectal ultrasound should be considered to rule out an abscess of the prostate.[2]

Management

Patients who have severe symptoms of illness, are not able to tolerate oral medications, have urinary retention, are at risk for antibiotic resistance, or are potentially septic should be admitted to the hospital for treatment.[2] Most patients with acute bacterial prostatitis can be managed as an outpatient. Empiric antibiotics should be prescribed initially, and later modified pending culture results. Consider the risk of *N. gonorrhoeae* and *C. trachomatis* and treat accordingly if these pathogens are suspected. Patients who are still febrile or who are not improving after 36 hours of treatment should be reassessed. Consideration should be given to abscess formation, septicemia, or inadequate pharmacologic treatment in these patients.

Recommendations for duration of antibiotic therapy range from 2 to 6 weeks, depending on the severity of symptoms, with 4 weeks being the most common. There is a concern for progression to chronic prostatitis with a shorter duration of treatment. A repeat urine culture is recommended 1 week after antibiotics have been completed to ensure resolution. Table 2.39 outlines recommended pharmacologic treatment for acute bacterial prostatitis. Patients should be encouraged to increase fluid intake and to take medication to control fever and pain.

TABLE 2.39 Outpatient Pharmacologic Management of Acute Bacterial Prostatitis

Drug Name	Common Dose	Comments
Ciprofloxacin	500 mg twice daily	Review FDA box warning
Levofloxacin	500–750 mg once daily	Review FDA box warning
Trimethoprim-sulfamethoxazole DS	160/800 mg twice daily	Check local resistance patterns

FDA, Food and Drug Administration.
Sources: Sharp VJ, Takacs EB, Powell CR. Prostatitis: diagnosis and treatment. *Am Fam Physician.* 2010;82:397–406; Coker TJ, Dierfeldt DM. Acute bacterial prostatitis: diagnosis and management. *Am Fam Physician.* 2016;93:114–120.

REFERENCES

1. Sharp VJ, Takacs EB, Powell CR. Prostatitis: diagnosis and treatment. *Am Fam Physician.* 2010;82:397–406.
2. Coker TJ, Dierfeldt DM. Acute bacterial prostatitis: diagnosis and management. *Am Fam Physician.* 2016;93:114–120.

PYELONEPHRITIS

Etiology

Pyelonephritis is an infection and inflammation of the kidney, most often due to an ascending urinary tract infection. *E. coli* is the most common pathogen, with estimates ranging from 80% to 90% of cases.[1,2] Other pathogens include those common to urinary infections, such as Enterobacteriaceae and enterococci.[1] It is often considered to be a complicated urinary tract infection.

Epidemiology

This condition is most common among young women, but it is also seen in infants and the elderly. It is less common in men and children. Although most patients can be treated as an outpatient, patients with pyelonephritis often require admission to the hospital for treatment.

Clinical Presentation

Fever and flank pain are the hallmark symptoms. Systemic symptoms such as malaise and nausea are common. Most, but not all, patients will also report irritative voiding symptoms such as dysuria and urinary frequency.

On examination, the presence of costovertebral angle tenderness is notable. A full abdominal, pulmonary, and cardiac examination should also be done. The patient may have suprapubic tenderness. Be attentive to abnormal vital signs. In women, a pelvic exam is recommended to rule out other causes of pain and fever such as pelvic inflammatory disease.

Diagnosis

The differential diagnosis of acute pyelonephritis includes appendicitis, cholecystitis, diverticulitis, nephrolithiasis, pancreatitis, pelvic inflammatory disease, or renovascular occlusion. In men, acute bacterial prostatitis should be considered.

A urinalysis will often show pyuria and leukocyte esterase. A positive urine culture confirms the diagnosis. Additional laboratory testing to consider includes a CBC with differential, electrolytes, renal function, hepatic panel, and blood cultures. These tests can assess for complications of pyelonephritis and help rule out other causes of flank pain and fever.

Imaging, in the form of ultrasound or CT scan, should be considered in patients with severe illness, who may have a renal stone, who are immunocompromised, or there is suspicion of abnormal anatomy or abscess formation.[1]

CLINICAL PEARL: Acute pyelonephritis can progress to bacteremia and sepsis. Be alert to signs and symptoms of these complications.

Management

The initiation of antibiotics, as seen in Table 2.40, should be done immediately and not delayed for urine culture results.

CLINICAL PEARL: Consider a one-time IV dose of a fluoroquinolone or ceftriaxone before starting oral therapy as an outpatient.

Patients who are generally healthy, hemodynamically stable, able to take oral medications, able to maintain hydration, and able to comply with followup can be treated as an outpatient. Supportive measures such as hydration and control of pain and fever are also indicated. Patients who do not improve in 24 to 48 hours should be reassessed to ensure the choice of antibiotic is appropriate and that they are free from complications such as bacteremia and renal abscess.

Inpatient management should be considered for those patients who have comorbidities or immunosuppression, cannot take oral medications, have abnormal electrolytes, concern for obstruction or abscess, have high fevers, or who are potentially septic.

TABLE 2.40 Outpatient Pharmacologic Treatment for Acute Pyelonephritis

Drug Name	Common Dose	Comments
Ciprofloxacin	500 mg twice daily × 7 days	Review FDA box warning
Levofloxacin	750 mg once daily × 7 days	Review FDA box warning
Trimethoprim-sulfamethoxazole DS	160/800 mg twice daily × 14 days	Check local resistance patterns

FDA, Food and Drug Administration.

Source: Gupta K, Hooton TM, Naber KG, et al. International clinical practice guidelines for the treatment of acute uncomplicated cystitis and pyelonephritis in women: A 2010 update by the Infectious Diseases Society of America and the European Society for Microbiology and Infectious Diseases. *Clin Infect Dis. 2011;*52:e103–e120. doi:10.1093/cid/ciq257

> **CLINICAL PEARL:** Emphasematous pyelonephritis is a severe, necrotizing infection of the kidney that should not be missed. It is more common in older people, particularly those who have diabetes.

REFERENCES

1. Colgan R, Williams M, Johnson JR. Diagnosis and treatment of acute pyelonephritis in women. *Am Fam Physician*. 2011;84:519–526.
2. Johnson JR, Russo TA. Acute pyelonephritis in adults. *N Eng J Med*. 2018;378:48–59. doi:10.1056/NEJMcp1702758

HEMATOLOGIC SYSTEM

ANEMIA

Etiology

Anemia is a deficiency in RBCs. This deficiency can result from defects in production as seen with aplastic anemia, destruction of cells, or acute/chronic blood loss. Etiologies are outlined in Tables 2.41 through 2.43. The hematopoietic system is highly susceptible to the influence of external factors due to its high rate of proliferation. Blood dyscrasias can be primary, when the disorder is intrinsic to the blood system, or secondary, due to an underlying systemic process such as chronic inflammation, rheumatologic disorder, infection, or malignancy. RBCs have a direct relationship with cardiac function, cognitive ability, exercise capacity, and quality of life. Disorders in these cells will result in signs and symptoms representing each of these organ systems, as well as the patient's morbidity and mortality.

TABLE 2.41 Anemia: Etiologies of Decreased Production of Red Blood Cells

Acquired	Inherited
1. Iron deficiency	1. Fanconi anemia
2. Folate deficiency	2. Shwachman–Diamond syndrome
3. B12 deficiency	3. Dyskeratosis congenita
4. Malignancy (leukemia, lymphoma, multiple myeloma)	4. Diamond–Blackfan anemia
5. Radiation, chemotherapy	5. Amegakaryocytic thrombocytopenia
6. Viral infections (hepatitis, EBV)	
7. Drugs	
8. Autoimmune disorders (lupus)	
9. Pregnancy	

EBV, Epstein–Barr virus.

TABLE 2.42 Anemia: Etiologies of Red Blood Cell Destruction

Acquired	Inherited
1. Immune hemolytic anemia (autoimmune, alloimmune antibodies, drugs [penicillin, acetaminophen, antimalaria medicines, levodopa])	1. Sickle cell anemia
	2. Thalassemia
2. Physical damage to RBCs (prosthetic valves, severe burns, preeclampsia)	3. Hereditary spherocytosis
	4. Hereditary elliptocytosis
3. Paroxysmal nocturnal hemoglobinuria	5. G6PD deficiency
4. Infection (malaria, tick-borne diseases)	6. Pyruvate kinase deficiency

G6PD, glucose-6-phosphate dehydrogenase; RBCs, red blood cells.

TABLE 2.43 Anemia: Etiologies of Blood Loss

Chronic	Acute
1. Heavy menstrual bleeding	1. Injuries
2. Heavy, frequent epistaxis	2. Childbirth
3. GI/GU bleeding	3. Ruptured blood vessel
4. Ulcers	4. Surgery
5. Malignancies (digestive tract, kidney, and bladder)	

GI/GU, gastrointestinal/genitourinary.

Epidemiology

Anemia is the most prevalent hematologic abnormality. Anemia of chronic disease is the most common red cell disorder seen in practice. Disorders of the RBCs can be acquired or inherited. You should approach anemia as a sign of an underlying disease. Anemia affects approximately 5.6% of the U.S. population. Anemia rates in men increase with age, whereas in women, anemia has a bimodal distribution affecting the 40- to 49-year-old and the 80- to 85-year-old age groups. The diagnosis of anemia is 6.4 times higher in Black women compared to the population average. Prevalence has almost doubled over the past decade.[1]

Clinical Presentation

- Depending upon the cause of anemia, patient symptoms will vary. Generally, patients will complain of fatigue, lightheadedness, shortness of breath, chest pain, and palpitations with exertion. They may experience headaches, cool hands and feet, greater susceptibility to infections, or restless leg syndrome. Complaints of diarrhea, nausea, weight loss, hematochezia, dark tarry stools, and upper abdominal pain can be seen with a GI cause. Left upper quadrant pain, jaundice, and dark urine can occur with hemolysis.
- The patient's overall appearance and nutritional status should be assessed. Vital signs may reveal tachycardia, tachypnea, hypotension, and orthostatic changes. Skin, nails, amd mucous membranes findings can include pallor, purpura, petechiae, telangiectasias, jaundice, glossitis, chelitis, amd brittle and spoon nails. Lymphadenopathy may be present with systemic infections or malignancy. Cardiac exam findings include tachycardia, irregular

rhythms, S_3 gallop, and a murmur. Positive findings on abdominal exam include tenderness, mass, or hepatosplenomegaly. Stool may be dark and heme positive, with the presence of blood on rectal exam. Tenderness over the sternum may be present. Abnormal neurological findings include sensory deficits such as stocking glove distribution, decreased vibratory sensation, muscle weakness, and/or an unsteady gait.

- Craving for nonfood substances, such as ice and dirt (pica), is present in some patients who are iron deficient.
- Swelling or soreness of the tongue is associated with vitamin B12 deficiency. They may describe a diet low in nutrients, iron rich foods, or a vegan diet.
- Pertinent past medical history:
  ○ Medications or supplements may be a cause of anemia. PPIs, metformin, and dilantin can be associated with B12 deficiency.
  ○ Exposure to certain chemicals, toxins such as pesticides, arsenic, or benzene that is toxic to the marrow.
  ○ Past medical history of gastric bypass, chronic illness, infections, inflammatory bowel diseases, celiac disease, Addison's disease, type 1 diabetes, Graves' disease, and vitiligo have also been associated with anemia. Family history of anemias, malignancies, and Northern European, Mediterranean, and African descent are important for genetic causes. G6PD deficiency is most common in men of African or Mediterranean descent (Thalassemias–Mediterranean descent).

Diagnosis

The blood work required may be extensive when working up a patient that is suspected of having a hematological disorder. There are several studies that are considered routine when working up the patient:

- CBC with differential and platelets to confirm the suspicion of anemia
- The peripheral smear is critical to determine the size, shape and physical characteristics of the cells, or fragmented cells. This test often provides the diagnosis and/or strategy for additional work-up
  ○ Heinz bodies on the smear support hemolysis (G6PD, SS): basophilic stippling is seen with beta-thalassemia
- Red cell indices can help with the differential diagnosis of anemia.
  ○ Mean corpuscular volume (MCV) reveals the size of the cells (micro- and macrocytosis) and mean corpuscular hemoglobin concentration (MCHC) details the chromicity of the red cells (hyper- and hypochromic), which allows for a quantitative measure of intracellular hemoglobin. Low indices are reflective of such conditions as iron deficiency and hereditary blood disorders, whereas high indices may be reflective of such disorders as hypothyroidism, or liver disease, and vitamin deficiencies (B12; folate).
  ○ Red cell distribution width (RDW) reflects the variety of sizes (volumes) of red cells values. It is helpful in diagnosing the cause of microcytosis and can be the earliest sign of iron deficiency. RDW values are increased in alcohol use disorder, iron, B12, folate deficiency, hemolysis, and post-transfusions. The RDW is normal with thalassemia, anemia of chronic disease, and acute blood loss.

- ○ The reticulocyte count measures the marrow response to anemia. Counts below 1% indicate a hypoproliferative marrow failure. Counts >4% are indicative of a hyperproliferative marrow that is hyperfunctioning and can be seen in conditions such as RBC destruction and acute blood loss. Reticulocytosis occurs within 3 to 4 days of initiating treatment.
- ○ Haptoglobin levels are low with hemolysis.
- Coombs' test identifies presence of antibodies directed against cells
- Labs confirming an iron deficiency (iron panel): Serum iron low, total iron binding capacity (TIBC) increased, unsaturated iron binding capacity (UIBC) increased, transferrin increased, and serum ferritin low
- B12 levels can be low in a macrocytic anemia: homocysteine and methylmalonic acid levels are elevated in pernicious anemia and there is a B12 deficiency
- Folate levels are low with a macrocytic anemia
- Hemoglobin electrophoresis: Identifies abnormal hemoglobin seen in SSA and thalassemias
- Pyruvate kinase: The absence of this kinase makes the red blood cell prone to hemolysis
- Hepatic panel: Elevated indirect bilirubin is seen with hemolysis
- Special testing for paroxysmal nocturnal hemoglobinuria (PNH) includes osmotic fragility of RBC and G6PD enzyme. When G6PD enzyme is deficient, hemolysis can occur
- Thyroid studies: Elevated TSH, low circulating T3 and T4 may cause anemia

Additional laboratory evaluation can reveal the cause of anemia, as outlined in Figure 2.9.

Additional investigations to consider include bone marrow aspirate, biopsy, cultures, iron stores, abnormal cells, blasts, and viruses to determine a cause. Endoscopy, colonoscopy, and capsule endoscopy may be indicated to identify the source of any GI blood loss when indicated.

Management

Routine therapy for the common causes of anemia is outlined in Table 2.44.

The main goals in treating any anemia include the following:

- Identify the underlying cause and manage accordingly
- Increase RBC count to improve the oxygen-carrying capacity
- Relieve the patient's symptoms and improve quality of life

Treatment options:

- Dietary changes and supplements include iron, cyanocobalamin, and folic acid
- Transfusions, plasmapheresis, IV gammaglobulin, and steroids may be indicated in immune-mediated hemolysis
- Medical therapy such as hydroxyurea in sickle cell anemia
- Surgery: Splenectomy, transplant if medical therapy has failed

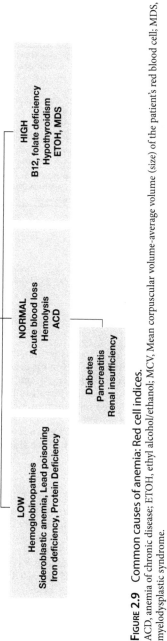

Figure 2.9 Common causes of anemia: Red cell indices.

ACD, anemia of chronic disease; ETOH, ethyl alcohol/ethanol; MCV, Mean corpuscular volume-average volume (size) of the patient's red blood cell; MDS, myelodysplastic syndrome.

TABLE 2.44 Treatment of Common Causes of Anemia

Condition	Iron Deficiency	B12 Deficiency	Folic Acid Deficiency
Medications	Ferrous sulfate 325 mg daily increased to three times daily × 3 months Take on an empty stomach, Vitamin C increases absorption	1,000 mcg sq weekly until normalized then 1,000 mcg sq every month *PO and sq equally effective	Folic acid 1–5 mg PO daily
Follow-up	Check reticulocyte count 7–10 days CBC 6–8 weeks	Check reticulocyte count 7–10 days CBC 6–8 weeks	Check reticulocyte count 7–10 days CBC 6–8 weeks
		Hypersegmented neutrophils disappear ≈ two week	Hypersegmented neutrophils disappear ≈ two week

CBC, complete blood count; PO, by mouth; sq, subcutaneously.

REFERENCES

1. Le CHH. The prevalence of anemia and moderate-severe anemia in the US population (NHANES 2003–2012). *PLOS ONE*. 2016;11(11):e0166635. doi:10.1371/journal.pone.0166635

FACTOR V LEIDEN MUTATION

Etiology

Activated protein C (APC) resistance is an inherited hypercoagulable state associated with thrombus formation within the central nervous system, coronary arteries, and deep veins of the lower extremities. APC impairs coagulation by degrading Factor Va. Patients resistant to the activity of APC have a mutation in the FV gene located on chromosome 1. This mutation renders FV protein resistant to degradation by APC. This defect results in the prolonged thrombogenic effects of factor V. Evidence to date is not clear whether homozygosity for factor V Leiden mutation is a risk factor for arterial thromboembolism.

Epidemiology

Factor V Leiden mutation occurs in 1 out of 17 individuals and is the most common inherited hypercoagulable state. This mutation is common among White populations of northern European ancestry. Family history can be positive for thrombotic events occurring before the age of 40 years; however, most events occur in carriers older than age 50 to 55 years. Homozygous carriers have an eightyfold greater risk of thrombosis.[1] Patients who are diagnosed with venous thrombosis have a 1.41-fold increased risk of recurrence, as well as an increased risk of fetal loss.[2] Factor V Leiden is the most common known genetic risk factor for venous thromboembolism.

Clinical Presentation

This condition must be considered in young patients who present with symptoms associated with, or a previous diagnosis, of a pulmonary embolism or deep venous thrombosis. These symptoms include shortness of breath, chest pain, and unilateral extremity edema. The factor V mutation does not appear to be associated with acute MI, CAD, or stroke. Patients may give a history of recurrent thrombosis without a defined precipitating event. The clots develop in uncommon sites, such as the arms, neck, and abdomen. Resistance to anticoagulation is also a feature of this disorder. Medications such as hormonal supplementation with estrogens will compound the risk of thrombosis in patients who have the factor V mutation.

Physical examination can be normal. The patient may be anxious, tachypneic, hypoxemic, or tachycardic. There may be unilateral extremity edema and calf/thigh tenderness suggestive of deep venous thrombosis.

Diagnosis

Laboratory studies include a D-dimer and/or a hypercoagulable workup to support the diagnosis of thrombus formation. The D-dimer levels are elevated in the presence of a clot. APC resistance assay may be abnormal. Genetic testing is done to identify the presence of the factor V Leiden (F5) R506Q mutation and to determine if the patient is hetero- or homozygous for the mutation.

Management

The approach is dependent upon whether the patient is symptomatic. Statistical evidence is insufficient to support prophylactic therapy if the patient is asymptomatic. Treatment of thrombosis includes warfarin, Low-molecular-weight heparin (LMWH), or newer agents used in treatment of thrombosis, such as direct thrombin inhibitors and factor Xa inhibitors.

General therapy for patients with thromboembolic risks:

- Avoid long periods of sitting (>2 hours), prolonged bed rest
- Avoid hormonal contraceptives, estrogen replacement therapy, smoking
- Notify providers of risk factors
- Maintain healthy weight

REFERENCES

1. Rosendaal FR, Koster T, Vandenbroucke JP, Reitsma PH. High risk of thrombosis in patients homozygous for factor V Leiden (activated protein C resistance). *Blood.* 1995;85(6):1504–1508.
2. vanDunné FM, Doggen CJM, Heemskerk M, et al. Factor V Leiden mutation in relation to fecundity and miscarriage in w omen with venous thrombosis. *Hum Reprod.* March 2005;20(3):802–806. doi:10.1093/humrep/deh640

LEUKEMIA

Etiology

Leukemia is a result of the uncontrolled clonal proliferation of hematopoietic stem cells within the bone marrow. In the primary care setting, the four most common subtypes seen are chronic lymphocytic (CLL), chronic myelogenous (CML), acute myelogenous (AML), and acute lymphoblastic (ALL).

Epidemiology

In 2018, it is estimated that there will be 60,300 new cases of leukemia, comprising 3.5% of all new cancers. Estimated deaths from leukemia are 24,370, 4% of all cancer deaths nationwide. Approximately 1.5% of men and women will be diagnosed with leukemia at some point during their lifetime. Rates for new leukemia cases have been rising on average 0.3% each year over the last 10 years, while death rates have been falling an average 1.5% each year over 2006 to 2015. The current 5-year relative survival rate is approximately 65%.[1,2]

The ALL cases are most often seen in the pediatric population, whereas CLL, CML, and AML are more commonly diagnosed in the adult population. AML is the most common subtype, comprising 80% of patients. Any patient that is suspected of having one of these blood disorders should be referred to the hematology oncology specialist. There are a number of known risk factors associated with the development of leukemia, which are outlined in Table 2.45.

Clinical Presentation

Between 20% and 50% of patients with CLL and CML remain asymptomatic. The diagnosis is often made incidentally on blood work that is obtained for some other reason. Constitutional symptoms are uncommon with the chronic leukemias, as only 15% to 30% with CLL will present with these symptoms.[3] Leukemia can affect all cell lines, and the patient's presentation may reflect abnormalities in red cells (oxygen carrying capacity) and platelets (control bleeding). Patients with leukemia may present with fevers, easy bruising, spontaneous bleeding episodes, epistaxis, fatigue, frequent infections, or night sweats. They may have a history of herpes zoster infection. Patients may find a painless enlarged lymph node. They may report shortness of breath, chest pain, and a decreased exercise tolerance. GI symptoms include anorexia, weight loss, upper abdominal pain, or discomfort. There may be a history of heavy bleeding with menses. Bone pain (back and long bones) may also be present. Central nervous system complaints can include headaches and mental status changes secondary to leukostasis.

Physical exam may reveal fever, tachycardia, and tachypnea with secondary infections. Pallor, ecchymosis, and petechiae can be found on skin exam with low red cell and platelet counts. Examination of the eyes will show conjunctival pallor. Diffuse lymphadenopathy may be present. Heart and lung exams are often normal. Hepatosplenomegaly (splenomegaly is found more often with CML) may be found on abdominal exam.

TABLE 2.45 Leukemia: Risk Factors for Leukemia

Genetic	Drugs, Toxins	Patient Characteristics
Down syndrome	Ionizing radiation	Obesity
Neurofibromatosis	Benzene (paint, plastic, petroleum, coal)	History of leukemia
Fanconi's anemia	Pesticides	Viral infections
	Chemotherapeutic agents	

CLINICAL PEARL: CLL should be suspected in older adults with a markedly elevated white blood cell count and an enlarged liver or spleen.

Diagnosis

The type of leukemia is determined by identifying the specific subsets utilizing special histochemical staining and immunophenotyping of the cells. Histochemical staining can identify the unique cytoplasmic or nuclear components of the abnormal cells, differentiating the type of leukemia. Immunophenotyping will detect the presence of specific cell membrane components that can further distinguish between the different types.

Blood work is critical in confirming the final diagnosis:

- A CBC can show marked leukocytosis >100,000 cells per μL, wihich is more common with the chronic leukemias, whereas the WBC counts with acute leukemias are often lower, approximately 20,000 cells per microliter. Platelet and RBC counts may be low. Nucleated RBCs can be present in the circulation, which is abnormal. Basophilia and eosinophilia can be seen with CML. Platelet counts can reach 1 million per cubic milliliter with CML.
- Abnormalities in the chemistry panel with electrolytes, uric acid, LDH, creatinine, BUN, potassium, phosphate, and calcium can help to determine the severity and burden of the disease.
- Hepatic panel may reveal a transaminitis and hyperbilirubinemia. Leukocyte alkaline phosphatase score will be low.
- Screening for disseminated intravascular coagulation with PT/PTT and fibrinogen should be obtained.
- Peripheral blood smear will show the morphology of the abnormal cells, presence of circulating >20% blast cells. The presence of Auer rods in the cytoplasm of myeloblasts support the diagnosis of AML. Greater than 50% of normal appearing lymphocytes on the smear is suspicious for CLL. Hypogammaglobulinemia can be seen in CLL.
- Special staining: Leukemias that do not express myeloperoxidase are M0 AML, M7 AML, and ALL.
- Bone marrow aspirate and biopsy with >30% blasts are consistent with acute leukemias. Chronic leukemias have <30% blasts in the marrow and more differentiation in the peripheral smear.
- Immunophenotyping by flow cytometry sorts and counts cells from blood or bone marrow by specific cell surface markers and is used to confirm an AML versus ALL. B cell counts of >5.0 × 10^9/L support a diagnosis of CLL.
- Cytogenetics examine the chromosomes to identify abnormalities specific to certain leukemia subtypes. For example, BCR-ABL1 fusion gene (Philadelphia chromosome) is seen in 95% of patients who have CML, and 20% of adults with ALL. MYC gene rearrangements are seen in Burkitt leukemia.
- Molecular testing looks for specific mutations at the DNA level.

Management

- Referral: To hematologist-oncologist
- Treatment options: Chemotherapy, radiation, monoclonal antibodies, and hematopoietic stem cell transplantation
- Tyrosine kinase inhibitors are specific for CML. They target the enzyme tyrosine kinase, responsible for the proliferation of these abnormal cells
- Primary care providers who are responsible for the management of patients who are in remission should monitor blood counts for otherwise unexplained leukocytosis, anemias, thrombocytopenias/cytosis. Be aware of physical exam findings of hepatomegaly, splenomegaly or lymphadenopathy, and unexplained symptoms of fever, fatigue, weight loss, and recurrent infections

CLINICAL PEARL: There is no standard staging system for leukemia. The disease is described as untreated, in remission, or recurrent.

Prognosis is dependent upon:

- Patient age
- Central nervous system involvement
- Genetic aberrancy, including the Philadelphia chromosome
- Whether the cancer has been treated before or has recurred

CLINICAL PEARL: Patients that are treated for leukemia are at an increased risk of developing a second malignancy.

REFERENCES

1. National Cancer Institute. SEER cancer statistics review 2006–2010. https://seer.cancer.gov/statfacts/html/leuks.html. Accessed June 9, 2018.
2. Noone AM, Howlader N, Krapcho M, et al. *SEER cancer statistics review, 1975–2015.* Bethesda, MD: National Cancer Institute. https://seer.cancer.gov/csr/1975_2015/, based on November 2017 SEER data submission, posted to the SEER web site, April 2018.
3. Yee KW, O'Brien SM. Chronic lymphocytic leukemia: diagnosis and treatment. *Mayo Clin Proc.* 81(8):1105–1129. doi:10.4065/81.8.1105; 2006

ELECTRONIC RESOURCES

Children's Oncology Group. Long-Term Follow-up Guidelines for Survivors of Childhood, Adolescent, and Young Adult Cancers.

http://www.survivorshipguidelines.org/

LYMPHADENOPATHY

Etiology

Lymphadenopathy is defined as a palpable lymph node larger than 1 cm. Lymph nodes in the supraclavicular, popliteal, iliac, and epitrochlear regions >5 mm in size are abnormal. Lymph nodes that are >3 cm are suggestive

TABLE 2.46 Important Causes of Lymphadenopathy: "MIAMI"

	Symptoms	Conditions
Malignancy	Fever, drenching night sweats, unexplained weight loss >10% of body weight	Kaposi sarcoma, leukemias, lymphomas, metastases, skin neoplasms
Infection	Fever, chills, fatigue, malaise	
Autoimmune	Skin rash, muscle weakness, arthralgias	Dermatomyositis, rheumatoid arthritis, Sjögren syndrome, Still disease, lupus erythematosus
Miscellaneous and unusual conditions		Histiocytosis, hyperthyroidism Kawasaki disease, sarcoidosis
Iatrogenic	Medications Serum sickness	Allopurinol, atenolol, captopril, carbamazepine, penicillins, dilantin, trimethoprim/sulfamethoxazole,

Sources: Bazemore AW, Smucker DR. Lymphadenopathy and malignancy. *Am Fam Physician. 2002;*6(11):2103–2110; Gaddey, H. I., and Riegel, A. M. (2016). Unexplained lymphadenopathy: Evaluation and differential diagnosis. *Am Fam Physician. 2016;*94(11):896–903.[1,2]

of neoplasia. Common conditions associated with lymphadenopathy can be grouped into five categories that are listed in Table 2.46.

Epidemiology

The incidence of malignant lymphadenopathy in primary care is <1%. Generalized adenopathy, the enlargement of two or more noncontiguous nodal groups, is most likely associated with systemic infections, autoimmune diseases, or malignancy and should be pursued with further testing. Most often the presence of lymphadenopathy represents a benign, self-limited condition. Children and young adults are most susceptible to reactive, hyperplastic lymph nodes.[3] Risk factors that are associated with malignant causes of lymphadenopathy include the older patient, nodal enlargement lasting longer than two weeks, and nodes that are located in the supraclavicular region.

Clinical Presentation

Patient age is important in determining the cause of adenopathy. Increased age (>40 years) carries greater concern for an underlying malignancy.[2] Consider the duration of lymphadenopathy. If present<2 weeks or >12 months *without any change,* malignancy is less likely. If present for more than 4 to 6 weeks, there is a greater suspicion for malignancy. The constellation of fevers, night sweats, weight loss, and finding of hepatosplenomegaly suggests lymphoma. Generalized adenopathy is more likely to be associated with infection, malignancy, or hypersensitivity. A history positive for recent infections, exposures (travel, animals, insects), immunizations, or medications suggests an infection or hypersensitivity reaction. A smoking history, exposure to UV radiation and occupational to exposure mining, masonry, and metallurgy (silicon, beryllium) raise concern for a neoplastic process. It is important to ask the patient about their sexual history. The presence of genital lesions/discharge

TABLE 2.47 Differential Diagnosis of Adenopathy by Region

Head and Neck	Trunk	Extremities
Preauricular nodes	Supraclavicular nodes	Epitrochlear nodes
Submandibular nodes	Infraclavicular nodes	Inguinal nodes
Anterior cervical nodes	Axillary nodes	
Posterior cervical nodes		
Associated infections:	Associated infections: Neck, chest,	Associated infections:
Scalp, URI, mononucleosis,	GI/GU tracts	Extremities, GU tract
toxoplasmosis, CMV, dental	Mycobacterial, fungal diseases of	Skin infections upper
disease	the chest, syphilis, mastitis	and lower extremities,
Neoplasms:	Neoplasms:	genital tract
Lymphomas, leukemias, skin,	Larynx, thyroid, breast, pul-	Neoplasms:
oral cavity, larynx	monary, gastrointesti-	Skin, genitourinary,
	nal/genitourinary tracts,	lymphomas
	non-Hodgkin's lymphoma,	
	melanoma	

CMV, cytomegalovirus; GI, gastrointestinal; GU, genitourinary; URI, upper respiratory infection.

or oral lesions may support an infectious etiology. You must inquire about a family history of autoimmune diseases or malignancies.

Physical exam is guided by the presenting symptoms and should focus on the affected system(s) and its lymphatic drainage. The location of adenopathy can be directly related to the cause. Regions are outlined in Table 2.47.

The patient may be febrile with an infection or lymphoma. Evaluate for regional or generalized adenopathy: firm, fixed, or matted lymph nodes may suggest malignancy or infection. Multiple small, hard lymph nodes are associated with reactive nodes seen with viral infections. Tender, fluctuant cervical adenopathy is most likely secondary to a strep or staph infection. Inguinal adenopathy of up to 2 cm can be present in the healthy adult. Epitrochlear adenopathy can be seen with melanomas and lymphomas. Isolated inguinal adenopathy is not commonly seen with lymphomas. Supraclavicular adenopathy is associated with a high risk of intrathoracic or abdominal neoplasms. The differential diagnosis of regional adenopathy is seen in Table 2.47.

Diagnosis

Laboratory testing may include CBC with manual differential to evaluate for leukocytosis. rapid plasma antigen (RPR), purified protein derivative (PPD), HIV, HCV, and HBsAg can help identify an underlying infection. ANA may be elevated in the presence of autoimmune disorders such as lupus. Monospot can be positive in mononucleosis.

Imaging options include ultrasound of the affected node in patients <14 years of age. CT of the affected area is recommended in patients >14 years of age. Fine-needle aspiration (FNA) can differentiate reactive versus malignant process with an accuracy of 90%, but is not accurate if there is concern for lymphoma. False-positive results are rare. Excisional biopsy is indicated with the suspicion of lymphoma. Choose the largest, most concerning, and most accessible node. Excisional biopsy is also recommended when the FNA is nondiagnostic.[2,4]

Management

Management focuses on primary treatment of the underlying disorder.

> **CLINICAL PEARL:** Corticosteroids should not be prescribed until a definitive diagnosis for the lymphadenopathy is made, as they may mask a diagnosis of leukemia or lymphoma.

REFERENCES

1. Bazemore AW, Smucker DR. Lymphadenopathy and malignancy. *Am Fam Physician*. 2002;66(11):2103–2110.
2. Gaddey HI, Riegel AM. Unexplained lymphadenopathy: evaluation and differential diagnosis. *Am Fam Physician*. 2016;94(11):896–903.
3. Rajasekaran K, Krakovitz P. Enlarged neck lymph nodes in children. *Pediatr Clin North Am*. 2013;60(4):923–936. doi:10.1016/j.pcl.2013.04.005
4. Chau I, Kelleher MT, Cunningham D, et al. Rapid access multidisciplinary lymph node diagnostic clinic: analysis of 550 patients. *Br J Cancer*. 2003;88(3):354–361. doi:10.1038/sj.bjc.6600738

POLYCYTHEMIA

Etiology

Polycythemia is a condition that results in an increased level of circulating RBCs in the bloodstream. Polycythemia is divided into two categories: primary and secondary. Primary polycythemia results from an inherent problem in the process of RBC production. Polycythemia vera (PV) is commonly associated with leukocytosis and thrombocytosis and the risk of myelofibrosis and acute myeloid leukemia. The associated hyperviscosity can affect organ perfusion and can result in angina, or HF. Splenomegaly and low erythropoietin levels are also seen with this disorder. Secondary polycythemia is associated with conditions causing systemic hypoxia, such as right to left shunting, severe pulmonary disease, and sleep apnea. It can also occur with conditions associated with increased erythropoietin production, such as hypernephromas, renal artery stenosis, and cystic kidney disease. Relative polycythemia can be seen with volume depletion.

Epidemiology

The incidence of PV in the United States is 44 to 57 per 100,000 and increases with age. Peak age at onset is 50 to 60 years.[1] Mutations in the JAK2 gene are associated with increased sensitivity to erythropoietin by premature erythrocytes that results in increased erythropoiesis. Primary familial and congenital polycythemia and PV are in this category. The prevalence of the secondary polycythemia is considered to be much higher but is difficult to quantify due to the various causes.[1,2]

Clinical Presentation

Patients with volume depletion may have a history of recent nausea, vomiting, or diarrhea. The patients may complain of unexplained bleeding, symptoms concerning for abnormal blood clotting, and pruritus. They may have a history of chest pain or shortness of breath. Hepatosplenomegaly can cause right or left upper quadrant pain/discomfort. Patients may complain of bone pain or a burning sensation in their hands or feet. Past medical history may be positive for HTN, kidney disease, and cardiopulmonary disorders. Inquire about a history of smoking. Review medications for diuretic use.

Begin the exam by observing for signs of volume depletion. Examine the skin and nails for cyanosis, digital clubbing, and ecchymosis. Perform a detailed cardiovascular exam to look for signs of underlying lung disease, right HF, or intracardiac shunting. Abdominal exam findings may reveal tender hepatomegaly, splenomegaly, which is more likely to be seen with PV, abdominal or pelvic masses, as seen with secondary causes.

> **CLINICAL PEARL:** If a patient is found to have an increased red cell mass, it is important to assess the patient's volume status and oxygen levels.

Diagnosis

- CBC reveals an elevated hemoglobin and hematocrit, and possibly leukocytosis and thrombocytosis, in the case of PV. Diagnostic criteria for polycythemia are defined in Box 2.4.
- Peripheral smear reveals an increase in RBCs, circulating blasts, and ringed sideroblasts associated with myelodysplasia; AML may be present.
- Red cell mass is elevated to levels >36 mL/kg for males and 32 mL/kg in females.
- Erythropoietin levels will be low in PV and should be followed up with a bone marrow biopsy. If levels are elevated, then the cause is less likely to be PV, but rather secondary polycythemia.

Box 2.4 World Health Organization criteria for polycythemia vera

Major Criteria

1. Hemoglobin: >16.5 in men; >16.0 in women

   Or
      Hematocrit: >49% in men; >48% in women
   Or
      Elevated red cell mass

2. Bone marrow biopsy: hypercellularity; erythroid, granulocyte, and megakaryocyte proliferation

3. Genetic: JAK2V617F or JAK2 exon 12 mutation

- Bone marrow aspirate and biopsy showing hypercellularity, megakaryocyte hyperplasia, and absent iron stores can be seen with PV.
- Oxygen saturation <94% is associated with secondary causes of erythrocytosis.
- Imaging may include CT scanning of the chest and abdomen and renal ultrasound to identify hydronephrosis, masses, or cardiopulmonary pathology.

Management

Goals of therapy are to normalize hemoglobin and hematocrit, keep platelet counts <300,000 per microliter, and reduce the risk of thrombosis.

- Referral: To hematologist
- General: Maintain moderate physical activity, avoid hot baths, which may worsen pruritus, protect extremities in cold weather, and avoid long periods of extremes in temperature
- Phlebotomy: Primary treatment; 1 unit of blood each week until H&H normalizes (HCT <45% men and <42% women)
- Medications: Primarily consist of cytotoxic and cytoreductive therapies. Hydroxyurea, ASA, interferon-alpha are more specific for the erythrocytes, whereas anagrelide and interferon are effective in controlling thrombocythemia, ultimately reducing the size of splenomegaly and the need for phlebotomy
- Radiation therapy: If medical therapy fails
- Ultraviolet light treatment: May improve pruritus

References

1. Keohane C, McMullin MF, Harrison C. The diagnosis and management of erythrocytosis. *BMJ*. 2013;347:f6667. doi:10.1136/bmj.f6667
2. Stuart BJ, Viera AJ. Polycythemia vera. *Am Fam Physician*. May 1, 2004;69(9):2139–2144.
3. Goroll AH, Mulley AG. *Primary Care Medicine. Office Evaluation and Management of the Adult Patient*. 6th ed. Lippincott Williams & Willkins; 2009:637–641.

Thrombocytopenia

Etiology

The normal coagulation system limits blood loss though the regulation of three divisions: circulating blood platelets, components of the vascular endothelium, and plasma proteins (clotting factors). Platelets are responsible for primary hemostasis through adhesion, activation, and aggregation. Secondary hemostasis is controlled by the plasma proteins. Thrombocytopenia can be defined by a platelet count of less than 150,000/μL. Platelet defects can be caused by many factors. Decreased production can be medication induced, occur as a result of marrow failure, or can be associated with metastasis. Sequestration occurs secondary to an enlarged spleen, cirrhosis, or portal HTN. Increased platelet destruction can be a result of drugs, such as heparin, or can also occur as a result of disorders such as lupus, lymphoma, and HIV. Disseminated intravascular coagulation should be a consideration. Finally, thrombocytopenia may be idiopathic.[1,2]

Epidemiology

Isolated thrombocytopenia can be inherited (less common) or acquired. Increased destruction (acquired) is the most common cause of thrombocytopenia. Idiopathic thrombocytopenia purpura (ITP), which is an example of accelerated platelet destruction, is commonly encountered in clinical practice. The patient develops antibodies to their own platelets, which are then cleared by the spleen. ITP is classified as acute or chronic. Acute ITP is common in children. It is usually preceded by a viral infection and is self-limiting, requiring no specific treatment. In adults, chronic ITP is more common, occurring more frequently in women 20 to 40 years old, lasting >6 months, and thought to be secondary to autoantibodies to platelet membrane surface proteins.

Clinical Presentation

Determine the significance of bleeding, when present, through history and physical examination. Ask the patient about fatigue, lightheadedness, shortness of breath, and chest pain. Patients may report easy bruising, predominately in the skin, mucous membranes, nose, GI, and genitourinary tracts. Patients can complain of blood in urine, with BMs, and heavier than normal menstrual bleeding resulting in iron deficiency. Bleeding with procedures can be immediate. Patients may have a medical history of chronic liver disease, cancer, autoimmune disorders, infections, and transfusion requirements with procedures. It is important to review the medication list as certain drugs can be associated with platelet destruction, such as chemotherapeutic agents, heparin, thiazides, sulfonamides, estrogens, and alcohol. There can be a family history of bleeding disorders.

Spontaneous bleeding is associated with platelet counts <10,000 to 20,000 /µL. Mild bleeding can present with skin manifestations, such as bruising and petechiae only. Moderate to severe bleeding, with counts <10,000 /µL, is associated with mucosal, GI or genitourinary bleeding, and intracranial hemorrhage.

The patient should be examined for volume depletion by checking orthostatic BP and heart rate. Check the oxygen saturation. Examine the skin for color and temperature. Petechiae, small pinpoint hemorrhages <3 mm, are commonly seen on the skin. Areas of small, superficial ecchymoses may be present. Bleeding into the joints and muscles is not associated with low platelets, but is more likely to be seen with clotting factor deficiencies. Regional or diffuse lymphadenopathy may be present. Positive findings on abdominal exam include hepatosplenomegaly and ascites.[3]

Diagnosis

- Examine the platelet count. On a normal peripheral smear there should be 1 platelet for every 20 red cells, 8 to 20 platelets per high-power field.
- The WBCs and RBCs are usually normal. Pancytopenia is suggestive of an underlying bone marrow condition.
- A prolonged bleeding time is associated with counts <100,000/µL.
- Patients should be tested for hepatitis C and HIV as these viruses are associated with an antibody-mediated platelet destruction.

- Antiplatelet antibodies can be seen with heparin-induced thrombocytopenia (HIT). HIT is classified as a hypercoagulable state.
- Phospholipids activate blood clotting, and when present in circulation these antibodies can inhibit the clotting process.
- Antinuclear antibodies can be seen in autoimmune conditions.
- Immunoglobulin levels are ordered to rule out common variable immune deficiency.
- Bone marrow biopsies may reveal pancytopenia; hypo-/hypercellular marrow may be indicated to rule out leukemia or tumor invasion.

Management

Identify and treat the underlying condition. The goal is to obtain adequate hemostasis, which does not necessarily mean a "normal" platelet count. In mild cases monitor blood work. Eighty percent of children will recover without therapy by 6 months. In moderate to severe cases, the goal is a target platelet count of $>20 \times 10^9$/L at 48 hours. Treatment responses are defined as a platelet count ≥ 30 but $<100 \times 10^9$/L, or a doubling from baseline.

Platelet transfusions will not help in autoimmune conditions because existing circulating antibodies will also attack transfused platelets. Transfusions may not help if there are circulating drugs that inhibit platelet function, such as clopidogrel or a glycoprotein IIb/IIIa receptor antagonist (abciximab) in the plasma.[4] Platelet transfusions are indicated in the following circumstances:

- Active bleeding with counts <50,000
- Individuals with underlying hematological disorders
- Transient chemotherapy-induced thrombocytopenia

MEDICAL TREATMENT OPTIONS
Adults:[5]

- Prednisone: 1 to 2 mg/kg orally for 21 days then tapered off
- IV immunoglobulin:1 to 2 g/kg × 1 with corticosteroids if a more rapid increase in platelet count is required
- Anti-D in Rh-positive, in individuals with their spleen, Pred IVIg contraindicated
- Rituximab and dexamethasone
- Thrombopoietin receptor agonists eltrombopag 50 mg po daily, romiplostim for chronic ITP unresponsive to earlier therapy
- Splenectomy is recommended for patients who have failed corticosteroid therapy
- In patients who require a rapid response to therapy, options include IVIG, platelet transfusion, and recombinant factor VIIa

Children:

- Prednisone 2 mg/kg/d for 2 weeks followed by a 21-day taper
- IV immunoglobulin: 0.8 to 1 g/kg as a single dose
- Anti-D immunoglobulin in certain pediatric cases
- Rituximab 375 mg/m²: weekly dose × 4 weeks
- Splenectomy (consider delaying × 1 year): response rate of approximately 70% to 80%
- Pneumococcal and meningococcal vaccination

> **CLINICAL PEARL:** To achieve adequate hemostasis quickly, IVIg has the most rapid onset of action

> **CLINICAL PEARL:** Septicemia is a complication of splenectomy. The most common agent is Streptococcus pneumonia and is associated with high mortality.

REFERENCES

1. Izak M, Bussel JB. Management of thrombocytopenia. *F1000 Prime Rep*. 2014;6:45. doi:10.12703/P6-45. http://f1000researchdata.s3.amazonaws.com/f1000reports/files/9008/6/45/article.pdf
2. Neutze D, Roque J. Clinical evaluation of bleeding and bruising in primary care. *Am Fam Physician*. 2016;93(4):279–286.
3. Gauer RL, Braun MM. Thrombocytopenia. *Am Fam Physician*. 2012;85(6):612–622. doi:10.1080/00207179.2012.669851
4. Kaufman RM, et al. Platelet transfusion: a clinical practice guideline. *Ann Intern Med*. February 2015;162(3):205–213. doi:10.7326/M14-1589
5. Neunert C, Lim W, Crowther M, et al. The American Society of Hematology 2011 evidence-based practice guideline for immune thrombocytopenia. *Blood*. 2011;117(16):4190–4207. doi:10.1182/blood-2010-08-302984

ELECTRONIC RESOURCES

Advancing Transfusion and Cellular Therapies Worldwide (AABB) Clinical Resources

> http://www.aabb.org/programs/clinical/Pages/default.aspx

MUSCULOSKELETAL SYSTEM

ADHESIVE CAPSULITIS

Etiology

Adhesive capsulitis, commonly referred to as a frozen shoulder, is a debilitating disorder with no clear etiology. Adhesive capsulitis has been attributed to capsular inflammation, thickening, and fibrosis.

Primary adhesive capsulitis is disproportionately idiopathic while secondary may develop after surgery, trauma, or continuous immobilization.

Epidemiology

Adhesive capsulitis has an incidence of 3% to 5% in the general population and about 20% in those with a history of diabetes. Women are more affected than men. Age prevalence is between 45 and 60 years old.[1,2]

Clinical Presentation

Pain quantification and localization can be difficult. Patients usually complain of sharp pain with attempted overhead motion and the pain may radiate down the arm. Range of motion (ROM) is often impaired, especially in forward flexion and abduction of the shoulder. It is not uncommon for patients to report weakness and/or abnormal sounds (crepitus) in the affected shoulder with movement. Adhesive capsulitis can mimic other shoulder pathologies such as impingement syndrome, rotator cuff disease, and calcific tendonitis.

In general, adhesive capsulitis consists of three stages:

1. Freezing: Gradual pain resulting in loss of shoulder motion over time. This stage can last from weeks to months.
2. Frozen: Reduction in pain and significantly decreased shoulder motion, which may affect activities of daily living such as dressing, grooming, bathing, employment, and homemaking. This stage usually lasts for about 6 months.
3. Thawing: Patients gradually regain normal shoulder motion and strength. This stage can take over a year to achieve.

Diagnosis

The diagnosis of adhesive capsulitis is made clinically, through history and physical examination. The hallmark signs are decreased active and passive ROM of the shoulder in all planes of motion compared to the unaffected side. Plain radiographs are normal. A MRI scan can aid in the diagnosis and clinical staging.

Management

There is a paucity of research on a consensus-based treatment algorithm for adhesive capsulitis. Treatment options include observation, subacromial or glenohumeral joint cortisone injections, NSAIDS, home exercise program (HEP), and extensive physical therapy. Transcutaneous electrical nerve stimulation (TENS) and interferential electrotherapy (IFE) have been used in conjunction with physical therapy to improve pain and ROM. Other treatment options include shoulder hydrodilatation (usually done by radiology), manipulation under anesthesia (MUA), and arthroscopic capsular release. The role of complementary alternative treatments such as acupuncture has not been well-established in the literature.[2-4]

> **CLINICAL PEARL:** Adhesive capsulitis can be treated successfully in primary care. Physical therapy with stretching exercises in combination with NSAIDS are the mainstay of treatment. Patients who are refractory to conservative treatment should be referred to an orthopedist. There is no role for narcotics in the treatment of adhesive capsulitis.

REFERENCES

1. Manske RC, Prohaska D. Diagnosis and management of adhesive capsulitis. *Curr Rev Musculoskelet Med.* 2008;1(3–4):180–189. doi:10.1007/s12178-008-9031-6

2. Manske RC, Prohaska A. Diagnosis and management of adhesive capsulitis. *Curr Rev Musculoskelet Med.* 2008;1(3–4):180–189.

3. Cvetanovich GL, Leroux T, Hamamoto JT, et al. Arthroscopic 360° capsular release for adhesive capsulitis in the lateral decubitus position. *Arthrosc Tech.* 2016;5(5):e1033–e1038. doi:10.1016/j.eats.2016.05.007

4. Martin D. Adhesive capsulitis: a reminder to treat the whole patient. *South Med Assoc.* 2008;101(6):578–579. doi:10.1097/SMJ.0b013e318172dd58

HERNIATED NUCLEUS PULPOSUS

Etiology

A herniated nucleus pulposus (HNP) occurs when there is a protrusion of an intervertebral disk through the annulus fibrosis.

Epidemiology

Precipitating factors include advanced age and stress. Most patients have pre-existing degenerative disk disease. Traumatic events such a fall, lifting, or even coughing may precipitate this condition. Risk factors include smoking, prior back problems, obesity, and poor fitness. Lumbar radiculopathy has a 3% to 5% lifetime incidence in adults, with males and females affected at equal rates.[1,2]

Clinical Presentation

HNP typically presents with an abrupt onset of low back pain followed by radiculopathy. The pain is relieved by rest. In lumbosacral disease, a straight leg raise will exacerbate the pain. The initial back pain is likely caused by direct mechanical pressure of the nerve root by the herniated nucleus pulposus, followed by the liberation of chemical factors that lead to radiculopathy. The signs of radiculopathy include sciatica, numbness, paresthesias, and weakness. Sciatica is pain along a specific dermatome. The specific nerve root findings are the following:

- L4: Weakness of quadriceps extension and anterior tibialis, pain in antero-lateral thigh and leg, numbness anterior thigh, diminished knee reflex, and weakness with arising from squat
- L5: Weakness with dorsiflexion of great toe, pain in posterolateral thigh and midfoot, numbness on top of midfoot, and weakness with heel walking. No reliable reflex abnormalities
- S1: Weakness in great toe flexor PF, pain in posterior calf, numbness lateral foot, diminished ankle reflex. Weakness with walking on toes

> **CLINICAL PEARL:** HNP is often asymptomatic.

Diagnosis

The diagnosis is made based on careful history and physical examination findings. Imaging studies are of questionable value initially. CT or MRI can identify the exact location of the lesion; however, these studies are usually reserved for patients that do not improve within four weeks of conservative therapy. Disk bulge can be seen in the absence of symptoms.[2]

Management

The initial management should be conservative, consisting of rest, ice, non-steroidal anti-inflammatory medications, and/or acetaminophen. Patients should avoid sitting and lifting. Narcotics are not typically recommended. Corticosteroid injections may offer temporary, albeit modest, relief of symptoms. Most patients with disk herniation will improve without surgery, as the pulposus reabsorbs over time. Surgical intervention is recommended if neurologic symptoms are progressive or severe, and may be considered if patients are unresponsive to at least 6 weeks of conservative therapy. Physical therapy is helpful to strengthen the paraspinal musculature and to help educate the patient on proper posture and lifting techniques.

You must be aware of the following alarm signs and symptoms:

- Cauda equina syndrome: Bilateral neurologic deficits, perineal numbness, leakage of stool or urine. This condition indicates spinal cord compression and warrants immediate imaging and referral
- Urinary retention
- Progressive neurologic deficit
- Symptoms that persist for >6 weeks
- Pain that awakens at night, especially associated with fever—this may signal possible infection

REFERENCES

1. Tarulli AW, Raynor EM. Lumbosacral radiculopathy. *Neurol Clin.* 2007;25:387. doi:10.1016/j.ncl.2007.01.008
2. Jensen MC, Brant-Zawadzki MN, Obuchowski N, et al. Magnetic resonance imaging of the lumbar spine in people without back pain. *N Engl J Med.* July 1994;331(2):69–73. doi:10.1056/NEJM199407143310201

LUMBOSACRAL STRAIN/SPRAIN

Etiology

More than 85% of patients presenting with back discomfort have "mechanical" low back pain only, with an absence of neurological findings. This presentation usually results from either acute or recurrent trauma, with no specific underlying condition identifiable.

Epidemiology

Low back pain is the second most common cause of disability among adults in the United States.[1] Risk factors include poor fitness, heavy or repetitive lifting, poor body mechanics, smoking, job dissatisfaction, and various psychosocial factors. Oftentimes, a specific traumatic event is not identified. The most commonly affected patient population is between 20 and 50 years of age.[2]

Clinical Presentation

Patients typically present with the acute onset of localized low back pain following a lifting injury. The pain may radiate to the gluteal region or the proximal thigh. Patients may have associated muscle spasm and postural abnormalities. Radiculopathy is characteristically absent.

Diagnosis

History and physical examination are vital to the diagnosis. A thorough history should include a description of pain location, radiation, onset, and provocative and palliative factors. Ask about radiation of pain below the knee and any associated numbness, tingling, or weakness. These are more often associated with HNP. Ask about perineal numbness and stool or urine leakage. These are worrisome for cauda equina syndrome. Ask about prior history/recent history of infection, IV drug use, MRSA, uncontrolled diabetes, pain at rest or that awakens at night, fever, or chills. These may suggest the possibility of spinal infection. A careful physical exam should include visual inspection, as well as testing of motor, sensory, and reflex at lumbosacral levels L4/L5/S1. Imaging is not recommended in the absence of a history suggestive of an alternative cause of the pain or focal findings on physical exam.[3]

CLINICAL PEARL: The differential diagnosis of low back pain is broad and should include a range of conditions including ankylosing spondylitis, abdominal aortic aneurysm, nephrolithiasis, multiple myeloma, drug-seeking behavior, a herniated disc, and an epidural infection.

Management

Rest, NSAIDS, acetaminophen, ice, and work modifications are the initial treatment recommendations for the first 3 to 5days. Avoid oral steroids, narcotics, and muscle relaxants. After the first 7 to 10 days, recommend physical therapy for treatment and education. This treatment may include modalities such as ice, heat, and electrical stimulation or ultrasound. However, more importantly, core strengthening exercises should be emphasized. Additionally, the patient should be educated on proper posture and body mechanics to reduce recurrence. Reevaluate the patient at four weeks. If they are unable to return to work or other activities, consider imaging, such as radiographs or MRI, or a referral to a physical medicine and rehabilitation specialist or a spine service if the patient is not improving.

REFERENCES

1. Centers for Disease Control and Prevention. Prevalence of disabilities and associated health conditions among adults—United States, 1999. *MMWR Morb Mortal Wkly Rep*. 2001;50(7):120.
2. Deyo RA. Descriptive epidemiology of low back pain and its related medical care in the United States. *Spine*. 1987;12:264. doi:10.1097/00007632-198704000-00013
3. Trafimow D, Trafimow JH. The shocking implications of Bayes' theorem for diagnosing herniated nucleus pulposus based on MRI scans. *Cogent Med*. 2016;3(1):1–7. Doi:10.1080/2331205X.2015.1133270

OSTEOARTHRITIS: KNEE

Etiology

Osteoarthritis (OA), often referred to as degenerative joint disease or "wear and tear" syndrome, is associated with a breakdown in hyaline joint cartilage and can lead to substantial morbidity. Modifiable and nonmodifiable factors attributing to the onset of knee OA include local joint and soft-tissue inflammation, mechanical forces, cellular processes, genetics, diet, obesity, sex, and age. Of these, obesity is the greatest modifiable risk factor for OA.

Epidemiology

According to the CDC, 54 million Americans have been diagnosed with some form of arthritis. OA is the most common arthritis and statistically affects women more than their male counterparts.[1-3]

Clinical Presentation

Depending on the severity of the knee OA, patients may present with joint stiffness and pain, antalgic gait, swelling, instability, decreased ROM, limb deformity, and crepitus. Patients with symptomatic knee OA often report insomnia, pain with activities of daily living, pain with prolonged standing and walking, start-up pain, and mechanical symptoms (locking, popping, or giving away of the knee). Mechanical symptoms may also be present in other knee pathologies, such as meniscal, cruciate, and collateral ligament tears.

Diagnosis

The diagnosis of knee OA is made through history and physical exam, in addition to relevant diagnostic testing. Plain x-rays (weight-bearing series), consisting of anteroposterior view, lateral, and sunrise views, are used to confirm the diagnosis and severity of knee OA. A MRI does not improve the diagnostic value in severe knee OA.

Management

The cure for knee OA remains elusive despite recent advancements in treatment. Prevention is key, through modification of risk factors. Conservative treatment options for knee OA include, but are not limited to, NSAIDS, weight loss coupled with exercise, physical and aquatic therapy, self-management programs, neuromodulation products, intraarticular corticosteroid injections, unloader bracing, and genicular nerve radiofrequency ablation.[4]

Surgical options for symptomatic knee OA include arthroscopy and unicompartmental versus total knee arthroplasty. Other options include steroid injection, viscosupplements, and arthroscop. General management considerations are outlined in Table 2.48.

TABLE 2.48 Treatment Options for Osteoarthritis

Modalities	Treatment Program	Length of Treatment
Physical therapy and HEP	Work on range of motion exercises, muscle strengthening, stretching exercises, soft tissue modalities, manual therapy, bracing and aquatic therapy	May require several months of therapy to improve symptoms.
Weight loss program BMI >30	Meet with nutritionist to discuss weight loss strategies	Depends on the individual needs of the patient

(continued)

TABLE 2.48 Treatment Options for Osteoarthritis (*continued*)

Modalities	Treatment Program	Length of Treatment
Injections	CSI are given every 3–4 months depending on the practice protocol. Exercise caution when administering to diabetics as CSI can cause abnormal blood glucose levels in these patients. CSIs should not be administered in patients with uncontrolled diabetes.	If used, should be in short duration. As stated earlier, there is a low level of evidence supporting the use of CSIs in knee osteoarthritis.
NSAIDS	Celecoxib, meloxicam, ibuprofen, diclofenac and naproxen have traditionally been used to address symptomatic knee osteoarthritis.	If used, should be administered in short duration. Consider the use of PPIs to reduce the risk of ulcerations from NSAIDS use.

BMI, body mass index; CSI, cortisone injections; HEP, home exercise program; NSAIDS, nonsteroidal anti-inflammatory drugs; PPIs, proton-pump inhibitors.

CLINICAL PEARL: Conservative treatment is the mainstay of treatment in most cases of knee arthritis. The use of opioid therapy in the treatment of moderate to severe chronic knee OA should be discouraged.

REFERENCES

1. Barbour KE, Helmick CG, Boring M, et al. Vital signs: prevalence of doctor-diagnosed arthritis and arthritis-attributable activity limitation - United States, 2013-2015. *MMWR Morb Mortal Wkly Rep.* March 10, 2017;66(9):246–253. doi:10.15585/mmwr.mm6609e1
2. Szoeke C, Dennerstein L, Guthrie J, et al. The relationship between prospectively assessed body weight and physical activity and prevalence of radiological knee osteoarthritis in postmenopausal women. *J Rheumatol.* 2006;33:1835–1840.
3. Hame SL, Alexander RA. Knee osteoarthritis in women. *Curr Rev Musculoskeletal Med.* 2013;6(2):182–187. doi:10.1007/s12178-013-9164-0
4. Kidd V. Genicular nerve radiofrequency ablation a novel approach to symptomatic knee osteoarthritis. *JBJS JOPA.* 2018;6(1):e10. doi:10.2106/JBJS.JOPA.17.00039

PLANTAR FASCIITIS

Etiology

The plantar aponeuroses is an important anatomic structure that spans the plantar aspect of the foot. It provides longitudinal support for the arch. Patients can develop plantar heel pain either acutely or chronically when this structure is subject to overuse. This overuse can lead to microtrauma where the body's ability to remodel and heal is overcome by repetitive force. Two common patient subsets are frequently seen:

- High-activity athletes, especially runners. Often there will be an associated history of change in training or activity regimen[1]
- Sedentary patients with high BMI[1,3]

In both categories, a resultant biomechanical overload occurs to the plantar aponeuroses that exceeds the body's attempt at healing.[4] Extrinsic factors may include Achilles tendinosis, Haglund's syndrome, stress fracture, rheumatoid arthritis, or diabetic neuropathy.[5]

Epidemiology

Plantar fasciitis is a common complaint in foot pain, accounting for over one million clinic visits a year in the United States.[6] The peak age at occurrence is between ages 40 and 60 and can be bilateral in one-third of cases.[7] The occurrence rate of plantar fasciitis in active athletes can reach 8% to 21% over their respective careers.[8]

Clinical Presentation

Patients will present with complaints of plantar heel pain that is either acute or chronic. The pain pattern can be variable. Some patients will have heel pain primarily when first arising out of bed that quickly improves during the day. Others will have either a recurrence or onset of heel pain as they progress with weight-bearing activities. In athletes, there is often a history of recent change in activity level or training prior to onset. The primary clinical features are complaints of heel pain that is reproduced with palpation of the origin of the plantar aponeurosis at the heel.

Diagnosis

According to a recent consensus statement by the Foot and Ankle Surgery Society, the diagnosis of plantar fasciitis is clinical and made on the findings of history and physical exam.[9] However, it is prudent to rule out other potential causes as listed under etiology earlier. Radiographic studies are not recommended unless there is a high index of suspicion for fracture.[9] Studies have shown an inconsistent relationship between a calcaneal spur and plantar fasciitis.[10]

Management

According to the 2017 Foot and Ankle Society consensus statement, the following are recommended for nonoperative care of plantar fasciitis:

- Rest, nonsteroidal anti-inflammatory medication
- Biomechanical foot supports
- PT/stretching
- Local corticosteroid injections as well as ice massage
- Night splints can be effectivem especially for patients whose symptoms are mainly related to the awakening period
- Other nonoperative therapy may include extracorporeal shockwave therapy
- Surgery is usually reserved for refractory cases where symptoms last for >6 months[9]

REFERENCES

1. Macintyre JG, Taunton JE, Clement DB, et al. Running injuries: a clinical study of 4,173 cases. *Clin J sports Med.* 1991;1:81–87. doi:10.1097/00042752-199104000-00002
2. Rano JA, Fallat LM, Savoy-Moore RT. Correlation of heel pain and BMI and other characteristics of heel pain. *J Foot Ankle Surg.* 2001;40:351–356. doi:10.1016/S1067-2516(01)80002-8

3. Van Leeuwen KD, Rogers J, Wizenberg T, et al. Higher body mass index is associated with plantar fasciitis; systematic review and meta-analysis of various clinical and imaging risk factors. *Br J Sports Med.* 2016;50:972–981. doi:10.1136/bjsports-2015-094695

4. Sarrafian SK. Functional characteristics of the foot and plantar aponeurosis under tibiotalar loading. *Foot Ankle.* 1987;8:4–18. doi:10.1177/107110078700800103

5. Wearing SC, Smeathers JE, Urry SR, et al. The pathomechanics of plantar fasciitis. *Sports Med.* 2006;36:585–611. doi:10.2165/00007256-200636070-00004

6. Riddle DL, Schappert SM. Volume of ambulatory care visits and pattern of care for patients diagnosed with plantar fasciitis; a national study of medical doctors. *Foot Ankle Int.* 2004;25:303. doi:10.1177/107110070402500505

7. Furey JG. Plantar fasciitis; The painful heel syndrome. *J Bone Joint Surg Am.* 1975;5:672. doi:10.2106/00004623-197557050-00016

8. Leach RE, Seavey MS, Salter DK. Results of surgery in athletes with plantar fasciitis. *Foot Ankle.* 1986;7:156. doi:10.1177/107110078600700305

9. AFCAS Clinical Consensus Statement , Schneider H, Baca J. American College of foot and ankle surgeons. Clinical consensus statement; diagnosis and treatment of adult acquired infracalcaneal heel pain. *J Foot Ankle Surg.* 2017;7:9.

10. Prichasuk S, Subhadrabandhu T. The relationship of pes planus and calcaneal spur tp plantar heel pain. *Clin Orthop Rel Res.* 1965;39:178.

SHOULDER IMPINGEMENT SYNDROME

Etiology

The shoulder is an inherently unstable joint but affords great ROM. The four muscles of the rotator cuff help to stabilize the glenohumeral joint and provide impressive ROM.

These include the following:

- Supraspinatus: Most commonly involved in impingement, it originates superior to the scapular spine and inserts onto the greater tuberosity of the proximal humerus. In transit it passes beneath the acromial arch. It is responsible for initiating abduction and forward elevation.
- Infraspinatus: Originates below the scapular spine and inserts on the greater tuberosity of the proximal humerus. It is mainly responsible for initiating external rotation.
- Teres minor: Arises from the inferior/medial scapular border and inserts on the lower portion of the humeral greater tuberosity. The major function is external rotation and to a lesser extent adduction.
- Subscapularis: Arises from the anterior surface of the scapula and inserts on the lesser tuberosity of the proximal humerus. The major function is to initiate internal rotation.

Shoulder impingement syndrome (SIS) occurs due to an impingement of the rotator cuff tendons under the acromion and a rigid coracoacromial arch. Several factors can lead to degeneration of the rotator cuff tendons, resulting in shoulder pain. These include increased humeral head translation, acromial morphology, and degenerative spurring of the acromioclavicular joint.[1] In 1972, Neer first presented SIS as a spectrum of disease, as opposed to a singular event, with three stages and proposed ages at which it is typically seen.[2]

- Stage I edema and hemorrhage usually <25 years old
- Stage II fibrosis/tendinitis ages 25 to 40 years
- Stage III Rotator cuff tear age >40 years

Neer further described three morphological types for acromial architecture which can lead to impingement and symptoms:[2]

- Type I: flat
- Type II: down sloping
- Type III: hooked or curved

Research has consistently shown an association with type III acromial morphology and rotator cuff pathology. Type III acromial morphology is associated with up to a 10 times greater incidence of impingement syndrome and rotator cuff tear.[3,4]

Epidemiology

SIS is the most common cause of shoulder pain affecting 16% to 34% of the general population in any given year[3] while presenting as the most common reason for treatment of shoulder pain.[5] Risk factors for SIS include repetitive use, overhead activities including sports, advancing age, and glenohumeral instability.[6]

Clinical Presentation

Typically, patients will present with pain over the anterolateral aspect of the affected shoulder. This pain may radiate laterally over the deltoid region. The onset may be insidious or acute. A precedent traumatic event may be identified in some cases. Pain at night is common and is often exacerbated by daily activities such as overhead activities and throwing.[7] Of note; patients who are younger and describe a specific traumatic event or are throwing athletes warrant consideration for rotator cuff tear. Acute pain and weakness are frequently seen in frank rotator cuff rupture.[8]

Diagnosis

A careful history should be undertaken to discover any factors that may implicate a frank tear. These include advanced age, specific trauma, acute onset, and weakness. A careful evaluation of active and passive ROM should be accomplished. A finding of impaired active ROM but intact passive ROM and weakness with muscle testing should raise suspicion for rotator cuff tear. Inspection should focus on signs of atrophy especially in patients with chronic symptoms. Motor testing of specific muscles will help to define pathology on an anatomic basis (see section "etiology"). Many provocative maneuvers have been described but data on their accuracy for most is lacking.

Significant diagnostic accuracy has been demonstrated by using the Hawkins and Neer impingement test.[9] For bursitis, the Neer sign demonstrates approximately 75% sensitivity while the Hawkins sign shows approximately 92% sensitivity. For rotator cuff tear, the Neer sign shows approximately 85% sensitivity while the Hawkins test shows approximately 88% sensitivity. The two tests also demonstrate a high negative predictive value; 96% for impingement and 90% for rotator cuff tear.[9]

DIAGNOSTIC IMAGING
- Plain radiographs: In general, plain radiographs are not recommended at the initial time of evaluation. Exceptions include associated

trauma, suspicion for fracture, or clinical findings of acute rotator cuff tear. Radiographs may be helpful in patients who present with chronic symptoms or are not responding to treatment. In addition to evaluation for fractures, plain radiographs may be helpful to evaluate for degenerative disease, superior migration of the humeral head (suggestive of large rotator cuff tear), and acromial morphology. The latter is best seen on the supraspinatus outlet view.[10] This view should be included in the shoulder series films when ordered.

- MRI: Can be useful to confirm full-thickness tendon tears. MRI sensitivity for identifying partial thickness tears is less reliable.[11] Clinical correlation is critical when diagnosing rotator cuff tear, including a careful evaluation for weakness. In one study MRI demonstrated rotator cuff tears in over 50% of asymptomatic patients over age 60.[12]

Management

The most common nonoperative modalities include rest, avoidance of overhead activity, NSAIDS, physical therapy, and subacromial corticosteroid injections.[13,14] In general, nonoperative care is recommended for a 3 to 6 month period of time. Studies have shown that a majority of patients will improve with nonoperative care that includes a shoulder -specific course of physical therapy.[15] Consideration for orthopedic referral should include a history of significant trauma, suspicion for fracture, a patient who is a high-level throwing athlete, strong suspicion for tendon tear, and failure to improve with nonoperative care.

REFERENCES

1. Van der Windt DA, Koes BW, de Jong BA, Bouter LM. Shoulder disorders in general practice: incidence, patient characteristics, and management. *Ann Rheum Dis.* 1995;54:959. doi:10.1136/ard.54.12.959
2. Neer CS. Anterior acromioplasty for the chronic impingement syndrome in the shoulder. A preliminary report. *JBJS.* 1972;54A:41. doi:10.2106/00004623-197254010-00003
3. Bigliani LU, Morrison DS, April EW. The morphology of the acromion and rotator cuff and its relationship to rotator cuff tears. *Orthopedic Trans.* 1986;10:228.
4. Balke M, Schmidt C, Dedy N, et al. Correlation of acromial morphology with impingement syndrome and rotator cuff tears. *Acta Ortho.* 2013;84(2):178–183. doi:10.3109/17453674.2013.773413
5. Urwin M, Symmons D, Allison T, et al. Estimating the burden of musculoskeletal disorders in the community: the comparative prevalence of symptoms at different anatomical sites, and the relation to social deprivation. *Ann Rheum Dis.* 1998;57:649. doi:10.1136/ard.57.11.649
6. Silverstein BA, Viikari-Juntura E, Fan ZJ, et al. Natural course of nontraumatic rotator cuff tendinitis and shoulder symptoms in a working population. *Scand J Work Environ Health.* 2006;32:99. doi:10.5271/sjweh.985
7. Sedeek SM. Sub acromial impingement syndrome: review article. *Hard Tissue.* September 28, 2013;2(4):39. doi:10.13172/2050-2303-2-4-949
8. Koester MC, George MS, Kuhn JE. Shoulder impingement syndrome. *Am J Med.* May 2005;118(5):542–545. doi:10.1016/j.amjmed.2005.01.040
9. MacDonald P, Clark P, Sutherland K. An analysis of the diagnostic accuracy of the Hawkins and Neer sub acromial impingement signs. *J Shoulder Elbow Surg.* July/August 2000;9(4):299–301. doi:10.1067/mse.2000.106918
10. Harrison MK, Flatow EL. Subacromial impingement syndrome. *J Am Acad Orthop Surg.* November 2011;19(11):701–708. doi:10.5435/00124635-201111000-00006

11. Gazzola S, Bleakney RR. Current imaging of the rotator cuff. *Sports Med Arthrosc.* 2011;19:300. doi:10.1097/JSA.0b013e3182189468

12. Sher JS, Uribe JW, Posada A, et al. Abnormal findings on magnetic imaging images of asymptomatic shoulders. *J Bone Joint Surg Am.* 1995;77:10. doi:10.2106/00004623-199501000-00002

13. Bigliani LU, Levine WN. Subacromial impingement syndrome. *J Bone Joint Surg Am.* December 1997;79(12):1854–1868. doi:10.2106/00004623-199712000-00012

14. Chang WK. Shoulder impingement syndrome. *Phys Med Rehab Clin N Am.* May 2004;15(2):493–510. doi:10.1016/j.pmr.2003.12.006

15. Morrison DS, Frogameni AD, Woodworth P. Nonoperative treatment of subacromial impingement syndrome. *J Bone Joint Surg Am.* May 1997;79(5):732–737. doi:10.2106/00004623-199705000-00013

NEUROLOGIC SYSTEM

ALZHEIMER'S DEMENTIA (NEUROCOGNITIVE DISORDER DUE TO ALZHEIMER'S DISEASE)

Etiology

Dementia is a progressive neurodegenerative disease. Among the subtypes of dementia, Alzheimer's dementia is the most common. Although the exact mechanism is unclear, it is characterized by the development of neurofibrillary tangles and plaques in the brain. These abnormalities hinder communication and metabolism of neurons, which result in neuronal death and an overall atrophy of the brain. The hippocampus is the most commonly affected location.

Epidemiology

In 2011, over four million Americans had Alzheimer's dementia, and by the year 2050, it is estimated that nearly 14 million Americans will have been diagnosed with it.[1] The prevalence of Alzheimer's dementia increases with age, which makes this the primary risk factor.[2] Early onset disease, although much less common, does occur. Women are affected more than men, but this is thought to be due to longevity. A family history of dementia is a strong risk factor for the development of dementia, especially if the case is of a first-degree relative. Other risk factors include sedentary lifestyle, history of vascular disease, hyperlipidemia, history of traumatic brain injury, HTN, and obesity.

Clinical Presentation

Memory difficulties are the most common symptom in Alzheimer's dementia, especially in the early stages. Classically, patients with Alzheimer's dementia will initially have difficulty with recent or "short-term" memory. This symptom may be reported by patients or their family, or it can be assessed during the neurologic exam via word recall. Problems with executive functioning and visuospatial deficits are also common in the early stages. Patients may experience trouble with organization or multitasking. As the disease progresses difficulties with language, behavior, and the ability to complete basic ADLs occurs. In some cases, patients may seem apathetic or depressed, while in others they may become agitated or violent. Problems with sleep are common.

Symptom onset is typically gradual, which can help differentiate it from other cognitive disorders, such as delirium.

> **CLINICAL PEARL:** It is common for patients to have poor insight into their own memory problems. It may be helpful to gather a history from family or caregivers.

Diagnosis

Although evidence of the histological changes of Alzheimer's dementia can be found on autopsy, most diagnoses are made clinically. In addition to ruling out other medical causes of a patient's symptoms, it is important to rule out other causes of neurocognitive decline when evaluating a patient with suspected Alzheimer's dementia.

Several validated instruments exist for office-based cognitive assessment. The most common are the Mini-Mental State Examination (MMSE), the Montreal Cognitive Assessment (MoCA), and the Mini-Cog. Each of these can generally be completed in less than 10 minutes.[3] In addition to a basic mental status exam, these instruments can support a diagnosis of dementia and assist in determining an individual's functional status. This knowledge of functional deficits may help inform treatment planning.

A complete history and physical examination should be performed with particular attention looking for neurologic deficits that may be due to another cause.

Diagnostic studies to consider include a blood count, a metabolic panel, thyroid testing, syphilis screening (if risk exists), and B12 levels. Imaging in the form of an MRI of the brain may help rule out reversible causes of dementia.

> **CLINICAL PEARL:** Emergent neuroimaging should always be performed in the cases of recent trauma, an acute onset of symptoms, or a rapid change in condition.

Management

There is no cure for Alzheimer's dementia. Pharmacologic and nonpharmacologic modalities can be used to slow the progression of the disease and improve function and quality of life.

NONPHARMACOLOGIC
- Exercise can improve physical function and depressive symptoms
- Cognitive stimulation such as puzzles, socialization, and leisure activities can help memory as well as quality of life
- Occupational therapy can assist with developing strategies to ease the completion of ADLs

PHARMACOLOGIC
There are no clear guidelines for duration of pharmacologic therapy. Table 2.49 outlines common pharmacologic treatments.

Table **2.49** Pharmacologic Treatment of Alzheimer's Disease

Drug Name(s)	Mechanism	Adverse Effects
Donepezil, galantamine, rivastigmine	Improves cholinergic function Improves cognitive symptoms and functional status Is not disease-modifying Common first-line therapy	Decreased appetite, AV block and other dysrhythmias, diarrhea, dizziness, headache, nausea/vomiting
Memantine	Protects neurons in the hippocampus Improves cognitive and functional status Used in moderate to severe disease	Dizziness, constipation, confusion. Rare— cerebrovascular event, acute kidney injury

Source: Epperly T, Dunay MA, Boice JL. Alzheimer disease: pharmacologic and nonpharmacologic therapies for cognitive and functional symptoms. *Am Fam Physician. 2017;95:771–778.*

Due to its progressive nature, patients with dementia will require increasingly skilled and complex care as their disease worsens. Estimating life expectancy for these patients is difficult. Issues such as advanced directives, educating patient/family on prognosis, and the use of palliative care are important. Patients with advanced dementia often have difficulty with feeding, infections, pressure ulcers, and frequent hospitalizations.[1] An interdisciplinary team, clear and compassionate family communication, and advanced care planning can improve the quality of life and preserve dignity at the end of life for patients with Alzheimer's disease.

References

1. Mitchell SL. Advanced Dementia. *N Eng J Med.* 2015;372:2533–2540. doi:10.1056/NEJMcp1412652
2. American Psychiatric Association, American Psychiatric Association. DSM-5 Task Force. *Diagnostic and Statistical Manual of Mental Disorders: DSM-5.* 5th ed. Arlington, VA: Author; 2013.
3. Epperly T, Dunay MA, Boice JL. Alzheimer disease: pharmacologic and nonpharmacologic therapies for cognitive and functional symptoms. *Am Fam Physician.* 2017;95:771–778.

Bell's Palsy

Etiology

Bell's palsy (facial palsy) is a peripheral nerve palsy of CN VII resulting in unilateral muscle weakness. It results from an inflammatory process that may lead to compression, ischemia, and loss of myelin. Bell's palsy has been associated with herpes simplex type 1, mononucleosis, CMV, adenovirus, rubella, mumps, influenza B, coxsackievirus, and Lyme disease.

Epidemiology

Facial nerve palsy does not favor one side or the other. It occurs at any age; however, peak incidence is in the 40s, affecting men and women equally. The annual incidence of Bell's palsy is 15 to 30/100,000 persons. Patients experiencing one episode have an 8% risk of recurrence.[1,2]

Clinical Presentation

Patients can present with rapid onset of unilateral mild weakness, drooping, difficulty smiling and frowning, drooling, numbness of the affected side, facial pain, and headache. They may report difficulty tasting and difficulty with tearing—making it difficult to close the eye. Hyperacusis may be present. Ear pain and fever are more consistent with Ramsay Hunt syndrome. There may be associated myalgias, joint pain, and swelling. The patient's past medical history (PMHX) may be positive for a recent URI, diabetes, sarcoidosis, Lyme disease, Guillain–Barré, or influenza vaccines.[3,4]

Positive exam findings include unilateral weakness and paralysis of the facial muscles. Disappearance of the nasolabial fold, facial creases, and folds may be noted in the forehead. Eyelids will not close, and the lower lid sags. On attempted closure, the eye rolls upward. Facial sensation will be preserved. The corner of the mouth droops. Inspect the ear canal, tympanic membrane, oropharynx for vesicular eruptions that will be seen with Ramsay Hunt. The skin should be examined for rashes. The neurological exam is otherwise normal.

It is usually a temporary condition and is rarely permanent. About 70% to 80% of patient symptoms improve spontaneously within a few weeks. Complete recovery is expected within approximately 6 months

> **CLINICAL PEARL:** The forehead is spared with a central (supranuclear) cause such as stroke, tumor, or multiple sclerosis.

Diagnosis

Often Bell's palsy is a clinical diagnosis and no testing is needed. Diagnostic workup may be required if the diagnosis is uncertain. Laboratory studies are patient specific and may include serum blood sugar, A1C levels to evaluate for presence of hyperglycemia, Lyme titers to rule out Lyme disease,[4] ESR if generalized inflammation is suspected, or angiotensin-converting enzyme (ACE) levels to R/O sarcoid.

Imaging studies can include electromyography (EMG) to confirm nerve damage, and MRI/CT scanning of the head to rule out a mass. Invasive procedures such as a lumbar puncture may be required if the diagnosis of Guillain–Barré or multiple sclerosis is being considered.

Management

Treatment is initiated to prevent permanent nerve damage, involuntary contraction of facial muscles, and vision loss in affected eye.

Medical therapy:[5–7]
Initiated within three days of symptom onset:

- Steroid taper: 10-day tapering course starting with prednisone 60 mg each day × 5 days, then taper for the remaining 5 days (take with food);
- Antivirals: Valtrex 1 g three times daily × 7 days

Supportive therapies:

- Physical therapy: To minimize contractures

- Eye protection: Lubricating drops, ointments, glasses during the day, patching at night
- Facial exercises: To relax muscles

> **CLINICAL PEARL:** There is no evidence to support beginning treatment earlier than 4 days after the onset of symptoms.

REFERENCES

1. Tiemstra JD, Khatkhate N. Bell's palsy: diagnosis and management. *Am Fam Physician.* 2007;76:997–1004–1002.
2. Albers JR, Tamang S. Common questions about bell palsy. *Am Fam Physician.* February 1, 2014;89(3):209–212.
3. Morris AM, Deeks SL, Hill MD, et al. Annualized incidence and spectrum of illness from an outbreak investigation of Bell's palsy. *Neuroepidemiology.* 2002;21:255–261. doi:10.1159/000065645
4. Makeham TP, Croxson GR, Coulson S. Infective causes of facial nerve paralysis. *Otol Neurotol.* 2007;28:100–103. doi:10.1097/01.mao.0000232009.01116.3f
5. Grogan PM, Gronseth GS. Practice parameter: steroids, acyclovir, and surgery for Bell's palsy (an evidence-based review): report of the Quality Standards Subcommittee of the American Academy of Neurology. *Neurology.* 2001;56:830–836. doi:10.1212/WNL.56.7.830
6. Hato N, Yamada H, Kohno H, et al. Valacyclovir and prednisolone treatment for Bell's palsy: a multicenter, randomized, placebo-controlled study. *Otol Neurotol.* 2007;28:408–413. doi:10.1097/01.mao.0000265190.29969.12
7. Gronseth GS, Paduga R. Evidence-based guideline update: steroids and antivirals for Bell palsy: report of the guideline development subcommittee of the American Academy of Neurology. *Neurology.* 2012;79:2209–2213. doi:10.1212/WNL.0b013e318275978c. https://www.aan.com/Guidelines/home/GuidelineDetail/573. Accessed July 15, 2018

HEADACHE: PRIMARY

Etiology

The International Headache Society (IHS) classifies the cause of headaches into primary and secondary types. Primary headaches are those for which the headache itself is the core condition.[1] Secondary headaches are headaches that are caused by other underlying conditions.

The neurologic origin of migraine headache pain is thought to come from the brain stem and hypothalamus and involves the vasculature as well as several neurotransmitters.[2] Tension-type headaches (TTH) have a different pathogenesis, thought to arise only from changes in pain modulation.[2] Because the severity of headaches can range from a minor inconvenience to a life-threatening emergency, you must be knowledgeable about the varying types of headaches and vigilant when looking for red flags that indicate a more serious condition.

Epidemiology

Of the primary headache types, tension-type headache is most common (69%) and migraine headache is the next most common (16%).[1] Among the general population, 30% to 78% will experience a tension-type headache at some point in their lives.[1] Migraine prevalence is about 15% in women and 6% in men per year.[2]

Clinical Presentation

Migraine headaches generally are unilateral, throbbing and associated with nausea and/or vomiting, and photophobia. The pain is most commonly in the frontal or temporal areas. Migraine pain can be bilateral in children. Pain can last from 4 to 72 hours.[1] It is common for migraine headaches to be familial. They can occur with or without an aura. An aura is an experience of temporary neurological symptoms, commonly visual or sensory, that precede a headache and resolve completely. Triggers can often be identified for migraine headaches. Common triggers include hunger, stress, hormonal changes due to menstruation, changes in sleep patterns, and alcohol.[2] Often the physical examination is completely normal, and a detailed history can prove the diagnosis. The physical examination must rule out other, more dangerous, causes of headache. A complete neurologic examination is recommended in addition to the general physical exam.

TTH, sometimes referred to as tension headaches or muscular contraction headaches, are common. Patients may complain of pain, pressure, or tightness in any area of the head, which can last from <1 hour to days. Unlike migraine headaches, TTH are not associated with nausea and/or vomiting, or photophobia. The physical examination will most often be normal, but some tenderness to palpation of the head over the area of pain may be seen with this type of headache. If tenderness is noted over the temporal artery areas, you must be sure to rule out giant cell arteritis.

Diagnosis

The IHS outlines the following criteria for diagnosis of migraine and TTH:[1]

Migraine: At least five attacks of pain meeting the criteria below

- Duration from 4 to 72 hours without effective treatment
- Pain has at least two of these characteristics: unilateral; pulsing/throbbing; moderate to severe in intensity; aggravated by normal physical activity or causes avoidance of normal physical activity
- At least one of the following occurs: nausea/vomiting; both photophobia and phonophobia

Tension-type headache: At least 10 episodes of pain meeting the following criteria:

- Duration from 30 minutes to 7 days
- Pain has at least two of these characteristics: bilateral; pressing/tightening (nonpulsatile); mild or moderate intensity; not aggravated by routine physical activity
- No nausea or vomiting
- Can have either photophobia or phonophobia, but not both

Management

Migraine headaches represent a chronic condition, and although they can be managed, patients will commonly have lifelong recurrences. From a nonpharmacologic standpoint, general healthy behaviors surrounding sleep, hydration, physical activity, and alcohol can minimize occurrences. Avoiding known migraine triggers is also helpful. Treatment for migraines can be divided into two categories: abortive and prophylactic.

Acetaminophen and NSAIDS are recommended as first-line treatment for acute mild to moderate migraines.[3] Other abortive therapy options include triptans such as rizatriptan and sumatriptan for moderate to severe episodes. These medications should be taken early, at the first sign of migraine pain, to be most effective. Triptans are effective and generally safe, but may be costly. Triptans are not recommended for use in patients with a history of CAD. Although they may have some moderate effect on migraine pain, opioids are generally not recommended. In addition to abuse potential, they may also negatively impact receptors that can make treatment more difficult.[3] Consider prescribing antiemetics for patients with migraines, if indicated. Patients with frequent migraines may benefit from prophylactic medications to help prevent recurrence of migraines. Treatment summary is outlined in Table 2.50.

TABLE 2.50 Migraine Pharmacotherapy

Abortive Therapy	Prophylactic Therapy
NSAIDS	Beta blockers (i.e., metoprolol, propranolol)
Tylenol + ASA + caffeine	Antidepressants (i.e., amitriptyline, venlafaxine)
Triptans	Anticonvulsants (i.e., valpropic acid, topiramate)
Ergotamine	

ASA, aspirin; NSAIDS, nonsteroidal anti-inflammatory drugs.

TTH are treated with a combination of pharmacologic and nonpharmacologic approaches. The same general healthy behaviors endorsed for migraine headaches can also be effective for TTH. An emphasis on stress reduction and relaxation is important. Pharmacologic treatment with acetaminophen and/or NSAIDS is recommended. Amitriptyline may be effective for chronic TTH.[2]

REFERENCES

1. Headache Classification Committee of the International Headache Society (IHS). The international classification of headache disorders, 3rd edition. *Cephalgia.* 2018;38(1):1–211. doi:10.1177/0333102417738202.
2. Friedman BW. Migraine and other primary headache disorders. In: Rowe BH, ed. *Evidence-Based Emergency Medicine.* Hoboken, NJ: Wiley-Blackwell; 2009: 493–502.
3. Mayans L, Walling A. Acute migraine headache: treatment strategies. *Am Fam Physician.* 2018;97(4):243–251.

PSYCHIATRY/BEHAVIORAL SCIENCE

ANXIETY: GENERALIZED ANXIETY DISORDER

Etiology

Although all people experience anxiety, feeling worried, or nervous, an anxiety disorder occurs when this worry is out of proportion to events or persists beyond appropriate boundaries. Anxiety differs from a phobia in that a phobia is a fear of a specific entity such as an object or situation. Panic attacks are instances of acute anxiety and fear and are limited events that last up to several minutes and resolve. Generalized anxiety disorder (GAD) is a persistent pattern of anxiety or worry that is impacted by, and occurs in, multiple areas of a patient's life.

Epidemiology

It is estimated that GAD occurs in about 3% of the U.S. population, and is seen in 7% to 8% of patients presenting to primary care settings.[1] Anxiety disorders are twice as common in women than in men.[2] Although substance abuse may coexist in any patient with GAD, men are more likely to experience substance abuse as a comorbidity of GAD than are women. GAD is more commonly diagnosed in individuals of European descent and in people from developed countries. There is a genetic predisposition to GAD.

Clinical Presentation

In addition to the following symptoms discussed, patients may have physical and somatic symptoms of anxiety, such as myalgias, trembling, muscle tension, sleep disturbance, nausea, diarrhea, headaches, and IBS. At times, the physical symptoms may be the only ones noted by the patient and reported to the clinician.

CLINICAL PEARL: The predominance of type of symptoms, cognitive versus somatic, may vary depending on a patient's culture.

Diagnosis

GAD can be diagnosed at nearly any time in a patient's life. Often symptoms of an anxiety disorder begin in childhood and can persist into adulthood. The diagnosis of GAD should be made according to the 5th edition, *Diagnostic and Statistical Manual of Mental Disorders* (DSM-5).

Symptoms consistent with GAD include excessive, pervasive worry and anxiety that persists for months, in addition to feelings of restlessness, fatigue, irritability, impaired concentration, and sleep disturbances. These symptoms will cause significant disturbances in functioning, and you must exclude alcohol, drugs, and medications as a source.[3]

The evaluation of GAD should include consideration of other psychiatric disorders, as well as medical causes of the patient's symptoms. Additional disease states to consider are seen in Box 2.5. Patients with GAD should also be screened regularly for substance abuse, depression, and suicidality. The GAD-7 is a seven-question scoring instrument that can be used to confirm the diagnosis of GAD and assess its severity.[1]

> **Box 2.5** Differential diagnoses of generalized anxiety disorder
>
> | **Medical differential diagnoses** |
> |---|
> | Hyperthyroidism |
> | Drug-induced, including caffeine |
> | Arrhythmia |
> | Pheochromoctytoma |
> | Hyperparathyroidism |
> | Temporal lobe epilepsy |
> | **Psychiatric differential diagnoses** |
> | Social anxiety disorder |
> | Illness anxiety disorder ("hypochondriasis") |
> | Posttraumatic stress disorder |
> | Adjustment disorder |

Management

The most successful treatment for GAD stems from a multifaceted approach.

LIFESTYLE RECOMMENDATIONS

- Educate the patient on the diagnosis and direct them to appropriate patient-oriented literature or other mediums[1]
- Encourage the patient to involve loved ones in their treatment as appropriate
- Limit or avoid stimulants such as tobacco and caffeine
- Appropriate sleep hygiene practices
- Regular physical activity

NONPHARMACOLOGIC TREATMENT

- Cognitive behavioral therapy[1]
  - First-line nonpharmacologic therapy
  - Can be individual, group, or computer based
- Mindfulness
- Applied relaxation therapies

PHARMACOLOGIC TREATMENT

The first-line pharmacologic treatment for GAD includes SSRIs and SNRIs. These medications generally achieve full effect after 4 to 6 weeks of treatment and should be continued for approximately 1 year before considering discontinuation.

Benzodiazepines also carry an indication for the treatment of GAD. These medications, however, have abuse potential, and you should therefore give careful consideration before prescribing benzodiazepines for anxiety. If they are used, the patient should be educated appropriately on the risk of abuse and dependence and there should be clear boundaries set regarding appropriate use and the duration of use. Generally, they are only recommended for a maximum duration of 3 to 6 months, and they are not a suitable long-term treatment.[1] Benzodiazepine use is contraindicated in a patient with a history of substance abuse.[1] They are inappropriate for elderly patients due to the risk of drug interactions and their sedating effects, which can increase the risk of altered consciousness and falls. Table 2.51 lists common medications used to treat anxiety.

TABLE 2.51 Medications Used to Treat Anxiety

Drug Class	Common Drug Names	Possible Adverse Effects
SSRIs	Citalopram, escitalopram, paroxetine, sertraline	Nausea, insomnia/somnolence, sexual dysfunction, headache, weight gain
SNRIs	Duloxetine, venlafaxine	Nausea, insomnia/somnolence, sexual dysfunction, headache, weight gain, hypertension
Benzodiazepines	Alprazolam, clonazepam, diazepam, lorazepam	Dizziness, somnolence

SNRIs, serotonin-norepinephrine reuptake inhibitors; SSRIs, selective serotonine reuptake inhibitors.
Sources: Stein MB, Sareen J. Generalized anxiety disorder. *N Eng J Med.* 2015;373:2059–2068; Locke AB, Kirst N, Shultz, CG. Diagnosis and management of generalized anxiety disorder and panic disorder in adults. *Am Fam Physician.* 2015;91:617–624.

CLINICAL PEARL: Children and adolescents who may benefit from pharmacologic treatment for GAD should be referred to psychiatry or a clinician with training and experience with pediatric psychiatry.

REFERENCES

1. Stein MB, Sareen J. Generalized anxiety disorder. *N Eng J Med.* 2015;373:2059–2068. doi:10.1056/NEJMcp1502514
2. Locke AB, Kirst N, Shultz CG. Diagnosis and management of generalized anxiety disorder and panic disorder in adults. *Am Fam Physician.* 2015;91:617–624.
3. American Psychiatric Association, American Psychiatric Association. DSM-5 Task Force. *Diagnostic and Statistical Manual of Mental Disorders: DSM-5.* 5th ed. Arlington, VA: Author; 2013.

ATTENTION DEFICIT HYPERACTIVITY DISORDER

Etiology

Attention deficit hyperactivity disorder (ADHD) is a neurodevelopmental disorder with an onset in childhood. Although the exact pathology is unknown, several genes, dopamine, serotonin, and impairment in connections of frontal-to-parietal structures are thought to play a role.[1] The intersection of environmental factors and genetic predisposition may increase a child's risk of developing ADHD.[2] Although ADHD can persist into adulthood, this section focuses on the pediatric and adolescent populations.

Epidemiology

The prevalence of ADHD in children and adolescents in the United States is estimated to be between 8% and 11%.[1,3,4] This condition is more common in men than in women and is highly heritable.[2]

Clinical Presentation

The cardinal symptoms of ADHD are inattention, hyperactivity, and/or impulsivity. These behaviors impact family relationships, friendships, and school performance. The presentation in children may be more inattentive or more hyperactive/impulsive. Parents may bring the concern for this condition to an office visit or, more often, it is noticed in school settings prompting teachers to contact parents with the concern. Common symptoms include seeming to not pay attention, constant movement, difficulty taking turns, interrupting conversations, or seeming to be careless or disorganized. If it is not recognized that these behaviors are stemming from a neurodevelopmental condition, essentially a medical problem, children can be disciplined harshly or be criticized frequently. Sometimes parents, teachers, or caregivers will mistakenly think these behaviors are ones that can be easily controlled by the child.

Diagnosis

ADHD can be diagnosed as early as 4 years old.[4] The diagnosis is made clinically and based on *DSM-5* criteria. It is important to solicit input from parents, teachers, and caregivers when determining whether sufficient diagnostic criteria are present. Children with ADHD will uniformly have some degree of inattention with or without hyperactivity that is pervasive and limits their ability to function in work or at school. Additional common symptoms include lack of organization and appropriate attention span, forgetfulness, failure to listen when spoken to, inability to follow through on tasks, and easy distractibility. Symptoms of increased activity can include excessive talking, inability to sit still or wait for a turn, frequent interruptions of others, and difficulty remaining seated. Be sure to inquire about the presence of symptoms before the age of 12, as is characteristic of this condition.[2]

The differential diagnosis of ADHD includes[2] the following:

- Oppositional defiant disorder (ODD)
- Intermittent explosive disorder
- Autism spectrum disorder
- A learning disorder—such as dyslexia
- Intellectual disability
- Mood disorder (anxiety, depression, bipolar)
- Personality disorder

CLINICAL PEARL: Although several of the differential diagnoses above can coexist with ADHD, it is important to know which is predominant. In these cases, referral to psychiatry is indicated.

Management

Successful treatment of ADHD minimizes symptoms, mitigates functional/relationship/social difficulties, and can improve school performance. The most successful management plans involve a team approach, including the clinician, parents/guardians, and teachers. Additional support in the academic setting can come in the form of educational accommodations, which can be outlined in a 504 plan or Individualized Education Plan (IEP).

Pharmacologic and nonpharmacologic treatments are available for ADHD, and the combination of both results in better outcomes.[3] A referral for behavioral therapy is indicated and will assist parents, caregivers, and teachers with developing structures and strategies to support children with ADHD. Pharmacologic therapy can be beneficial. The decision to medicate children on nonschool days (weekends, holiday breaks, summers) should be individualized and informed by input from the clinician, parents, and the therapist.

Pharmacologic Treatment Options for ADHD[1]
Amphetamine stimulants:

- Mixed amphetamine salts (e.g., amphetamine and dextroamphetamine)
- Dextroamphetamine

Methylphenidate stimulants:

- Methylphenidate (e.g., methylphenidate hydrochloride, methylphenidate)
- Dexmethylphenidate (e.g., dexmethylphenidate hydrochloride)

Norepinephrine-reuptake inhibitors:

- Atomoxetine

You should pay particular attention to the duration of action of each medication in order to provide adequate coverage for the school day and homework or activities in the evening, but not interfere with sleep onset. Dosing frequency is also important; long-acting agents may be preferred to avoid the need for dosing during the school day.

Prior to beginning therapy with stimulant medications, inquire about the patient's and family's history of cardiovascular disease, syncope, and sudden cardiac death.[1] Patients who have neurologic tics may experience an increase in these symptoms when taking these medications. Common side effects of ADHD medications include appetite suppression (weight should be monitored), headache, delayed onset of sleep, and nausea.[1] Side effects that are less common but potentially more serious include increased BP, elevated heart rate, anxiety, and slowed rate of growth.[1] For atomoxetine, less common side effects can include liver abnormalities and suicidal ideation.[1]

After starting pharmacologic treatment, regular monitoring is recommended, with the initial follow-up appointment 1 month after initiating the medication.[1] Subsequent visits can be every 1 to 3 months thereafter and should include an evaluation of symptoms, height, weight, BP, and mood.[1]

References

1. Feldman HM, Reiff MI. Attention deficit–hyperactivity disorder in children and adolescents. *N Eng J Med.* 2014;370:838–846. doi:10.1056/NEJMcp1307215
2. American Psychiatric Association, American Psychiatric Association. DSM-5 Task Force. *Diagnostic and Statistical Manual of Mental Disorders: DSM-5.* 5th ed. Arlington, VA: Author; 2013.

3. Felt BT, Biermann B, Christner JG, et al. Diagnosis and management of ADHD in children. *Am Fam Physician.* 2014;90:456–464.
4. Sonnack M, Brenneman A. Treatment strategies for ADHD in preschool and school-age children. *J Am Acad Physician Assist.* 2014;27:22–26. doi:10.1097/01.JAA.0000453859.08958.31

DEPRESSION: MAJOR DEPRESSIVE DISORDER

Etiology

Major depressive disorder is often a chronic condition and relapses are common. Although not completely understood, the neurotransmitters serotonin, norepinephrine, dopamine, and GABA, in addition to changes in the hypothalamic–pituitary–adrenal axis and other factors, seem to have a role in the disease.

Epidemiology

Risk factors for depression include genetics, low self-esteem, trauma during childhood, and lack of social support.[1] Depression is more common in those with medical comorbidities such as neurologic disorders, cardiac disease, DM, vitamin D deficiency, IBS, and neoplastic syndromes. Those at greatest risk for major depressive disorder include women, people aged 18 to 44 years, those with a family history of depression, and those who are separated or divorced. Depression is one of the leading causes of disability in adults. There is a significant personal and public burden associated with depression. All adolescents and adults should be screened for depression in the primary care setting.

Clinical Presentation

Patients with major depressive disorder will experience symptoms every day for most of the day. Although some patients may present with awareness of their cognitive symptoms of depression, others may present instead with somatic symptoms such as fatigue or sleep problems. The key symptom is either depressed mood or anhedonia. Appetite problems, psychomotor agitation or slowing, difficulty making decisions, weight changes, and changes in bowel habits are often present. Many people also feel guilt or worthlessness. Other symptoms include problems with concentration or attention which may lead to difficulties at school or work.

All patients with depressive symptoms should be screened for suicidality.[1,2] Patients with depression may experience passive thoughts of suicide or may have true suicidal ideation with intent and a plan. Patients with depression should always be considered to be at risk for suicide.[1,2] Men, single people, and those who live alone or have strong feelings of hopelessness have increased risk.[2] Those who have attempted suicide in the past, or who have made threats of suicide, are also at significant risk.[1,2]

Diagnosis

Screening tools that can be used for depression include the Patient Health Questionnaire-9 (PHQ-9), Beck Depression Inventory, and the Hamilton Depression Rating Scale. The diagnosis of major depressive disorder should be made according to the *DSM-5*.

The most significant symptoms that suggest major depressive disorder (MDD) include depressed mood and/or loss of interest. Other supporting symptoms include significant changes in interest of pleasure in activities, changes in sleep patterns, fatigue, feelings of worthlessness or guilt, trouble concentrating, and recurrent thoughts of death including suicidal ideations. These symptoms typically cause significant problems in day-to-day functioning and are not due to another cause such as medications or a coexisting medical condition. Manifestations are pervasive, occurring over the majority of a 2-week period.[1] Alternative diagnoses to consider are seen in Box 2.6.

Box 2.6 Differential diagnosis of major depressive disorder

Differential Diagnoses

Attention deficit hyperactivity disorder
Depressive disorder due to a medical condition
Bipolar disorder
Adjustment disorder
Substance-/medication-induced depressive disorder
Neurocognitive disorder

CLINICAL PEARL: Consider substance use disorders as a potential comorbidity.

Management

- Nonpharmacologic treatment
  - Psychotherapy should be recommended to all patients with major depressive disorder. Cognitive behavioral therapy is most common, but there are several other types of therapy available. Patients may also benefit from family and/or couples' counseling as well. Relaxation techniques, mindfulness, and exercise may also help mitigate the symptoms of depression.
- Pharmacologic treatment
  - Antidepressants are more effective than placebo in treating symptoms of depression. SSRIs and SNRIs are most commonly used as first-line pharmacologic therapy for major depressive disorder (see Table 2.52). The choice of which medication to use should be based on the side effects profile, cost, and patient preference. These medications take 4 to 6 weeks to have a full effect, and should be continued for at least one year. The most common reason patients discontinue medication for depression is due to an adverse effect.

TABLE **2.52** Medications Used to Treat Major Depressive Disorder

Drug Class	Common Drug Names	Possible Adverse Effects
SSRIs	Citalopram, escitalopram, fluoxetine, paroxetine, sertraline	Nausea, insomnia/somnolence, sexual dysfunction, headache, weight gain
SNRIs	Duloxetine, venlafaxine	Nausea, insomnia/somnolence, sexual dysfunction, headache, weight gain, hypertension
Dopamine/norepinephrine agonist	Bupropion	Agitation, GI upset, hypertension
Tricyclic antidepressants	Amitriptyline, imipramine, nortriptyline	Anticholinergic effects, sedation, weight gain

GI, gastrointestinal; SNRIs, serotonin-norepinephrine reuptake inhibitors; SSRIs, selective serotonin reuptake inhibitors;

Source: Kovich H, Dejong A. Common questions about the pharmacologic management of depression in adults. *Am Fam Physician.* 2015;92:94–100.

> **CLINICAL PEARL:** Serotonin syndrome is characterized by tremor, delirium, neuromuscular rigidity, and hyperthermia. It is a serious condition that can occur with SSRI/SNRI overdose or when other medications are combined with these antidepressants.

> **CLINICAL PEARL:** Patients who are have suicidal ideation, suicide attempts, or who are suspected of having bipolar disorder should be referred to psychiatry for evaluation and treatment.

REFERENCES

1. American Psychiatric Association, American Psychiatric Association. DSM-5 Task Force. *Diagnostic and Statistical Manual of Mental Disorders: DSM-5.* 5th ed. Arlington, VA: Author; 2013.
2. Bono V, Amendola CL. Primary care assessment of patients at risk for suicide. *J Am Acad Physician Assist.* 2015;28:35–39. doi:10.1097/01.JAA.0000473360.07845.66.

INSOMNIA

Etiology

Inadequate or poor-quality sleep can be a significant issue in a patient's life leading to difficulties with mood, work performance, and attention, as well as contribute to health problems like obesity, HTN, diabetes, and cardiovascular disease. Hyperarousal is thought to be a cause of insomnia, with many patients reporting worry or racing thoughts interfering with sleep.[1] Hyperarousal can also lead to excessive cortisol levels and elevated BP.[1]

Epidemiology

Insomnia is the most common of all the sleep-related disorders and may exist in up to 15% of the population.[2] It occurs more often in women, in those who have disabilities, and those who are shift workers. Half of patients who have insomnia also have another psychiatric diagnosis such as a mood disorder.[1] People who have insomnia are more likely to develop major depressive disorder.

Clinical Presentation

People with insomnia generally report trouble initiating sleep, maintaining sleep, or returning to sleep after waking earlier than desired. Difficulty maintaining sleep is the most commonly experienced feature. The symptoms must occur regularly for at least 3 months to meet diagnostic criteria.[2] Patients also experience the effects of insomnia during the daytime as well, reporting fatigue or problems with performance, concentration, and/or memory.[3] Patients may also develop unhealthy patterns and behaviors related to sleep due to their efforts to correct the insomnia, including alcohol use as means of self-medication.

Diagnosis

Patients with insomnia report dissatisfaction with either falling asleep, staying asleep, or waking too early. Sleep disturbences results in impairments in other areas of life such as school or work. These symptoms occur often during the week and this pattern lasts months at a time or more. Similar to with other behavioral medicine disorders, you must rule out medications, substances, and comorbid conditions as a cause.[2] Consider differential diagnoses, as seen in Box 2.7, as potential causes of sleep-related complaints.

Box 2.7 Differential diagnoses of insomnia disorder

Restless leg syndrome
Narcolepsy
Major depressive disorder
Situational insomnia
Substance/medication-induced sleep disorder
Obstructive sleep apnea
Generalized anxiety disorder
Normal sleep variation

CLINICAL PEARL: Polysomnography is generally not recommended as a diagnostic study for insomnia disorder unless you suspect sleep apnea, restless leg syndrome, or another sleep-related disorder as the cause of the patient's symptoms.[1]

Management

Nonpharmacologic treatment modalities are recommended as first-line therapies for those with insomnia. Pharmacologic therapy carries the risk of adverse drug effects and is only effective when drugs are used. The effects of lifestyle changes and other nonpharmacologic treatments can have longer lasting and farther-reaching effects contributing to a patient's overall wellness.[4]

NONPHARMACOLOGIC TREATMENT

- Sleep restriction: Limit time in bed to time spent sleeping[4]
- Stimulus control: Only go to bed when actually sleepy and avoid doing other activities such as watching television or reading in bed. If unable to fall asleep after 20 minutes, leave the bedroom; wake at the same time every morning regardless of how much sleep was had the night before; avoid napping
- Sleep hygiene practices: Maintain a regular sleep schedule; keep the bedroom dark and quiet; avoid stimulants such as caffeine; do not eat before bed; exercise regularly; and avoid screens and bright lights before bed
- Cognitive behavioral therapy: Highly recommended and well studied; refer for the specific subtype of cognitive behavioral therapy (CBT) for insomnia
- Relaxation training: These techniques may include breathing exercises, muscle contraction/relaxation, or mindfulness.

PHARMACOLOGIC TREATMENT

Pharmacologic treatment options, as seen in Table 2.53, should be tailored to individual needs and based on the safety profile of each medication. Patients should be counseled on the effects and precautions with these medications. If the initial choice of treatment is ineffective, you may try a different drug in the same class, or try a different class of medication. Patients with sleep-disordered breathing or hypoxia due to lung disease should be evaluated by a sleep medicine specialist before prescribing sedating medications.

TABLE 2.53 Pharmacologic Treatment of Insomnia

Drug Class/Names	Effects/Adverse Effects	Comments
Benzodiazepines quazepam temazepam triazolam	Sedation Decreased anxiety Muscle relaxation Retrograde amnesia Caution in hepatic/renal impairment	Promotes sleep onset and maintenance Schedule IV medications Vary in onset and duration; be attentive to this May negatively impact sleep quality Not recommended for geriatric patients Significant risk for physical dependence and rebound insomnia after cessation

(continued)

TABLE 2.53 Pharmacologic Treatment of Insomnia (*continued*)

Drug Class/Names	Effects/Adverse Effects	Comments
Z-drugs *eszopiclone* *zaleplon* *zolpidem*	Dizziness Disinhibition GI upset Hallucinations Somnambulism *These effects can be dose dependent*	Some promote sleep onset and some promote sleep onset and maintenance Schedule IV medications Counsel patients about the possibility of somnambulism
Melatonin agonists *Rozerem*	Dizziness Dysgeusia	Promotes sleep onset
Tricyclic antidepressants *doxepin*	Anticholinergic effects—avoid in patients with urinary retention or glaucoma Potentiates the effects of alcohol	Only one medication in this class is FDA approved for insomnia; others are used off-label Promotes sleep maintenance
Antihistamines *diphenhydramine* *doxylamine*	Anticholinergic effects—avoid in patients with urinary retention or glaucoma	Available over the counter Recommended only for insomnia that is pregnancy related
Orexin receptor antagonists *suvorexant*	Daytime drowsiness	Promotes sleep onset and maintenance Schedule IV medication High cost Not first line

FDA, Food and Drug Administration; IV, intravenous.

CLINICAL PEARL: Melatonin, purchased OTC, may be as effective for insomnia as some prescription medications. However, it is not FDA-regulated so quality and purity may vary among brands.

REFERENCES

1. Winkelman JW. Insomnia Disorder. *N Eng J Med.* 2015;373:1437–1444. doi:10.1056/NEJMcp1412740
2. American Psychiatric Association, American Psychiatric Association. DSM-5 Task Force. *Diagnostic and Statistical Manual of Mental Disorders: DSM-5.* 5th ed. Arlington, VA: Author; 2013.
3. Maness DL, Khan M. Nonpharmacologic management of chronic insomnia. *Am Fam Physician.* 2015;92:1058–1064.
4. Taylor K, Bilan N, Tsytsyna N, et al. A nonpharmacologic approach to managing insomnia in primary care. *J Am Acad Physician Assist.* 2017;30:10–15. doi:10.1097/01.JAA.0000525905.52107.20

Pulmonary System

Asthma

Etiology

Asthma is an obstructive airway disease characterized the following triad:

- Chronic airway inflammation
- Bronchial hyperreactivity
- Obstruction of airflow that can be reversible by bronchodilators

The inflammation leads to airway narrowing and increased mucus production. Asthma can be both intrinsic (nonallergic) and extrinsic (allergic). Most of the cases are extrinsic, in which symptoms are triggered by an allergic reaction. In extrinsic asthma, patients produce immunoglobulin E (IgE) to environmental antigens, such as pollen, house dust, mold, animals, infections, cold air, smoke, medications, and exercise.[1] This type of asthma may be associated with atopy and eczema, and this constellation of symptoms is generally present at a young age.

Epidemiology

Asthma affects about 8% of the U.S. population and can be as high as 11% among low-income communities. The incidence is increasing. According to the CDC, one in 12 people had asthma in 2009, compared with 1 in 14 in 2001.[2] Asthma tends to be more prevalent in the 5- to 19-year-olds age group, but can begin at any age.[3,4] Children in the Western world are more likely to develop asthma than children born outside the Western world.[5]

Clinical Presentation

The common signs and symptoms include cough, dyspnea, chest tightness, and expiratory wheezing. The severity of these symptoms may vary but are typically worse at night. Patients with an acute asthma exacerbation may have tachycardia, tachypnea, diffuse wheezing, use of accessory muscles, and intercostal retractions. On physical examination, the most common finding is wheezing, but not all wheezes are due to asthma.

Intrinsic asthma is less likely to be related to environmental triggers or atopy, but is suggested by the presence of nasal polyps and diminished forced expiratory volume in one second (FEV_1) by spirometry, and tends to present after childhood.

Diagnosis

The diagnosis is made based on clinical and laboratory findings. Key elements of the history when diagnosing asthma should include specific details on history of wheezing, shortness of breath, cough frequency, and character of sputum. Ask about alleviating/exacerbating symptoms such as exercise. A chronic night cough lasting several months may be the only symptom. You should also ask about risk factors such as smoking exposure and personal and family history of asthma. A thorough lung examination for wheezing, prolonged expiration, increased resonance to percussion, and flattened diaphragm should be conducted.

You can distinguish nonallergic asthma from allergic based on negative skin tests to the typical allergens. A positive skin test shows a tendency to produce IgE antibodies in response to low doses of allergens, predisposing to atopy.

Pulmonary function tests may show a decreased FEV_1 or may be normal in asthma patients. An increase in FEV_1 of at least 12% after bronchodilator therapy supports a diagnosis of asthma. Peak expiratory flow rate is also used to measure air flow obstruction. Patients can use peak flow meters at home to monitor their asthma control, and readings should be compared to their baseline.[5-8]

- Normal range is about 450 to 650 L/min (men) and 350 to 500 L/min (women)
- Mild obstruction is >300 L/min
- Moderate to severe obstruction is >100 to 300 L/min
- Severe obstruction is <100 L/min.

CXRmay show hyperinflation and ABG studies may show respiratory alkalosis, hypoxemia, and metabolic acidosis.

Management

The goal of treatment is to minimize chronic symptoms, prevent attacks, and improve quality of life. The following components of asthma management have been recommended by the National Heart, Lung, and Blood Institute Expert Panel.[6]

- Manage/avoid triggers and other factors that contribute to asthma severity
- Objective measurement of lung function for diagnosis, severity classification, and assessing response to therapy
- Utilize pharmacology therapy to control lung inflammation
- Patient education and partnership in asthma care.

Asthma should be managed as a chronic disease. Self-management is critical for long-term success. An asthma action plan is an important component of self-management, and you should provide a written set of instructions for the patient to follow.[6]

Medications

Various drugs used in asthma fall in one these categories: bronchodilators, inhaled corticosteroids, and anticholinergics. Treatment is governed by severity of disease, which is determined based on patient symptoms and the results of testing. Medication options are outlined in Table 2.54.

- Inhaled beta-2 agonists are available as:
  - Short-acting beta-2 agonists (SABA) such as albuterol, which are often used for rescue acute attacks
  - Long-acting beta-2 agonists (LABA) such as salmeterol, generally used to prevent nighttime symptoms
- Inhaled corticosteroid (ICS) for moderate to severe asthma
- Montelukast-leukotriene modifiers
- Cromolyn sodium

TABLE **2.54** Asthma Classification and Recommended Medication in Adults

Severity Classification	Symptoms/Spirometry Findings	Asthma Medications for Adults
Intermittent	**Symptoms** Daytime symptoms ≤ twice a week Night symptoms ≤ twice a month No interference with normal activity **Lung function** FEV_1 is normal FEV_1/FVC is normal (≥85%)	SABA as needed
Mild persistent	**Symptoms** Daytime symptoms >twice a week Night symptoms three to four times a month Minor limitation in normal activity **Lung function** FEV_1 is ≥80% FEV_1/FVC is normal ((≥ 80%)	Low- to medium-dose ICS
Moderate persistent	**Symptoms** Daily daytime symptoms Daily use of inhaled beta-2 agonists Night symptoms >once a week but not nightly Some limitation in normal activity **Lung function** FEV_1 is 60%–80% FEV_1/FVC is reduced 5%	Medium-dose ICS + LABA Alternatives: Medium-dose ICS + montelukast sodium High-dose ICS + LABA or montelukast sodium
Severe persistent	**Symptoms** Continued daytime symptoms Frequent night symptoms Extremely limited activity **Lung function** FEV_1 is <60% FEV_1/FVC is reduced >5%	High-dose ICS + LABA + oral corticosteroid AND consider omalizumab for patients who have allergies (elevated IgE)

FEV_1, forced expiratory volume in one second; FEV_1/FVC, ratio of a timed forced expiratory volume to the forced vital capacity; ICS, inhaled corticosteroid; LABA, long-acting beta-2 agonists; SABA, short-acting beta-2 agonists.

REFERENCES

1. Asthma and Allergy Foundation of America. http://www.aafa-md.org/asthma_basics.htm.
2. Centers for Disease Control and Prevention. Asthma in the US. https://www.cdc.gov/vitalsigns/asthma/index.html
3. Ziyab AH, Abul AT. Trends in asthma hospital admissions and mortality in Kuwait, 2000-2014: a national retrospective observational study. *BMJ Open.* 2018;8(5):e021244. doi:10.1136/bmjopen-2017-021244
4. Akinbami LJ, Bailey CM, Johnson CA, et al. Trends in asthma prevalence, health care use, and mortality in the United States, 2001–2010. *NCHS Data Brief.* 2012;94:1–8.
5. Sloane PD. *Essentials of Family Medicine.* Philadelphia, PA: Lippincott Williams & Wilkins; 2008.

6. National Asthma Education, Prevention, Program (National Heart, Lung, & Blood Institute). Second Expert Panel on the Management of Asthma. *Guidelines for the Diagnosis and Management of Asthma (No. 90)*. DIANE Publishing; 1997.

7. Asthma care quick reference (National Heart, Lung, & Blood Institute). https://www.nhlbi.nih.gov/files/docs/guidelines/asthma_qrg.pdf

8. Richter DC, Joubert JR, Nell H, et al. Diagnostic value of post-bronchodilator pulmonary function testing to distinguish between stable, moderate to severe COPD and asthma. *Int J Chronic Obstruct Pulm Dis*. 2008;3(4):693. doi:10.2147/COPD.S948

CHRONIC OBSTRUCTIVE PULMONARY DISEASE

Etiology

COPD is a common, preventable, and treatable disease that is characterized by persistent respiratory symptoms and airflow limitation that is due to airway and/or alveolar abnormalities usually caused by significant exposure to noxious particles or gases.[1,2]. Tobacco smoking is the main risk factor for COPD, but other environmental exposures such as biomass fuel exposure and air pollution may contribute. Host factors such as genetic makeup, abnormal lung development, and accelerated aging also predispose individuals to develop COPD.

COPD presents in two forms: chronic bronchitis and emphysema. Chronic bronchitis is characterized by excessive secretion of bronchial mucus with a productive cough that lasts for three months or more per year for at least 2 consecutive years, with no other disease that might account for these symptoms. Emphysema is characterized by abnormal permanent enlargement of air spaces distal to the terminal bronchioles, accompanied by the destruction of alveolar walls and without obvious fibrosis.

Epidemiology

COPD is among the leading causes of morbidity and mortality worldwide. The estimated global prevalence is approximately 11.7% and is expected to rise over the next 30 years due to continued exposure to COPD risk factors and aging of the population.[1-5]

> **CLINICAL PEARL:** COPD is more prevalent in smokers and ex-smokers compared to nonsmokers. It often manifests in patients who are ≥40 years and tends to be more prevalent in men than women. In countries where the major risk factor is biomass smoke, COPD starts early in life and may be more prevalent in women.

Clinical Presentation

The most common respiratory symptoms include dyspnea, cough, and/or sputum production (Box 2.8). Clinical features are similar to other cardiopulmonary diseases (Box 2.9), and therefore a thorough history and physical examination should be performed in order to rule out concomitant disorders. COPD may be punctuated by periods of acute worsening of respiratory symptoms, called exacerbations.

Box 2.8 Features suggestive of COPD

- Mid-life onset
- Slowly progressive
- History of tobacco/smoke
- Productive cough, exertional dyspnea, fatigue, rhonchi/wheezing, central cyanosis, hypoxia,
- Weight loss, tripod position, severe dyspnea, minimal to no cough, increased AP chest diameter, hyperresonance, decreased air movement, and decreased breath
- Dyspnea that is progressive over time, worse with exercise, or persistent
- Chronic cough: Intermittent /may be unproductive
- Recurrent wheeze
- Chronic sputum production
- Recurrent lower respiratory infections
- Risk factors: Genetics, smoking, or cooking with biomass fuels; pollutants
- Family history of COPD, child hood factors such as low birth weight or infections

COPD, chronic obstructive pulmonary disease.

Box 2.9 Differential diagnosis of COPD

- Asthma
  - Early onset, symptoms vary widely from day to day
  - Symptoms worse at night/early morning
  - Often associated with allergy, rhinitis, eczema
- COPD
  - Mid-life onset
  - Slowly progressive
  - Hx tobacco/smoke
- Infection (TB)
  - Chest x-ray shows infiltrate
  - High local TB prevalence
- HF
  - Chest x-ray shows dilated heart
  - Pulmonary edema
  - PFT = volume restriction not obstruction
- Bronchiectasis
  - Large volume of purulent sputum
  - Associated with bacterial infection
  - Chest x-ray shows bronchial dilation, bronchial wall thickening

- Other intrathoracic conditions
  - Lung cancer
  - Interstitial lung disease
  - Cystic fibrosis
  - Idiopathic cough
- Other extrathoracic conditions
  - Medications (e.g., ACE inhibitors)
  - Chronic allergic rhinitis
  - Postnasal drip syndrome
  - GERD

ACE, angiotensin-converting enzyme; COPD, chronic obstructive pulmonary disease; GERD, gastroesophageal reflux disease; HF, heart failure; PFT, pulmonary function test; TB, tuberculosis

A thorough and focused history is essential for discerning between COPD and other pulmonary diseases. The key history components that are critical in making a diagnosis include dyspnea, cough, onset and duration, pattern of symptom development, duration and timing of symptoms, associated symptoms, and presence or absence of risk factors. COPD symptoms often start in the fourth decade of life. Patients often complain of fatigue and decreased exercise tolerance. Inquire about a family history of COPD.

A focused and thorough physical examination, particularly of the lungs, is indicated in narrowing down the differential diagnosis. Note the general appearance, body habitus, sitting position, breathing patterns, and skin/mucus membrane color. Chronic bronchitis patients (blue bloater) are often obese, cough productively, wheeze, display exertional dyspnea and hypoxia, and may have central cyanosis. Emphysema patients (pink puffers) typically present with weight loss, tripod position, severe dyspnea, minimal to no cough, increased AP chest diameter, hyperresonance, decreased air movement, and decreased breath. A thorough cardiac exam should be performed to rule out HF.

CLINICAL PEARL: Differentiating Asthma from COPD can be difficult. They can both have wheezing and cough, and are both obstructive diseases. Airflow limitation is reversible in asthma but not in COPD. The persistent and chronic progressive nature of COPD is also helpful in differentiating the two conditions.

Diagnosis

COPD should be suspected in any patient with dyspnea, chronic cough, sputum production, and/or history of risk factor exposure. The dyspnea in COPD is often progressive over time, persistent, and worse with exercise. The cough is chronic, intermittent, and may be productive or unproductive. Depending on the subtype of COPD (chronic bronchitis vs. emphysema), the predominant symptoms and signs may vary. Spirometry is required to make a definitive diagnosis.

Common diagnostic studies include the following:

- PFTs: Evaluate for obstructive pattern with reduced FEV1/FVC
- ABG: May be consistent with hypoxemia, hypercarbia
- CBC: Polycythemia may be present
- EKG: May show right axis deviation, right ventricular hypertrophy
- CXR: Increased vascular markings; bronchiectasis may be present

Making the diagnosis requires a combination of pertinent findings from the history, physical, and spirometry data.

The GOLD Criteria for COPD Diagnosis

- A postbronchodilator FEV1/FVC ratio of <0.70 is considered diagnostic for COPD.[4]
- The Global Initiative for Chronic Obstructive Lung Disease (GOLD) system categorizes airflow limitation into stages
  - ○ Stage I: Mild COPD, FEV_1/FVC <0.70, FEV_1 ≥80%
  - ○ Stage II: Moderate COPD, FEV_1/FVC <0.70, FEV_1 50% to 79%
  - ○ Stage III: Severe COPD, FEV_1/FVC <0.70, FEV_1 30% to 49%
  - ○ Stage IV: Very severe COPD, FEV_1/FVC <0.70, FEV_1 <30% or <50% with chronic respiratory failure present. Chronic respiratory failure is defined as PaO_2 <60 mmHg or $PaCO_2$ >50 mmHg while breathing air at sea level

While airflow limitation staging is still performed as a predictor of mortality and to determine nonpharmacological treatment options, the main focus for medical treatment is now based on degree of dyspnea and exacerbation history. The new GOLD Criteria, updated in 2018, employs an ABCD scale based on dyspnea and exacerbations rather than airflow limitation (FEV_1 values) to guide treatment. Exacerbation history and dyspnea levels have a stronger correlation to functional limitations and quality of life.

Patients with obstructive lung disease and limited symptoms and exacerbations over the past year are placed into Group A. If more symptomatic (more short of breath than people of the same age, or need to stop when walking at own pace on level ground), but fewer than two exacerbations and none that lead to hospitalizations, the patient is classified as a Group B patient. When two or more exacerbations are present over the last year, the patient is elevated to either a Group C or D assignment depending on the degree of symptoms. Group C is for less symptomatic patients and Group D for patients who are more short of breath than people of the same age or need to stop when walking on level ground at own pace.

Management of Stable COPD

Management of COPD requires both pharmacologic and nonpharmacologic approaches to reduce symptoms, treat comorbidities, prevent exacerbation, and improve quality of life.[3] Patients should be managed according to the their exacerbation history over the past year and level of dyspnea. An overview of COPD medications can be found in Appendix C, Asthma and Chronic Obstructive Pulmonary Disease Inhalation Formulations.[4]

Group A: (All groups must have confirmed obstructive patterns on PFT [FEV_1/FVC ratio <70%])

- Smoking cessation
- Vaccinations (influenza and pneumococcal)
- A bronchodilator (SABA or LABA) versus long-acting muscarinic antagonists (LAMA)

Group B:
- All of the abovementioned plus
- Begin with a bronchodilator (LAMA or LABA) and add on to create a LAMA + LABA if persistent symptoms
- Pulmonary rehabilitation

Group C:
- Begin with a LAMA and add a LABA if further exacerbations. Consider a LABA and ICS if the patient has asthma or elevated eosinophil levels
- Oxygen if needed (PaO_2 <55 mmHg or SaO_2 <88%)

Group D:
- Begin with a LAMA + LABA and add an ICS if further exacerbations. If exacerbations persist, consider the addition of roflumilast (FEV_1 <50% predicted and chronic bronchitis) or daily macrolide therapy
- Consider surgical treatment

> **CLINICAL PEARL:** Each pharmacologic treatment regimen should be individualized and guided by the severity of symptoms, risk of exacerbations, side effects, comorbidities, drug availability and cost, and the patient's response, preference, and ability to use various drug delivery devices.

Ongoing management and monitoring:

- Provide influenza and pneumococcal vaccination to decrease the incidence of lower respiratory tract infections
- Offer pulmonary rehabilitation to improve symptoms, quality of life, and physical and emotional participation in everyday activities
- In patients with severe resting chronic hypoxemia, long-term oxygen therapy improves survival
- In patients with stable COPD and resting or exercise-induced moderate desaturation, long-term oxygen treatment should not be prescribed routinely. However, individual patient factors must be considered when evaluating the patient's need for supplemental oxygen
- Monitor for a decline in FEV_1 by spirometry performed at least once a year
- Monitor symptoms such as cough and sputum, breathlessness, fatigue, activity limitation, and sleep disturbances at each visit
- Monitor the frequency, severity, type, and likely causes of all exacerbations
- Image lungs if there is a clear worsening of symptoms
- Assess current and past smoking status and smoke exposure and follow with appropriate action

Management of COPD exacerbation:

COPD exacerbation is defined as an acute worsening of respiratory symptoms that result in additional therapy, and can be classified as:

- Mild (treated with short-acting bronchodilators only [SABD])

- Moderate (treated with SABDs plus antibiotics and/or corticosteroids)
- Severe (patient requires hospitalization or visits the emergency room)

The cornerstones of treatment for a COPD exacerbation include supplemental oxygen, bronchodilators, steroids, and antibiotics. Indications for noninvasive positive pressure ventilation (NPPV) include severe dyspnea, acidosis (pH ≤ 7.35) and/or hypercapnia (PCO_2 >45 mmHg), and respiratory rate >25 breaths/min. After their acute COPD exacerbation has resolved, patients should undergo PFTs (if not done recently) to stage their COPD, and they should be treated according to the stage of COPD that is found:

- Short-acting inhaled beta-2 agonists, with or without short-acting anticholinergics, are recommended as the initial bronchodilators to treat an acute exacerbation.
- In patients hospitalized with an exacerbation of COPD and acute respiratory failure, Noninvasive Positive –Pressure Ventilation (NPPV is the standard of care for decreasing morbidity and mortality.

REFERENCES

1. Hu G, Zhou Y, Tian J, et al. Risk of COPD from exposure to biomass smoke: a meta-analysis. *Chest*. 2010;138(1):20–31. doi:10.1378/chest.08-2114
2. van Gemert F, Kirenga B, Chavannes N, et al. Prevalence of chronic obstructive pulmonary disease and associated risk factors in Uganda (FRESH AIR Uganda): a prospective cross-sectional observational study. *Lancet Global Health*. 2015;3(1):e44–e51. doi:10.1016/S2214-109X(14)70337-7
3. Yawn B, Kim V. Treatment options for stable chronic obstructive pulmonary disease: current recommendations and unmet needs. *J Fam Practice*. 2018;67(2):S28–S28. doi:10.3949/ccjm.85.s1.05
4. Global Initiative for Chronic Obstructive Lung Disease. *Global Strategy for the Diagnosis, Management, and Prevention of Chronic Obstructive Pulmonary Disease 2019 Report*. Fontana, WI: Author; 2019. https://goldcopd.org/wp-content/uploads/2018/11/GOLD-2019-v1.7-FINAL-14Nov2018-WMS.pdf. Accessed January 6, 2019
5. World Health Organization. Chronic obstructive pulmonary disease. https://www.who.int/news-room/fact-sheets/detail/chronic-obstructive-pulmonary-disease-(copd). Published December 1, 2017

COMMUNITY-ACQUIRED PNEUMONIA

Etiology

Pneumonia is an important condition that affects both adults and children, which results from the infection of the lung parenchyma by viruses, bacteria, fungi, or mycobacteria.[1,2] Quite often, the offending pathogen is not identified. In one study, approximately 23% of the cases were caused by viruses, 11% by bacteria, 3% by both viruses and bacteria, and 1% by fungi or mycobacteria.[2] Pneumonia may be broadly classified into five different categories depending on where the infection was acquired, namely community-acquired pneumonia (CAP), aspiration pneumonia (AP), hospital-acquired pneumonia (HAP), and ventilator-associated pneumonia (VAP). The discussion of bacterial CAP will be the focus in this chapter.

In the adult population, the most frequently seen viruses that cause pneumonia are *rhinovirus* and *influenza*. Meanwhile, the bacteria frequently associated with CAP are *S. pneumoniae, Haemophilus influenza, Moraxella,*

Chlamydophila pneumoniae, and *Mycoplasma pneumoniae.* Although *S. aureus* and *Enterobacteriaceae* may be present at a lower rate, they are commonly seen in patients requiring admission to ICU. The less common bacteria include *Mycobacterium tuberculosis, Legionella sp.,* and *P. aeruginosa.*[1]

Epidemiology

The incidence of CAP in the United States for adults is estimated at 24.8 per 10,000 people and the rate of increases are parallel with age when patients reach 65 or older.[2,3] A survey in 2014 found that 800,000 hospitalizations and 400,000 emergency room visits for both adults and children in the United States were due to pneumonia.[1] It is one of the most expensive disease states treated in the hospital, with estimated total medical costs exceeding $10 billion in 2011 and $9.5 billion in 2013.[1,2] In general, the economic burden of CAP is estimated to be more than $17 billion yearly in the United States.[4]

Clinical Presentation

Patients with pneumonia often present with the acute onset of chills or fever accompanied by a productive purulent cough, although a nonproductive cough may also occur. Other frequently seen symptoms include fatigue, anorexia, weight loss, and pleuritic chest pain. Patients who are immunocompromised may present with fewer overt symptoms, such as lethargy, weakness, altered mental status, headaches, or other GI symptoms. Patients may also develop tachypnea and hypotension, which will require urgent interventions. On physical exam, patients may have reduced breath sounds with positive rales or crackles, rhonchi, tactile fremitus, or egophony.[1,3]

Diagnosis and Assessment of Severity of Pneumonia

The diagnosis of pneumonia is primarily based on both clinical presentation and chest radiographic studies. The medical history of recent travel as well as a history of lung disease or smoking are important to aid in the diagnosis. CXR is usually requested for patients who have a temperature >100°F, heart rate >100 bpm, or respiratory rate >20 per minute.[1]

When infiltrations are present in lung tissue and other diagnoses have been ruled out, the diagnosis of pneumonia may be confirmed. Sputum and blood cultures may be obtained prior to the start of treatment; however, they often provide low yield information while their costs may be relatively expensive. Nevertheless, when the culture and sensitivity data become available, they may help you tailor appropriate therapies to treat the patient more effectively.

There are multiple tools used to assess the severity of pneumonia and predict 30-day mortality. The most frequently used tool in pneumonia assessment is CURB-65, which also estimates the 30-day mortality risk. This tool utilizes five parameters to stratify patients with pneumonia: confusion, blood urea, respiratory rate, BP, and age >65. One point is assigned to each of these variables. A score of 0 to 1 indicates low risk of mortality; therefore, patients with that score may be managed in the outpatient settings. Patients with a CURB-65 score of 2 or greater must be admitted and managed in the hospital. See Table 2.55.

TABLE **2.55** Pneumonia Severity Assessment: CURB-65 Scoring

Criteria	Point assigned
Age ≥ 65 years old	1
Confusion	1
Uremia (BUN >19 mg/dL)	1
RR >30/min	1
BP <90/60	1
Total score	= 1 → treat outpatient
	> 1 → hospitalize (higher score, higher mortality)

BUN, blood urea nitrogen; CURB-65, confusio, urea, respiratory rate, blood pressure plus age ≥65 years.

Management

The empiric management of pneumonia may be grouped into two broad categories, the low-risk patient who can be managed as an outpatient, and the high-risk patient who should be hospitalized (see Table 2.56). When the diagnosis of pneumonia is confirmed and the CURB-65 score of the patient is 1 or less, the patient may be managed in the outpatient settings with oral antibiotics.

- The first-line agents are macrolide antibiotics such as azithromycin, clarithromycin, or erythromycin. Alternatively, a tetracycline, namely doxycycline, may be considered. These agents target *S. pneumoniae*.
- If the patient has a recent use of antibiotics within the previous 3 months, the risk for resistant *S. pneumoniae* may be high; therefore, a respiratory fluoroquinolone such as levofloxacin, moxifloxacin, or gemifloxacin may be used.
  - Alternatively, initiate dual therapy with a macrolide or doxycycline with:
    - A beta-lactam (such as high-dose amoxicillin or amoxicillin-clavulanate)
    - A second-generation cephalosporin (such as cefuroxime)
    - A third-generation cephalosporin (such as cefdinir or cefpodoxime)[1,5]

Evaluate the patient for other comorbidities such as DM, COPD, HF, or immunosuppression. When these conditions are present, the risk of multidrug-resistant bacteria is high; consequently, a respiratory fluoroquinolone or dual therapy (i.e., a macrolide together with a beta-lactam) should be considered first. While there are no significant differences in efficacy between various antibiotic drug classes, the side effect profile of each class of antibiotics may be very different.[1,6] The duration of antibiotic therapy should be a minimum of 5 days or until resolution of symptoms; however, for patients with higher severity, the therapies may be continued for 7 to 10 days or until there is improvement in the outpatient setting.

When the patient is admitted to the hospital under a non-ICU setting, a respiratory fluoroquinolone is recommended or alternatively dual therapy of a macrolide or doxycycline together with a preferred beta-lactam, namely cefotaxime, ceftriaxone, or ampicillin. Ertapenem may also be considered for a selected group of patients.[1,5] If the patient is ill enough to require admission to the ICU, the risk of multidrug resistant infection must be considered.

TABLE 2.56 Summary of Infectious Diseases Society of America Guidelines for Community-Acquired Pneumonia in Adults, 2007

	Comorbidities	Drug Classes	Level of evidence	Recommended Agents
Outpatient Empirical Therapy	None	Macrolide	I	Azithromycin
				Clarithromycin
				Erythromycin
		Tetracycline	III	Doxycycline
	Chronic heart, lung, liver, renal diseases	Fluoroquinolone	I	Moxifloxacin
	Diabetes			Gemifloxacin
	Alcoholism			Levofloxacin
	Malignancies	Beta-lactam	I	HD Amox + Macrolide
	Asplenia	+ Macrolide or		HD Amox/Clav (Augmentin)+ Macrolide
	Immunosuppression	+ Doxycycline (level II evidence)		Ceftriaxone + Macrolide
	Use of antibiotics within the previous 3 months			Cefpodoxime + Macrolide
				Cefuroxime + Macrolide
Inpatient (non-ICU) Empirical Therapy		Fluoroquinolone	I	Moxifloxacin
				Gemifloxacin
				Levofloxacin
		Beta-lactam	I	Cefotaxime + Macrolide
		+ Macrolide or		Ceftriaxone + Macrolide
		+ Doxycycline (level III evidence)		Ampicillin + Macrolide
				Ertapenem + Macrolide

Inpatient ICU	Pencillin Allergy	I	Cefotaxime + Fluoroquinolone
	Beta-lactam + Fluoro-quinolone + Macrolide (level II evidence)		Ceftriaxone + Fluoroquinolone
			Ampicillin/sulbactam + Fluoroquinolone
		n/a	
	Monobactam + Fluoroquinolone		Aztreonam + Fluoroquinolone
	Pseudomonas Infection	III	Piperacillin/tazobactam + Ciprofloxacin or Levofloxacin
	Antispseudomonal Antibiotics + quinolone		Cefepime + Ciprofloxacin or Levofloxacin
			Imipenem/cilastatin + Ciprofloxacin or Levofloxacin
			Meropenem+ Ciprofloxacin or Levofloxacin
	Antispseudomonal Antibiotics + Aminoglycoside + Azithromycin		
	Antispseudomonal Antibiotics + Aminoglycoside + Fluoroquinolone		
	MRSA Infection	III	
	Add Vancomycin or Linezolid		

MRSA, methicillin-resistant *Staphylococcus aureus*.

According to a Cochrane review in 2011, the use of corticosteroids was found to shorten the time to resolve symptoms of pneumonia. However, this practice has not been widely recommended in various reputable guidelines.[1,5,7]

Monitoring of therapeutic responses while treating pneumonia is prudent. There is a growing body of literature that suggests procalcitonin (PCT) level as a biomarker in diagnosis and monitoring of patients with bacterial infections. Not only does PCT help to distinguish between bacterial versus viral or noninfectious inflammatory conditions, it may guide effective antimicrobial stewardship.[8] The normal serum PCT level in humans is <0.1 ng/mL. When this level >0.25 ng/mL, it may imply an existence of a bacterial infection. Furthermore, when infection is resolved, PCT levels decline as patients clinically recover. Consequently, the trending of PCT levels may be used to monitor the clinical progression of the patient. Studies have shown PCT levels begin to elevate within 3 to 4 hours after the onset of a bacterial infection and peak after 12 to 24 hours.[1,8] In pneumonia, when PCT levels have dropped by 80% to 90%, or the serum concentration has reduced <0.25 ng/mL, the antibiotic therapy may be discontinued if the patient is clinically stable. Repeat PCT levels are suggested to be drawn every 1 to 2 days.[8]

REFERENCES

1. Grief SN, Loza JK. Guidelines for the evaluation and treatment of pneumonia. *Prim Care*. 2018;45(3):485–503. doi:10.1016/j.pop.2018.04.001
2. Jain S, Self WH, Wunderink RG, et al. Community-acquired pneumonia requiring hospitalization among U.S. adults. *N Engl J Med*. 2015;373(5):415–427.
3. Regunath H, Oba Y. Pneumonia, community-acquired. In: *StatPearls*. Treasure Island, FL: StatPearls Publishing; 2018.
4. File TM Jr, Marrie TJ. Burden of community-acquired pneumonia in North American adults. *Postgrad Med*. 2010;122(2):130–141. doi:10.3810/pgm.2010.03.2130
5. Mandell LA, Wunderink RG, Anzueto A, et al. Infectious Diseases Society of America/American Thoracic Society consensus guidelines on the management of community-acquired pneumonia in adults. *Clin Infect Dis*. 2007;44(suppl 2): S27–72.
6. Pakhale S, Mulpuru S, Verheij TJ, et al. Antibiotics for community-acquired pneumonia in adult outpatients. *Cochrane Database Syst Rev*. 2014;(10):CD002109. doi:10.1002/14651858.CD002109.pub4
7. Chen Y, Li K, Pu H, et al. Corticosteroids for pneumonia. *Cochrane Database Syst Rev*. 2011;(3):CD007720. doi:10.1002/14651858.CD007720.pub2
8. Covington EW, Roberts MZ, Dong J. Procalcitonin monitoring as a guide for antimicrobial therapy: a review of current literature. *Pharmacotherapy*. 2018;38(5):569–581. doi:10.1002/phar.2112
9. Fine MJ, Auble TE, Yealy DM, et al. A prediction rule to identify low-risk patients with community-acquired pneumonia. *N Engl J Med*. 1997;336(4):243–250. doi:10.1056/NEJM199701233360402
10. Shehata SM, Sileem AE, Shahien NE. Prognostic values of pneumonia severity index, CURB-65 and expanded CURB-65 scores in community-acquired pneumonia in Zagazig University Hospitals. *Egy J Chest Dis Tuberc*. 2017;66(3):549–555. doi:10.1016/j.ejcdt.2017.01.001
11. Marcos PJ, Restrepo MI, Gonzalez-Barcala FJ, et al. Discordance of physician clinical judgment vs. pneumonia severity index (PSI) score to admit patients with low risk community-acquired pneumonia: a prospective multicenter study. *J Thorac Dis*. 2017;9(6):1538–1546. doi:10.21037/jtd.2017.05.44

WOMEN'S HEALTH

ABNORMAL UTERINE BLEEDING

Etiology

AUB is defined as abnormal menstrual bleeding in quality, duration, and timing in reproductive-aged women. A normal menstrual cycle is defined as 24 to 38 days with a 4- to 8-day flow. The two types of abnormal uterine bleeding (AUB) include heavy menstrual bleeding and intermenstrual bleeding. PALM-COEIN is a mnemonic used in the classification of AUB. Rather than defining the type of bleeding, this device classifies the AUB by structural or nonstructural etiology.[1]

PALM: Structural, COEIN: Nonstructural[2]
PALM-COEIN[1]

> **P:** polyps (endometrial or cervical)
> **A:** adenomyosis
> **L:** leiomyoma (uterine fibroids)
> **M:** malignancy
> **C:** coagulopathy
> **O:** ovulatory dysfunction
> **I:** iatrogenic
> **N:** not yet classified

Causes of heavy bleeding may include[3] the following:

- Leiomyoma
- Endometrial polyps
- Cervical polyps
- Coital and postcoital bleeding
- Adenomyosis
- Coagulopathy
- Long-acting reversible contraception (LARC) such as intrauterine device (IUD [copper]) and progestin [levonorgestrel], progestin dermal implant (etonogestrel), and IM (medroxyprogesterone). Progestin IUD can be used to also treat AUB due to ovulatory dysfunction.
- Endometrial hyperplasia
- Thyroid disease
- Gynecological malignancy: Endometrial adenocarcinoma, cervical cancer
- Trauma: Assault, foreign body in vagina, pelvic trauma, straddle injury

Causes of irregular bleeding are often due to ovulatory dysfunction such as:

- Anovulation
- PCOS
- Hyperprolactinemia
- Thyroid disease
- Perimenopause
- Postmenopausal bleeding

Heavy bleeding (menorrhagia) that requires additional evaluation includes the following:
- Soaking greater than one pad or tampon/hour over several hours
- Menses requiring double protection, such as a tampon and a pad
- Passing of clots quarter size or larger
- Awakening in the middle of night to change hygiene product
- Disruption of daily activities/quality of life
- Symptoms of anemia such as fatigue and shortness of breath

> **CLINICAL PEARL:** Heavy bleeding should prompt urgent evaluation when there is a drop in hemoglobin/hematocrit and symptoms of hypotension/hypovolemia, such as near syncope.

Epidemiology

AUB affects approximately 14% to 25% of reproductive age women in the United States, and treatment of AUB can greatly improve quality of life.[3]

Clinical Presentation

Key history components to ascertain in the patient with AUB are outlined in Table 2.57.
- If a patient presents with more than one cycle of abnormal vaginal bleeding, clarify the following pertinent information:
    - Intermenstrual bleeding, coital bleeding, changes in cycle length, flow (light, lack of, or heavy) based on number of pads/tampons used.
    - Inquire about symptoms of anemia including fatigue, dizziness, pallor, and shortness of breath. Vasomotor symptoms can be present in perimenopausal AUB (ovulatory dysfunction). Symptoms of endocrine dysfunction and pregnancy symptoms may also be present.

Physical Examination

- Assess for signs of PCOS, such as hirsutism and acanthosis nigricans; hyperprolactinemia, such as galactorrhea and visual changes; and coagulopathy, such as ecchymosis or easy bruising
- Thyromegaly may be noted, with or without nodules
- A thorough pelvic exam should be performed including an external genital examination for evidence of trauma, such as fissures, fistulas, abrasions, and lacerations
- The vagina should be examined for discharge and lesions, and the cervix for polyps, lesions, mucopurulence, and lesions. The bimanual exam should include an assessment of uterine size, shape, mobility, tenderness, and presence or absence of a Chandelier sign
- Palpate for adnexal masses and tenderness

Diagnosis

Laboratory evaluation: Should evaluate for potential causes of AUB, both primary and secondary:
- HCG
- CBC

TABLE 2.57 Key History Components in Abnormal Uterine Bleeding

Menstrual	LMP, perimenopause, menopause
Family history	Fibroids, endometriosis, adenomyosis, members of family with hysterectomy for bleeding
Pregnancy status	Presenting with a positive pregnancy test or retained POC
Contraception	Progestin-based contraception: irregular bleeding and amenorrhea
	Progesterone only IUD: irregular bleeding and history of amenorrhea
	Nonhormonal IUD (copper): heavy, long, and painful periods
	Noncompliance with contraception
Medications	Systemic corticosteroids
	Anticoagulant therapy
	Thyroid medication
	Antibiotics, if using with combined hormonal contraception (CHC), may cause breakthrough ovulation and pregnancy
	Tamoxifen may cause postmenopausal bleeding
	Antipsychotic medications may cause amenorrhea
Medical history	Coagulopathy
	Thyroid disease
	Severe liver disease
	History of thrombotic events
ROS with pertinent associated condition	PID/infection: fever, chills, pelvic pain, coital bleeding
	Endometriosis/adenomyosis: dysmenorrhea/dyspareunia
	Endocrine: galactorrhea, headaches, and visual changes which can be associated with a pituitary disorder
	Thyroid: weight changes, heat or cold intolerance, tachypalpitations, and skin changes which can be associated with a thyroid disorder
	Leiomyoma may be associated with bowel or bladder changes

CHC, combined hormonal contraception; IUD, intrauterine device; IUD, intrauterine device; LMP, last normal or abnormal menstrual periods; PID, pelvic inflammatory disease; POC, products of conception; ROS, review of systems.

- Prolactin, thyroid panel
- FSH, LH, estradiol
- Testosterone
- Coagulation panel: von Willebrand disease/factor (vwf)
- Cervical cultures: *N. gonorrhoeae*, *C. trachomatis*, trichomonas, HSV, Pap smear

Diagnostic imaging:

Pelvic ultrasound to evaluate for:
- Leiomyoma (fibroids)
- Endometrial polyps
- Adenomyosis
- Measure endometrial lining, only in postmenopausal women: abnormal >4 mm

Procedures may include the following:

- Endometrial biopsy
- Sonohysterography

Diagnostic and therapeutic options include the following:

- D&C hysteroscopy, with or without polypectomy

  MRI and CT may be utilized as additional diagnostic modalities.

Management

The management of AUB is based on the etiology, contraceptive needs, and fertility preservation desires. Specific options are outlined in Table 2.58. Additional management should target the etiology and/or sequelae of the bleeding:

- Anemia: Determine the cause and manage appropriately. Order iron studies to rule out iron deficiency
- Dysmenorrhea/heavy flow: Low-dose combination hormonal contraceptive therapy or progestin therapy is the mainstay of treatment. If estrogen is contraindicated or undesired, such as in a patient with a history of or at risk for venous thromboembolism, treat with nonsteroidal anti-inflammatories or consider tranexamic acid (antifibrinolytic)
- Endocrine: Thyroid dysfunction, hyperprolactinemia, hyperandrogenism—treat appropriately or refer to endocrinology. PCOS is an etiology that should be considered
- Coagulopathy: von Willebrand disease (VWD) is more common in adolescents; these patients are typically referred to hematology

> **CLINICAL PEARL:** Contraindications to estrogen should always be considered, as estrogen increases risk of venous thromboembolism, cerebrovascular accident, and transient ischemic attacks.

TABLE 2.58 Management Options in Abnormal Uterine Bleeding

MEDICAL	SURGICAL
Heavy bleeding IUD decrease flow/ovulatory dysfunction—first line when contraception is desired and no contraindications exist	**Endometrial ablation:** heavy menstrual bleeding
OCHC—regulates and decreases flow (estrogen/progestin combination). Cyclic progestin (medroxyprogesterone acetate or norethindrone)	**Uterine artery embolizaton:** fibroids
GnRH agonist (leuprolide) fibroids and endometriosis	**Myomectomy:** in certain types of fibroids
Tranexamic acid: may help decrease flow but is not a contraceptive	**Hysterectomy**
NSAIDs: decrease flow and dysmenorrhea, do not provide contraception	

GNRH, gonadotropin releasing hormone; IUD, intrauterine device; NSAIDs, nonsteroidal anti-inflammatory drugs; OCHC, oral contraceptives.

> **CLINICAL PEARL:** Contraception must be utilized in reproductive-aged women as they should not get pregnant after ablation.

REFERENCES

1. Munro MG, Critchley HOD, Broder MS, et al. FIGO classification system (PALM-COEIN) for causes of abnormal uterine bleeding in nongravid women of reproductive age. *Int J Gynecol Obstet*. 2011;113:3–13. doi:10.1016/j.ijgo.2010.11.011
2. American College of Obstetricians and Gynecologists. ACOG committee opinion no. 557: management of acute abnormal uterine bleeding in nonpregnant reproductive-aged women. *Obstet Gynecol*. 2013;121:891. doi:10.1097/01.AOG.0000428646.67925.9a
3. Whitaker L, Critchley HOD. Abnormal uterine bleeding. *Best Pract Res Clin Obstet Gynaecol*. 2015;2016(34):54–65. doi:10.1016/j.bpobgyn.2015.11.012

BREAST MASS

Etiology

Benign breast disease includes fibroadenomas and breast cysts and occurs as a result of hormonal changes in breast development, pregnancy, and age. Estrogen and progesterone play significant roles in these breast changes. Exogenous hormones such as estrogen-containing systemic contraception agents and menopausal hormone therapy (particularly estrogen) often contribute to breast changes. Menopause causes atrophic changes in the breast tissue.

Epidemiology

Benign breast disease affects approximately one million women in the United States annually. Benign breast disease is commonly diagnosed during the onset of reproductive years. Changes to breast morphology will occur during early to mid reproductive years as well as postreproductive.[1] Additional changes in breast morphology will occur during pregnancy and lactation. Fibroadenomas are common in women ages 15 to 35 and are found in 10% of all women.[2] While the majority of breast masses are benign, you should consider the possibility of malignancy and inquire about risk factors for malignancy, as outlined in Table 2.59.

Clinical Presentation

Patients may present with a new onset of a breast lump, abnormal nipple discharge, or breast pain. It is not uncommon for a patient to state that her breast may feel different and use descriptors such as heavy, full, lumpy, or note a discrepancy in size of breasts. Additional historical questions include the following:

- Menstrual: Menarche, last normal menstrual period (lnmp), menopause status, breast changes during ovulation and menses
- Obstetric: Number of pregnancies, most recent pregnancy, breastfeeding status if applicable
- Prior breast imaging/procedures: Breast ultrasound, mammogram, biopsies

TABLE 2.59 Risk Factors for Breast Malignancies

Age	50–69 years old (1 in 44) 60–69 years old (1 in 29) 70 years old and older (1 in 15)
Sex	Female
Race	Caucasian. Black women are more likely to be diagnosed with more invasive disease.
Weight	BMI >30, perimenopausal weight gain is a risk factor
BMD	Higher BMD because bone has estrogen receptors and may be more sensitive to circulating endogenous and exogenous estrogen levels.
Family history	Breast malignancy, specifically BRCA mutations that increase breast cancer risk. Ashkenazi Jewish descent increases BRCA risk.
Exogenous hormone use	OCHCs and HRT/ERT
Menarche	Early (prior to 13 years)
Obstetric history	Nulliparity
Age at first pregnancy	>35 years of age
Social	Early tobacco use (include duration and pack history), daily and greater than moderate use of alcohol increases risk

BMD, bone mineral density; BMI, body mass index; CHCs, combined hormonal contraceptive; ERT, estrogen replacement therapy; HRT, hormone replacement therapy.
Source: McLaughlin M. Fibroadenoma. *Gale Ency Med. 2011;3:*1723–1724.

- Medical history: Benign breast cysts, fibroadenomas, mastitis, history of malignancy such as breast, colon, or uterine cancer
- Family history: Breast cancer, premalignant lesions, any family history of malignancy such as ovarian, pancreatic, or colon cancer
- Medications/hormones: Bioidentical hormones
- Review of systems: Breast pain, breast skin changes, palpable breast mass, heaviness or fullness of breast, nipple discharge, weight loss, fatigue, fever, bone pain

Physical Examination

- Clinical breast exam (CBE) in all four quadrants and tail of Spence in the sitting and supine position. The exam must include inspection and palpation with attention to skin changes, symmetry, nipple inversion, or other visible or palpable findings. Attempt to express nipple discharge, or have the patient attempt expression, and note the color, consistency, and amount of discharge present. Consider sending the fluid to pathology in a formalin jar
- Palpate for axillary and supra and infraclavicular lymphadenopathy bilaterally
- Palpate the chest wall to assess for the presence of bony pain

Diagnosis

The diagnostic evaluation should include a thorough breast exam and complete history. If the patient states the nodularity or palpable mass resolves after menses, offer reassurance and monitoring. In any woman with a breast mass, assess breast cancer risk using a breast cancer risk assessment tool. The Gail Model uses a patient's medical, personal, reproductive, and breast cancer history of first-degree relatives to estimate breast cancer risk. This tool is available at https://www.bcrisktool.cancer.gov.

Imaging is warranted when a breast mass does not resolve after menses, or if there are risk factors present for breast cancer. Imaging laterality in most cases is limited to the affected breast unless risk factors, prior breast diagnoses, and/or updated breast surveillance warrant bilateral.

The definitive diagnosis requires a tissue sample. Breast density is a radiological, not a physical, finding. Breast density limits the sensitivity of mammography detection of small cancers. Benign breast lesions are histologically classified in three groups: nonproliferative, proliferative without atypia, and atypical hyperplasia (AH).[1,3] Breast density is classified using the Breast Imaging Reporting and Data System (BI-RADS):[4]

> 1/A: Fatty
> 2/B: Scattered fibroglandular
> 3/C: Heterogeneoulsy dense (may obscure small lesions)
> 4/D: Extremely dense (lowers sensitivity of mammogram)

Tissue sample consistent with nonproliferative:

- Normal cells
- No increased risk for breast malignancy
- Simple breast cyst/benign lesion
- Fibrocystic changes/disease, cystic mastitis, and mammary dysplasia are all terms associated with nonproliferative lesions

Tissue sample consistent with proliferative without atypia:

- Increased number of normal cells
- 1.5- to 2-fold increased risk of breast malignancy[3]
- Fibroadenoma: Carries a risk of breast cancer only if complex
- Ductal hyperplasia
- Intraductal papillomas:
  - Solitary B bloody nipple discharge common

Tissue sample consistent with AH:

- Increase in abnormal cells
- Increased risk for breast cancer, requires surgical excision
- Atypical ductal hyperplasia (ADH): 3- to 4-fold increase in breast malignancy[5]
- Atypical lobular hyperplasia (ALH): 3- to 4-fold increase in breast malignancy[5]
- Flat epithelial atypia
- Ductal carcinoma in situ (DCIS)
- Lobular carcinoma in situ (LCIS)

Fibroadenomas often require additional attention as these can be benign or carry a risk of breast cancer. Fibroadenomas are discrete, solid, noncancerous masses that are firm, rubbery, and painless (2). Simple fibroadenomas are those that measure <3 cm. Complex fibroadenomas are larger, tend to occur in older patients, and are associated with a slight increase in the risk of breast cancer. A phyllodes tumor is uncommon and begins as a benign fibroadenoma which undergoes rapid growth which can increase risk for breast malignancy.[6]

> **CLINICAL PEARL:** Extensive patient education on breast health needs to be undertaken and documented in the chart. Patients with breast masses should be reassessed within 3 to 6 months. In general, most patients over 35 years with any mass (regardless of its relationship to the menstrual cycle) should receive a diagnostic evaluation.

Diagnostic imaging is indicated in the following scenarios:

- Women 40 years of age or older: Diagnostic mammogram or diagnostic digital breast tomosynthesis is appropriate[7]
- Women younger than 30 years of age: Breast ultrasound is appropriate[7]
- Women 30 to 39 years of age: Breast ultrasound, diagnostic mammogram, and digital breast tomosynthesis all are appropriate[7]
- A radiologist will recommend additional imaging or biopsy if warranted, such as galactography (ductography)

Procedural/Surgical: Recommended by radiologist or breast specialist/surgeon
- Percutaneous ultrasound-guided biopsy

Management

Management is based on radiological findings, histology, and pathology. In most cases, a breast specialist will manage care as these patients are generally referred. Management can include surveillance with more frequent imaging or surgical excision for high-risk lesions with SERMs (selective estrogen receptor modulators). Fibroadenomas will regress spontaneously in patients younger than 35 years of age in most cases. If fibroadenomas change in size or occur in women over the age of 35 years old, then excision is recommended. Surveillance every 6 to 12 months is appropriate.

REFERENCES

1. Schnitt S, Collins L. Pathology of benign breast disorders. *Dis Breast*. 2014:71–88.
2. McLaughlin M. Fibroadenoma. *Gale Ency Med*. 2011;3:1723–1724.
3. Dyrstad SW, Yan Y, Fowler AM, et al. Breast cancer risk associated with benign breast disease: systematic review and meta-analysis. *Breast Cancer Res Treat*. 2015;149:569–575. doi:10.1007/s10549-014-3254-6
4. Timmers JMH, van Doorne-Nagtegaal HJ, Zonderland HM, et al. The Breast Imaging Reporting and Data System (BI-RADS) in the Dutch breast cancer screening programme: its role as an assessment and stratification tool. *Eur Radiol*. 2012;22(8):1717–1723.
5. Hartmann LC, Degnim AC, Santen RJ, et al. Atypical hyperplasia of the breast—Risk assessment and management options. *N England J Med*. 2015;372:72–89. doi:10.1056/NEJMsr1407164
6. Nassar A, Visscher DW, Degnim AC, et al. Complex fibroadenoma and breast cancer risk: a mayo clinic benign breast disease cohort study. *Breast Cancer Res Treat*. 2015;153:397–405. doi:10.1007/s10549-015-3535-8
7. Moy L, Heller SL, Bailey L, et al. ACR appropriateness criteria palpable breast masses. *J Am Coll Radiol*. 2017;14:S203–S224. doi:10.1016/j.jacr.2017.02.033

DYSMENORRHEA

Etiology

Dysmenorrhea is caused by prostaglandins that are released by the endometrium. Endometrial thickness is directly proportional to the release of prostaglandins. Secondary dysmenorrhea occurs as a result of a reproductive organ disorder. The differences between primary dysmenorrhea and secondary dysmenorrhea are outlined in Table 2.60.

Epidemiology

Approximately 16% to 91% of reproductive age women have some form of dysmenorrhea, which improves with age.[1]

Clinical Presentation

Patient history should include the assessment of menstrual cycle length, duration, and flow. Determine the timing of pelvic discomfort, medications used, and any prior assessment by a medical professional. Inquire if the pain started with menarche. A complete review of symptoms to assess for secondary causes of dysmenorrhea should also include asking about dyspareunia. Physical exam should include a complete pelvic exam assessing for areas of tenderness/pain, size and shape of uterus, and assessment of ovaries for size and tenderness.

Diagnosis

Primary dysmenorrhea is often a clinical diagnosis. Transvaginal ultrasound is indicated for secondary dysmenorrhea. Refer patient to an obstetrician/gynecologist (ob/gyn) when supportive and medical management fails, such as NSAIDS and/or hormonal contraceptives.

Management

The management options are outlined in Table 2.61.

TABLE 2.60 A Comparison of Primary and Secondary Dysmenorrhea

Primary Dysmenorrhea	Secondary Dysmenorrhea
Begins within the first few years of menarche and is responsive to NSAIDs	Dysmenorrhea occurs later in the underlying disease process
Occurs as a result of prostaglandins from within the endometrial lining and is worst within the first couple days of menses	Pain may be present
	Can be due to endometriosis, adenomyosis, leiomyomas[a]
Associated with lower abdominal, pelvic, low back, and thigh pain	Associated with crampy lower abdominal pain, typically recurrent, but can also cause daily pelvic pain

NSAIDs, nonsteroidal anti-inflammatory drugs.
[a]**Endometriosis:** condition where endometrial implants are located outside of the uterus. **Adenomyosis:** endometrial lining invades the uterine muscle. **Leiomyomas:** benign growths arising from the uterine muscle.

TABLE 2.61 Management of Dysmenorrhea

Primary Dysmenorrhea	Secondary Dysmenorrhea
Supportive: heating pad, exercise, relaxation methods **Pharmacological:** NSAIDs, hormonal contraceptives (continuous dosing is most effective)	Treat underlying cause: **Endometriosis:** hormonal suppression, lysis of adhesions, hysterectomy **Uterine fibroids:** uterine artery embolization, myomectomy, hysterectomy **Adenomyosis:** hysterectomy **Supportive therapies** and NSAIDs for symptom relief

NSAIDS, nonsteroidal anti-inflammatory drugs.

CLINICAL PEARL: If there is no resolution of primary dysmenorrhea symptoms in 3 months consider secondary dysmenorrhea and referral to ob/gyn.

REFERENCES

1. Ju H, Jones M, Mishra G. The prevalence and risk factors of dysmenorrhea. *Epidemiol Rev.* 2014;36:104–113. doi:10.1093/epirev/mxt009

INCONTINENCE: URINARY

Etiology

Urinary incontinence in women is an involuntary loss of urine that is classified as stress urinary incontinence (SUI), urgency incontinence (urge), mixed incontinence, and overflow incontinence.

Specific etiologies include the following:

SUI
- Involuntary leakage due to increase in intra-abdominal pressure—sneezing, coughing, jumping, running
- Urethral hypermobility
- Intrinsic sphincteric deficiency

URGE
- Overactive bladder
- Urge to void is present preceding or with involuntary leakage
- Drops of urine to complete emptying of bladder
- Detrusor overactivity—involuntary detrusor muscle contractions during bladder filling

MIXED
- Symptoms of both SUI and urge

OVERFLOW
- Continuous urine leakage, weak stream, hesitancy, and nocturia
- Detrusor muscle underactivity

- Bladder outlet
- Genitourinary syndrome of menopause (GSM)
- Stroke
- Parkinson's disease
- Diabetic autonomic neuropathy

Epidemiology

Urinary incontinence affects about 10% to 17% of nonpregnant women over the age of 20; however, that number increases as women age. It is estimated that about 30% of women over the age of 60 have experienced urinary incontinence.[1-3] Specific risk factors include the following:

- Age: Urge incontinence
- Obesity: SUI, associated with a 50% improvement with weight reduction[4]
- Increased parity and vaginal delivery predispose to pelvic organ prolapse (POP) risk and urinary incontinence
- High-impact activities such as running and jumping: SUI
- Tobacco use
- Caffeine use
- GSM and vaginal atrophy
- Hysterectomy
- Pelvic radiation

Clinical Presentation

Patients are often hesitant to discuss urinary leakage. All women over the age of 65 need to be assessed by history. Urinary incontinence can be classified by both history and the use of a simple three question test, the 3IQ.[5] The 3IQ has a sensitivity of 0.75 and specificity of 0.77 for urge incontinence and 0.86 and 0.60, respectively, for stress incontinence and is therefore helpful in differentiating between the two.[6]

1. During the last 3 months have you leaked urine?
   - Yes
   - No, if no do not proceed
2. During the last 3 months, did you leak fluid? (check all that apply)
   - **A.** When you were performing a physical activity such as coughing, sneezing, lifting, or exercise
   - **B.** When you had the urge or need to empty your bladder, but could not get to the toilet fast enough
   - **C.** Without physical activity and without a sense of urgency
3. During the last 3 months, did you leak urine most often? (check only one)
   - **A.** When you were performing a physical activity
   - **B.** When you had the urge or the feeling that you needed to empty your bladder
   - **C.** Without physical activity and without a sense of urgency
   - **D.** About equally as often with physical activity as with a sense of urgency

Answer response to question 3:

   A = Stress or stress dominant
   B = Urge or urge dominant

C = Other causes

D = Mixed

Other important history questions can include the following:

- Onset, duration, frequency of symptoms, impact to patient's quality of life, social activities, sexual activity, hygiene
- Assess for symptoms of UTI: fever, dysuria, pelvic pain, and hematuria
- Changes in bowel function (constipation)
- Symptoms related to underlying neurologic conditions
- Medication, diet (caffeine and ETOH) and activity triggers
- Obstetrical history: parity, mode of delivery, infant birth weight, length of second phase of labor
- Use of pad or protective products

Pelvic exam should include assessment for POP, GSM/vaginal atrophy, and pelvic masses. Perform a neurological exam if neurological symptoms present or sudden onset of urgency.

Avoiding diary can be used to assess if fluid intake and particular types of fluids may be triggers. This record may also help to assess incontinence severity and assist with bladder training. Recording can be done over 24 hours or 3 days. Please see www.augs.org (American Urogynecological Society) for more information about voiding diaries.

Diagnosis

- Urinalysis
- Urine culture if there is concern for UTI or if hematuria is present
- Bladder stress test can diagnose SUI: A patient with a full bladder should stand while the provider asks the patient to perform a valsalva maneuver in order to assess for leakage of urine from the urethra
- Urodynamic testing is typically performed by a urogynecologist or urologist, and is typically reserved for failed treatment or an uncertain diagnosis
- Urethral mobility evaluation may be performed by a urogynecologist or a urologist

Management options are outlined in Table 2.62.

TABLE 2.62 Management of Urinary Incontinence

SUI	URGE	Mixed	Overflow
Lifestyle modifications: Pelvic floor exercises (Kegel) Bladder training Weight loss	Lifestyle modifications: Pelvic floor exercises (Kegel) Bladder training	After lifestyle modifications are ineffective treat based on predominant symptoms: SUI or urge	Lifestyle modifications: Pelvic floor exercises (Kegel)

(continued)

TABLE 2.62 Management of Urinary Incontinence (*continued*)

SUI	URGE	Mixed	Overflow
Pharmacologic: Topical/vaginal estrogen therapy (GSM) **Support Devices:** Continent pessaries **Surgical:** Mid-urethral sling-specialist	**Pharmacologic:** Antimuscarinic such as oxybutynin, beta-3 adrenergic agonist such as mirabegron, or topical/vaginal estrogen therapy **Referral:** To urogynecologist if medication ineffective		**Referral:** If impaired bladder emptying is not improved with lifestyle refer to urogynecology

GSM, genitourinary syndrome of menopause; SUI, stress urinary incontinence.

REFERENCES

1. Wu JM, Vaughan CP, Goode PS, et al. Prevalence and trends of symptomatic pelvic floor disorders in US women. *Obstet Gynecol.* 2014;123:141–148. doi:10.1097/AOG.0000000000000057
2. O'Halloran T, Bell RJ, Robinson PJ, et al. Urinary incontinence in young nulligravid women: a cross sectional analysis. *Ann Intern Med.* 2012;157:87. doi:10.7326/0003-4819-157-2-201207170-00005
3. Al-Mukhtar OJ, Akervall S, Milsom IAN, et al. Urinary incontinence in nulliparous women aged 25-64 years: a national survey. *Am J Obstet Gynecol.* 2017;216:149 e11. doi:10.1016/j.ajog.2016.09.104
4. Subak LL, Wing R, West DS, et al. Weight loss to treat urinary incontinence in overweight and obese women. *N Engl J Med.* 2009;360:481. doi:10.1056/NEJMoa0806375
5. Nature Review. The 3IQ test is an accurate and simple way to classify incontinence. *Nature Clin Pract Urol.* 2006;3:402–402. doi:10.1038/ncpuro0538. https://www.nature.com/articles/ncpuro0538

MASTALGIA

Etiology

Breast pain is classified as cyclical, noncyclical, or extramammary.[1] Cyclical pain is related to normal physiological changes of the menstrual cycle and can be bilateral and diffuse. Noncyclical pain is unrelated to the menstrual cycle and can be unilateral. Extramammary pain is that which is referred and can be due to irritation from nerves T3 to T5, as well as musculoskeletal, trauma, pulmonary, cardiac, and esophageal disorders.

Physiological hormonal fluctuations associated with menstrual cycle, mastitis, trauma, breast cysts of abrupt onset, breast cancer (inflammatory breast cancer), ill-fitting bra, caffeine, and large breasts can all contribute to mastalgia. Hormone replacement therapy is associated noncyclical mastalgia.[1]

Epidemiology

Mastalgia is a common condition, with 50% to 70% of women reporting breast pain at some point.[2]

Clinical Presentation

In order to narrow the differential diagnosis, it is most important to note if breast changes are associated with menses and ovulation, laterality, breast or chest wall trauma, or infection. Inquire about the use of hormone medications to include combined hormonal contraceptives and hormone replacement therapy. Obtain a thorough family history of breast malignancy or premalignant lesions and of personal breast surveillance/biopsies, and perform a breast cancer risk assessment tool with https://bcrisktool.cancer.gov

A thorough breast, lymph node, and chest wall examination should be performed.

Diagnosis

- Cyclical: No imaging required[3]
- Noncyclical: Imaging recommended. Imaging is also recommended for a unilateral breast mass that is not extramammary
- If the patient is under 30 years of age, perform a breast ultrasound. Proceed to mammogram if the ultrasound is abnormal or if risk factors are present for breast malignancy
- If the patient is 30 years of age or older, perform diagnostic mammogram or diagnostic digital tomosynthesis and breast ultrasound
- Extramammary: Workup is based on suspected etiology

CLINICAL PEARL: Mammography is pursued in cases when a woman has significant risk factors for breast malignancy.

Management

- Pharmacological[4]
  - First line: Acetaminophen, NSAIDs, diclofenac gel. Consider change in current hormone management. Allow a minimum of 6 months of treatment before starting second-line pharmacologic treatment
  - Second line: Danazol 200 mg QD. Advise patient of possible androgen side effects
- Nonpharmacological
  - Correct ill-fitting bra to provide good breast support
  - Decrease caffeine, apply warm or cold compresses as needed

CLINICAL PEARL: If symptoms do not improve with first-line treatment, consider referral to ob/gyn.

REFERENCES

1. Iddon J, Dixon JM. Mastalgia. *BMJ*. 2013;347:f3288. doi:10.1136/bmj.f3288
2. Scurr J, Hedger W, Morris P, et al. The prevalence, severity and impact of breast pain in the general population. *Breast J*. 2014;20:508–513. doi:10.1111/tbj.12305
3. Jokich PM, Bailey L, D'Orsi C, et al. ACR appropriateness criteria breast pain. *J Am Coll Radiol*. 2017;14:S25–S33. doi:10.1016/j.jacr.2017.01.028
4. Kataria K, Dhar A, Srivastava A, et al. A systematic review of current understanding and management of mastalgia. *Indian J Surg*. 2014;76:217–222. doi:10.1007/s12262-013-0813-8

MASTITIS

Etiology

Mastitis is defined as a painful, swollen, and erythematous breast presenting in breastfeeding women. Lactational mastitis is due to prolonged engorgement, poor milk drainage, blockage of milk duct, infrequent feeding, poor infant latch, and rapid weaning. The most common cause of lactational mastitis is *S. aureus*.[1]

CLINICAL PEARL: Abscess formation is common with delayed or ineffective treatment.

Epidemiology

Lactational mastitis occurs in about 2% to 10% of lactating women.[2] Risk factors include poor latching, missed breastfeeding, milk stasis, poor maternal nutrition, and infection.

Clinical Presentation

- Lactational mastitis: Engorgement, pain, red swelling seen within the first 3 months, resolves within 12 to 24 hours
- Infective lactational mastitis: Pain, red, tender fever >38.3°C, malaise, flu-like symptoms lasting >24 hours

Diagnosis

Diagnosis is typically clinical and based on a suggestive history and focal tenderness of the affected breast(s) with or without fever.

Management

- Lactational mastitis:[3]
  - Symptomatic management: NSAIDs, cold compresses, encourage complete emptying of breasts: frequent feeding, pumping, manual expression
- Infective lactational mastitis: Symptomatic measures with the addition of one of the following:
  - Dicloxacillin 500 mg QID × 7 days (first line)
  - Cephalexin 500 mg QID × 7 days
  - Clindamycin 300 mg TID × 7 days

REFERENCES

1. Kvist LJ, Larsson BW, Hall-Lord ML, et al. The role of bacteria in lactational mastitis and some considerations of the use of antibiotic treatment. *Int Breastfeed J*. 2008;3:6. doi:10.1186/1746-4358-3-6
2. Committee on Health Care for Underserved Women, American College of Obstetricians and Gynecologists. ACOG committee opinion no. 361: breastfeeding: maternal and infant aspects. *Obstet Gynecol*. 2007;109:479. doi:10.1097/00006250-200702000-00064
3. Jahanfar S, Ng CJ, Teng CL. Antibiotics for mastitis in breastfeeding women. *Sao Paulo Med J*. 2016;134:273–273. doi:10.1590/1516-3180.20161343T1

3

Diagnostic Testing in Family Medicine

The clinical value of a given test is governed by specificity and sensitivity in addition to the pretest probability of the disease being tested. The specificity of a test refers to the ability to correctly identify those individuals who do not have the disease being tested. Tests with high specificity have a low percentage of false-positive results. The sensitivity of the test is the ability to correctly identify those individuals who truly have the disease. Tests with high sensitivity have a low percentage of false-negative results. Specificity is helpful to rule in a given disease, while sensitivity is helpful to rule out a given disease.

Commonly encountered labs in family medicine are outlined in Table 3.1. This chapter also presents an overview of diagnostic imaging indications and findings in family medicine, including CT, MRI, plain radiography, and ultrasound.

LABS

TABLE 3.1 Commonly Encountered Labs in Family Medicine

Name	Normal Reference Range	Indication	Interpretation
A1C (glycated hemoglobin	4.0%–5.6%	Screening and monitoring for diabetes	Evaluates the average amount of glucose in the blood over the last 2–3 months by measuring the percentage of glycated (glycosylated) hemoglobin. ≥6.5% is diagnostic for diabetes
ANC	(ANC) 2,000–8,250/μL	Suspected infection	ANC is derived by multiplying the WBC count times the percent of neutrophils in the differential WBC count. Below normal suggests neutropenia

(continued)

TABLE 3.1 Commonly Encountered Labs in Family Medicine (*continued*)

Name	Normal Reference Range	Indication	Interpretation
ACTH, plasma	10–60 pg/mL	Signs and symptoms suggesting excess or deficient cortisol production	ACTH is elevated during hypocortisolism due to primary adrenal insufficiency. In patients with Cushing's syndrome, elevated ACTH suggests pituitary adenoma
Albumin, serum	3.5–5.5 g/dL	Evaluation of liver and kidney function	Albumin is essential in keeping fluid balance (maintaining colloidal osmotic pressure) in the vascular and extravascular spaces. Increased albumin concentration is seen during dehydration. Decreased levels are seen during infection, chronic inflammation, cirrhosis, and nephrotic syndrome
Aminotransferase, serum alanine (ALT, SGPT)	10–40 U/L	Diagnoses liver diseases and monitor treatment outcomes. Differentiates between hemolytic jaundice and jaundice due to liver diseases	Increased ALT levels may be associated with hepatocellular abnormalities, alcoholic cirrhosis, metastatic liver, infections, obstructive jaundice, and trauma
Aminotransferase, serum aspartate (AST, SGOT)	10–40 U/L	Indicated to evaluate liver and heart tissue damage	AST levels are usually increased in myocardial infarction and liver disease. AST is more sensitive for alcoholic liver disease than ALT
Bicarbonate	22–29 mEq/L	Evaluation of acid–base balance; measures amount of CO_2 in blood	Decreased in acute metabolic acidosis, increased in acute metabolic alkalosis
BUN, serum or plasma	8–20 mg/dL	Suspicion of renal disease, confusion, and convulsions	Increased BUN implies impaired renal function (acute and chronic). Decreased BUN levels may signal liver failure, malnutrition
B-type natriuretic peptide, plasma	<100 pg/mL	Consider a BNP for a patient with dyspnea and suspected heart failure	Increased BNP levels imply heart failure, diastolic dysfunction, decreased left ventricular ejection fraction
Chloride	98–106 mEq/L	Evaluation of the acid–base balance and assessment of hydration	Rarely evaluated beyond calculation of the acid–base balance

(*continued*)

TABLE 3.1 Commonly Encountered Labs in Family Medicine (*continued*)

Name	Normal Reference Range	Indication	Interpretation
Cholesterol, serum	Total desirable <200 mg/dL	Evaluating risk of atherosclerosis, coronary arterial occlusion, and MI	Total cholesterol levels predict coronary disease risk. Levels >239 mg/dL are considered high
HDL	≥50 mg/dL (female) ≥40 mg/dL (male)	Evaluating risk of atherosclerosis, coronary arterial occlusion, and MI	Elevated HDL levels are cardio-protective and low levels may be atherogenic
LDL	<100 mg/dL	Evaluating risk of atherosclerosis, coronary arterial occlusion, and MI	Increased levels of LDL may be caused by familial hypercholes-terolemia, diet, hypothy-roidism, hepatic disease, diabetes, and chronic renal diseases
Cortisol, plasma	8 a.m. = 5–25 μg/dL 4 p.m. = less than 10 μg/dL 1 hour after cosyntropin = 18 μg/dL or greater Overnight suppression test (1 mg) = <1.8 μg/dL Overnight suppression test (8 mg) = >50% reduction in cortisol	Screening for Addison's disease and Cushing's syndrome	Evaluates adrenal hormone function. Decreased cortisol levels occur in Addison's dis-ease. Increased levels occur in Cushing's syndrome
Creatinine	0.6–1.2 mg/dL	Evaluation of renal func-tion	Elevation can be seen in renal injury
Erythrocyte sedimen-tation rate (Wester-gren)	Female: 0–20 mm/hr; male: 0–15 mm/hr	Signs and symptoms suggesting chronic inflammation such as temporal arteritis, systemic vasculitis, polymyalgia rheumat-ica, rheumatoid arthri-tis, unexplained weight loss, and joint stiffness	Increased levels are found in collagen disease, infections, inflammatory diseases, car-cinoma, acute heavy metal poisoning. Extreme levels seen in malignant lympho-carcinoma of colon or breast, myeloma, and rheumatoid arthritis

(continued)

TABLE 3.1 Commonly Encountered Labs in Family Medicine (*continued*)

Name	Normal Reference Range	Indication	Interpretation
Glucose, CSF	50–75 mg/dL	Signs and symptoms of CNS infection	Assess impaired transport of glucose from plasma to CSF, CNS infection. Decreased levels signal bacterial meningitis, tuberculosis, and subarachnoid hemorrhage. Increased CSF glucose may imply diabetic hyperglycemia
Glucose, plasma (fasting)	70–99 mg/dL	Diabetes testing	Fasting blood sugar ≥ 126 mg/dL implies a diagnosis of diabetes
Iron studies serum	Serum levels: 50–150 μg/dL Transferrin: 250–425 mg/dL TIBC: 250–310 μg/dL	Symptoms of iron deficiency or iron poisoning	These tests help in the differential diagnosis of anemia. Increased iron is seen in hemolytic anemia. Decreased iron occurs in iron deficiency anemia. Increased transferrin is associated with iron deficiency while decreased transferrin is seen in microcytic anemia of chronic disease. Increased TIBC is found in iron deficiency
Leukocyte count	4,000–11,000 per microliter	Evaluation of infectious causes	Evaluate the number of WBC in the blood. Elevation of leukocyte count may mean infection. Significant elevation or reduction can be seen in blood cancers
Osmolality, urine	38–1,400 mOsm/kg H_2O	Precise measurement of urine concentration and monitoring course of renal disease	Increased osmolality is observed in dehydration, hyponatremia prerenal azotemia HF, Addison's disease. Decreased osmolality occurs in compulsive water drinking, acute renal failure, diabetes insipidus, hypokalemia, hypernatremia
Platelet count	150,000–450,000 per microliter	Assessing bleeding disorder	Increased numbers suggest thrombocythemia, leukemia, myeloproliferative diseases. Decreased levels may signal thrombocytopenic purpura, anemia, infections, or drug toxicity

(*continued*)

TABLE 3.1 Commonly Encountered Labs in Family Medicine (*continued*)

Name	Normal Reference Range	Indication	Interpretation
Potassium	3.5–5.1 mEq/L	Cardiac arrhythmias, most critical conditions	Hyperkalemia can predispose to bradyarrhythmia. Hypokalemia can predispose to ventricular arrhythmias, particularly polymorphic ventricular tachycardia
Prolactin, serum	<20 ng/mL	Symptoms such as amenorrhea, galactorrhea, and infertility. Suspicion of prolactin-secreting tumor	Abnormalities in prolactin levels generally imply a disease in the hypothalamus and pituitary
PSA	<2.5 ng/mL	Screen for prostate cancer in men ≥50 years, men who report prostate symptoms. Used in conjunction with the DRE	Often elevated in men with prostate cancer and benign prostatic hypertrophy, but the test lacks specificity and sensitivity to be considered a gold standard for prostate cancer diagnosis
Reticulocyte count	0.5%–1.5% of red cells	To differentiate anemia caused by bone marrow failure from anemia caused by hemorrhage or hemolysis. Test is also indicated to monitor treatment outcomes	Young, immature, nonnucleated red blood cells found circulating in the blood. Increased reticulocyte count suggests increased red blood cell production, such as in hemolytic anemia. Decreased reticulocyte count suggests that bone marrow is not producing enough erythrocytes such as in iron deficiency anemia
Sodium	135–145 mEq/L	Evaluate and monitor fluid and electrolyte balance and therapy	Levels indicate inverse relationship between free body water and sodium. Symptoms of hyponatremia occur generally at sodium levels <125 mEq/L
SG, urine	1.002–1.030	Evaluation of kidney function	Assess the ability of the kidneys to concentrate or dilute urine (renal dysfunction). Low SG occurs in diabetes insipidus, glomerulonephritis. Increased SG may be associated with dehydration, fever, vomiting, diarrhea glycosuria, infections

(continued)

TABLE 3.1 Commonly Encountered Labs in Family Medicine (*continued*)

Name	Normal Reference Range	Indication	Interpretation
TSH, serum	0.5–4.0 μU/mL (0.5–4.0 mU/L)	Screening for thyroid disorder and monitoring treatment	Assess thyroid function. High TSH implies hypothyroidism and low TSH implies hyperthyroidism
T_4, serum	Total: 5–12 μg/dL Free: 0.8–1.8 ng/dL	Screening for thyroid disorder and monitoring treatment	When combined with TSH levels, T_4 provides additional diagnostic value in assessing thyroid function. T_4 is elevated in Graves' disease and decreased in hypothyroidism
Triglycerides, serum (fasting)	$\leq$100 mg/dL	Assess atherosclerosis risk and body's ability to metabolize fat	Triglycerides are increased in hyperlipoproteinemia, liver disease, alcohol use disorder, renal disease, and in hypothyroidism. Triglycerides are decreased in some congenital, malnutrition and malabsorption disorders

ANC, absolute neutrophil count; BNP, brain natriuretic peptide; BUN, blood urea nitrogen; CNS, central nervous system; CSF, cerebrospinal fluid; DRE, digital rectal exam; HDL, high-density lipoprotein; LDL, low-density lipoprotein; MI, myocardial infarction; PSA, prostate-specific antigen; SG, specific gravity; T_4, thyroxine; TIBC, total iron-binding capacity; TSH, thyroid-stimulating hormone; WBC, white blood cell.

DIAGNOSTIC IMAGING STUDIES

- **CT imaging** is produced by passing a rotating fan beam of x-rays through the patient and measuring the transmission at thousands of points. The absorption of the x-ray beam is measured and an image is created at multiple locations. The images produced are presented as a series of slices of tissue, offering two-dimensional images of multiple areas. The areas can be enhanced by intravenous or oral contrast as needed.[1,2]
  - Contrast is used to differentiate between organs and improve lesion detection. In the lungs, contrast is useful to define abnormalities involving the mediastinum (e.g., mediastinal adenopathy). Contrast offers an improved view in most circumstances.

CLINICAL PEARL: Nephrolithiasis, intracranial hemorrhage, and details of the lung parenchyma are best seen without contrast as abnormalities can be seen simply by the relative density difference in surrounding structures. In some cases (acute hemorrhagic stroke), contrast can obscure pertinent findings.

  - You should consider ordering a CT scan when the diagnosis is not clear on plain films or when additional details are needed.

> **CLINICAL PEARL:** Some common indications for CT scans include acute stroke, closed head injury, diffuse lung disease, renal disease, pancreatitis, and suspected pulmonary embolism.

- **MRI** is produced by applying varying magnetic fields to the body tissues, which causes alignment of atoms. As the field is released, radio waves are generated, which occurs at different levels depending on the tissue it is penetrating. Computer analysis of this data creates the images obtained from this study.[1,2]
  - ○ MRI offers greater details of soft tissue and inflammation than CT. It is also superior in the detection of tumors. Contrast is often not needed, due to the natural contrast that occurs between blood vessels and other tissues. CT scan can offer more detail regarding bony structures.

> **CLINICAL PEARL:** MRI is often a study of choice in the evaluation of the central nervous system, neck, and back due to the fine details the images offer.

  - ○ A major benefit of MRI over CT is that it uses no radiation.
  - ○ Significant disadvantages of MRI over CT include the following:
    - Higher cost, longer study requiring the patient to remain motionless, contraindications in patients with some types of metal implantable devices, and risk of claustrophobia

> **CLINICAL PEARL:** If time is crucial, consider CT scan.

- **Plain radiography** is the most common imaging examination performed. For this test, x-ray beams are passed through the patient, with absorption of different structures occurring at different amounts. A small percentage of the x-ray beam passes through the patient and strikes a fluorescent screen, creating light that exposes the film image.[1,2] Common indications for plain films include the following:
  - ○ Trauma: The primary diagnostic imaging modality of choice in most cases of trauma, plain films can diagnose bony fractures, subcutaneous emphysema, and free air in the abdomen.
  - ○ Joint and spine disease: Plain films are commonly ordered in the assessment of joint and spine disease and should always be considered prior to advanced imaging techniques.
  - ○ Abdominal pain: Plain films can often identify suspected bowel obstruction, perforation, foreign body, and renal calculi.

> **CLINICAL PEARL:** Plain films are less helpful in imaging soft tissue structures.

❍ Cardiopulmonary disease: The chest radiograph should be the first imaging test ordered in the evaluation of dyspnea. This study can identify common abnormalities such as pleural effusions, pneumonia, nodules/masses, atelectasis, pneumothorax, pulmonary vascular congestion, heart failure, and cardiomegaly. Additional abnormalities can include vague descriptions of the amount of x-ray that is absorbed. Denser objects absorb more x-rays and appear lighter on the film. When this occurs, the abnormalities may be referred to as opacities, infiltrates, or consolidation. The clinical scenario often helps guide the diagnosis when these terms are included in a report and may require additional imaging modalities for a conclusive diagnosis. Pertinent findings with associated clinical condition are detailed in Table 3.2.

TABLE 3.2 Chest X-Ray Findings and Their Associated Condition

Condition	Findings
Acute respiratory distress syndrome	Bilateral diffuse pulmonary infiltrate
Asbestos-related disease	Bilateral calcified pleural plaques
Asthma	Severe cases show hyperinflation
Enlarged cardiac silhouette	Heart has a globular contour
COPD	Air trapping leading to hyperinflation, flattened diaphragm, enlarged retrosternal space. The lungs also appear more lucent (dark), with decreased vascular markings
ILD	Reticular or reticular nodular diffused changes, ground glass, honeycombing (scarred shrunken lung)
Mesothelioma	Unilateral irregular nodular and diffuse pleural thickening
Nodule	Single well-circumscribed (rounded) densities
Pancoast tumor	Unilateral apical opacity
Pleural effusion	Silhouette sign, atelectasis, blunting of costophrenic angle
Pneumonia	Opacities, consolidation, fluffy clouds
Pneumothorax	Increased lucency, atelectasis
Pulmonary aspergillosis	Round mass (aspergilloma or fungus ball) with adjacent crescent-shaped air space
Pulmonary hypertension	Enlarged pulmonary arteries; dilated right ventricle and clear lung fields
Sarcoidosis	Bilateral hilar lymphadenopathy
Silicosis	Eggshell calcifications
Solitary pulmonary nodule	Single discrete pulmonary opacity with no adenopathy
Tuberculosis	Upper lobe or diffuse infiltrate with cavitation; hilar and paratracheal lymphadenopathy

COPD, chronic obstructive pulmonary disease; ILD, interstitial lung disease.

- **Ultrasound imaging** (US) is produced by measuring the echoes that are produced by utilization of high-frequency sound waves. The echoes are created based on the different densities of the structures that are being passed. Ultrasound utilization has increased significantly due to the lack of ionizing radiation that is needed to create these images.[1,2]
  - Ultrasound offers excellent views of internal organs and vasculature. Therefore, it is an optimal first study in the evaluation of conditions affecting organs such as the liver, gallbladder, spleen, pancreas, kidneys, bladder, heart, and thyroid.
  - There is also a prominent role for ultrasound in procedures such as fine-needle biopsy in the diagnosis and staging of cancers.
  - Doppler US images allow for determination of blood flow and velocity and can demonstrate arterial plaque and stenosis in the vasculature.

> **CLINICAL PEARL:** US is the study of choice for most acute complaints in the pregnant patient due to its safety and lack of ionizing radiation.

PLAIN RADIOGRAPHY: CHEST X-RAY

- This section will focus on the specifics of the chest x-ray (CXR), as this is the most commonly ordered diagnostic imaging study in family medicine. Indications include the following:
  - Identification of nodules
  - Infection, such as pneumonia
  - Disorders of mediastinum, bony thorax, and major trauma
  - Acute chest pain
  - Asthma/bronchiolitis that is difficult to diagnose or refractory to treatment
  - Evaluation of acute and chronic dyspnea
  - Evaluation of hemoptysis
  - Assessment of a suspected mass, metastasis, or lymphadenopathy
  - Presence of foreign body
  - Heart failure
- When ordering and interpreting a CXR:
  - Obtain both posteroanterior (PA) and lateral views if possible
  - Assess for the film quality/penetration
  - Assess if film was taken in full inspiration
  - If possible, compare current and previous x-rays
  - Use a systematic approach for reading the x-ray

COMPUTED TOMOGRAPHY

Head

> **CLINICAL PEARL:** The most appropriate diagnostic test for a patient with head trauma and altered mental status is a noncontrast CT scan of the head. A contrast-enhanced head CT is discouraged in trauma situations because the contrast can mask hemorrhage.

- Alteration in mental status: A head CT is particularly important in patients with neurologic changes such as those with abnormal scores on the Glasgow Coma Score or Mini-Mental State Examination.
  - Pertinent Findings: Alteration of mental status may be secondary to intracranial injury, cerebral infarction, intracranial hemorrhage, and tumors, which will be detected by the CT. Findings consistent with space-occupying lesions should generally be followed by MRI.
- Cerebrovascular disease and stroke:
  - To identify or exclude hemorrhage as the cause of stroke
  - To identify extraparenchymal hemorrhages, neoplasms, abscesses, and other conditions presenting like a stroke
  - Pertinent findings: Arterial hyperdensity due to a thrombus inside the artery[3]
- Head trauma:
  - In trauma, CT is indicated to evaluate intracranial hemorrhage, cerebral contusion, and skull fractures.
  - Pertinent findings: Hemorrhage appears as white (hyperdense) areas on a CT image.[4] A contusion will appear as a hypodense area, commonly found in the anterior portion of the temporal lobes and in the inferior portions of the frontal lobes.[5]
  - Fractures appear as dark lines running the white-colored skull.
- Mass effect:
  - Pertinent findings: Space-occupying lesions such as tumors, abscesses, and hematoma may push the brain away (slide or herniate), causing loss of normal symmetry or displacement of brain structures.
- Severe chronic rhinosinusitis
  - Pertinent findings: Mucosal thickening, secretions, and opacification of sinuses[6]
  - In fungal sinusitis, CT scan show high soft-tissue attenuation (areas of increased density).

Neck

- Neck cancer: Most common sites of head and neck cancer are the vocal cords, the pterygopalatine fossa, cavernous sinus, and the nasopharyngeal soft tissues.[6]
  - In general, tumors disrupt the normal anatomic spaces and vascular relationships.
  - Pertinent Findings: In case of a carcinoma of the pterygopalatine fossa, a neck CT will reveal a large mass in the pterygopalatine.
  - Parotid gland tumors may push the carotid artery posteriorly or medially.
- Retropharyngeal abscess
  - Pertinent findings: On a CT scan, the abscess may be visualized as a mass impinging on the posterior pharyngeal wall. Other findings include soft-tissue swelling and mass effect.
- Carotid or vertebral artery dissection or stenosis
  - Pertinent findings: Dissection is often accompanied by hemorrhage.[2,7–9]

- Traumatic injury of the neck: CT commonly follows plain radiography imaging.
  - Pertinent findings: Can identify high-risk injuries, in spinal cord trauma, or in patients with altered cognition[7,10]
  - Parapharyngeal gas and fat stranding are some of the signs of pharyngoesophageal perforation on a CT.

Cardiac

- Aortic dissection
  - Pertinent findings: Evaluate for contrast filling a true lumen and a false lumen[7]
- Coronary artery calcification
  - Pertinent findings: Calcium present in the left anterior descending artery proximal to its point of bifurcation into the LAD and circumflex arteries. Abnormalities are identified using the left vessels only.[7]

Chest

- Pulmonary nodules and neoplasm
  - A suspected lung tumor is an indication for CT scanning, which helps in the diagnosis, staging, and defining the location as parenchymal, mediastinal, or pleural.
  - Pertinent findings: Lung adenocarcinoma appears as peripheral mass (>5 cm) or nodule (<5 cm) with spiculated borders (spikes or points on the surface).[6]
  - Squamous cell carcinoma generally occurs in the walls of a central bronchus and presents with bronchial obstruction. Small cell will appear as a central mass.
  - For pulmonary nodules, CT may show growth rate, density, shape, and malignancy potential. Lesions <5 mm are considered benign, but must be followed depending on the patient's age, growth rate, and density of the lesion.[7]
- Dyspnea
  - CT scan is useful in evaluating dyspnea in conditions such as increased reticular markings on a CXR, hyperinflation, pleural effusion, anatomic abnormalities, and enlarged or abnormal heart contour on a chest radiograph.
  - Pertinent findings: For acute dyspnea, CT may show filling defects within pulmonary arteries, commonly at the bifurcation of an artery[7]
  - For chronic dyspnea, CT may show ground-glass opacities, with possible effusions, atelectasis, pleural thickening.[7]
- Sarcoidosis
  - Pertinent findings: Chest CT is essential in defining the extent of lymphadenopathy secondary to sarcoidosis.
- Thoracic trauma
  - Following a traumatic event, CT scan should be ordered whenever there is high clinical suspicion for internal organ injury.
  - Pertinent findings: Evaluate for mediastinal hematoma and aortic lacerations[7]
  - In case of an aortic rupture, CT scan will show aortic wall irregularity.

- Pulmonary thromboembolism
  - ○ On a CT, chronic pulmonary embolism manifests as peripheral filling defects within the walls of pulmonary arteries

Abdomen

- Abdominal mass
  - ○ Pertinent findings: Dilation of the outer diameter of the aorta >3 cm is diagnostic for abdominal aortic aneurysm (AAA). Intimal flap with true and false lumen is diagnostic of aortic dissection.[7]
- Acute abdominal pain, fever
  - ○ Pertinent findings: Evaluation for peritonitis. For appendicitis, most commonly CT demonstrates distended appendix of >6 mm in diameter, thickened walls, and periappendiceal changes with fat stranding.[7,11]
- Abdominal injury and blunt trauma
  - ○ Pertinent findings: Diagnostic study of choice in patients with blunt abdominal trauma. Evaluate for signs of peritoneal-free fluid[7,12]
- Bowel obstruction, suspected
  - ○ Pertinent findings: CT reveals site of obstruction, inflammation, or neoplasia. Dilated loops of small bowel filled with gas and fluid are the most common radiological findings.
- Flank pain
  - ○ Pertinent findings: Unilateral hydronephrosis, possible urinary tract calcification (calculus)[7]
- Jaundice
  - ○ Pertinent findings: Evaluate for biliary obstruction with findings of a dilated bile duct. Etiologies may include gallstones, tumor, stricture, and pancreatitis.[7,13]
- Pancreatitis
  - ○ Pertinent findings: CT provides a definitive diagnosis of pancreatitis with findings such as edema, inflammation, fluid, and dilatation. Focal or diffuse enlargement of the pancreas, with decreased density of the pancreatic parenchyma, may be noted.[7]
- Crohn's disease
  - ○ Pertinent findings: Wall thickening of the terminal ileum. On further examination by colonoscopy, areas of thickened mucosa with skip lesions, deep rose-thorn ulcerations, strictures, and fistulae are common findings.
- Diverticulitis
  - ○ Pertinent findings: CT can reveal colonic wall thickening, inflammation, and pockets of extraluminal gas (in case of perforation).[14]

Pelvis

- Abnormal uterine bleeding
  - ○ CT may be performed if ultrasound suggests mass. CT findings of endometrial carcinoma include a mass, dilation, and fluid in the endometrial canal.
- Hematuria: CT abdomen should be included
  - ○ Pertinent findings: Evaluate for hydronephrosis, renal calculi, and bladder carcinoma, which will appear as a focal thickening of the bladder wall or soft-tissue mass projecting into the bladder.[7]

- Nephrolithiasis
  - ○ Pertinent findings: Renal calculi appear as high attenuation on a CT. Other findings include calcification of the associated collecting system.
- Ovarian mass, suspected cancer
  - ○ Pertinent findings: Cystic mass with thick, irregular walls, internal septations, and prominent soft-tissue components[7]
- Pelvic inflammatory disease
  - ○ Pertinent findings: Thickening of the uterine tubes and enlargement of the ovaries.[5] Pyosalpinx has the appearance of uterine tube filled with high-attenuation fluids and debris in the adnexa.[7]
- Prostate carcinoma
  - ○ Pertinent findings: Evaluate the degree of involvement of various pelvis structures. Prostate cancer appears as an enlargement with nodules and/or stranding densities in the periprostatic fat as well as asymmetric enlargement of seminal vesicles.[7]

Musculoskeletal

- Malignant bone neoplasms
  - ○ Pertinent findings: If bone neoplasms are suspected on plain films, CT and MRI imaging should be ordered to identify additional areas.
- Trauma: Hip/pelvis fracture
  - ○ Pertinent findings: CT is indicated when evaluating for loose bodies or when a position of a fragment needs to be determined. CT may also be necessary when plain films do not clearly show all the abnormalities or if the clinical picture suggests fracture in light of a negative plain film.[7,10]
- Sacroiliac joints
  - ○ Pertinent findings: Sacroiliac joint sclerosis and erosions in ankylosing spondylitis[7,10]
- Trauma: Thoracic/lumbar spine
  - ○ Pertinent findings: Compression deformity of a spinal level[7,10]

MAGNETIC RESONANCE IMAGING

Head

- Acoustic schwannoma
  - ○ Pertinent findings: MRI with gadolinium is the imaging modality of choice for acoustic schwannoma and will show a brightly enhancing mass in the internal auditory canal (IAC)[15]
- Dizziness
  - ○ Pertinent findings: Sequelae of bleeding or mass including mass effect, acute cerebrovascular accident, or parenchymal disease[1,2,7]
- Headache
  - ○ Pertinent findings: Sequelae of bleeding or mass including mass effect, vascular density, and activity of the tumor[1,2,7,16]
- Infection
  - ○ Pertinent findings: White matter changes of the brain parenchyma indicating acute infection[1,2,7]

- Multiple sclerosis
  - ○ Pertinent findings: MRI lesions suggestive of multiple sclerosis may be seen in the periventricular area, corpus callosum, centrum semiovale, and basal ganglia. Hyperintensity is seen on T2-weighted studies; hypointensity is seen on T1 weighting.[1,2]
- Brain neoplasms
  - ○ Pertinent findings: MRI will show small enhanced lesions
- Seizure
  - ○ Pertinent findings: Evaluation of fine cerebral anatomy, often used in preparation for surgery[1,7]
- Stroke
  - ○ Pertinent findings: MRI will show decreased perfusion, most commonly in the distribution of the middle cerebral artery.[7,17] MRI with diffusion-weighted imaging is very sensitive and specific in diagnosing strokes. It reveals an area of high signal intensity in the affected territory of the stroke.

Neck

- Brachial plexus injury
  - ○ Pertinent findings: Direct visualization of the nerves constituting the brachial plexus[7]
- Carotid disease
  - ○ Pertinent findings: Evaluation of the entire internal carotid artery is possible with this modality. Imaging can determine size, composition, and the presence of plaque inflammation.[18] Bright lumen signals along the distribution of the carotid artery are considered positive.[7–9]
- Cervical adenopathy
  - ○ Pertinent findings: Size and morphology can be estimated by MRI. Biopsy is still needed.[2,7,19]

Chest

- Mesothelioma
  - ○ Pertinent findings: Low intensity signal on T1 weighting. Hyperintensity seen on T2 weighting[7]

Abdomen

- Aortic disease
  - ○ Pertinent findings: Used in cases when echocardiogram is nondiagnostic[1,7]
- Biliary colic with jaundice
  - ○ Pertinent findings: Magnetic resonance cholangiopancreatography (MRCP) can be used to assess the intrahepatic and extrahepatic bile ducts and pancreatic duct. It is used to assess for biliary obstruction, cholangiocarcinoma, and malignant lesions of the biliary system.[1,2,7]
- Renal artery stenosis
  - ○ Pertinent findings: MRA used to assess proximal renal artery stenosis[7,9]
- Tumors/cysts of the adrenals, kidneys, liver, pancreas, and spleen
  - ○ Pertinent findings: Used if indeterminate findings on other imaging studies, such as ultrasound or CT[2,7]

Pelvis

- Bladder mass
  - ○ Pertinent findings: Used to determine the extent of damage to the bladder wall, muscular involvement, and local lymphatic metastasis for staging in the presence of bladder cancer[7]
- Ovarian or uterine mass
  - ○ Pertinent findings: Used to assess if other screening modalities are indeterminate, such as CT or ultrasound. Some evidence suggests that the presence of calcifications in the uterine mass is more likely to be leiomyomatous disease.[7]
- Prostate cancer
  - ○ Pertinent findings: Used in staging and metastasis of prostate cancer[7]

Musculoskeletal

- Back pain
  - ○ Pertinent findings: Most sensitive for early detection of disk injuries, metastatic lesions, and neuropathic disease
- Herniated disk/HNP
  - ○ Pertinent findings: Localizes the area of nerve impingement and stenosis[7]
- Infection including osteomyelitis
  - ○ Pertinent findings: Marrow edema and enhancement. Evaluate for abscess, sinus tract, and skin ulcers.[7]
- Multiple sclerosis
  - ○ Pertinent findings: MRI lesions suggestive of multiple sclerosis may be seen in the periventricular area, corpus callosum, centrum semiovale, and basal ganglia. Hyperintensity is seen on T2-weighted studies; hypointensity is seen on T1 weighting.[7]
- Neuropathy/radiculopathy
  - ○ Pertinent findings: Evaluation of disk herniation as well as intraspinal pathologies, inflammatory disorders, metastatic lesions, and vascular anomalies[7]
- Trauma to the cervical, thoracic, or lumbar spine
  - ○ Pertinent findings: Used if CT unavailable. Evaluation of the spinal cord is best performed with MRI if neurologic findings present. Underestimates the presence of bony injuries[2,7]
- Osteomyelitis
  - ○ Pertinent findings: MRI enables visualization of lytic cortical lesions and spread of infection to other structures.

ULTRASOUND

Head and Neck

- Head and neck sonograms are used to evaluate carotid or vertebral artery stenosis
  - ○ Pertinent findings: Normal carotid appears as two thin bright lines with a hypoechoic layer in between. In atherosclerotic disease, ultrasound allows plaque identification, visualization of intimal thickness, and luminal narrowing.[18]

- Lymphadenopathy.
  - Pertinent findings: Enlarged benign nodes demonstrate hypoechoic outer cortex and hyperechoic inner medulla. Numerous and large nodes are likely to be lymphoma.[18]
- Salivary gland masses
  - Pertinent findings: Warthin's tumors are benign tumors of the parotid gland. They appear complex, mixed solid, and cystic masses. Pleomorphic adenomas appear in the superficial part of the glands and appear solid, hypoechoic, and homogenous with some detectable vascularity.[18]
  - In case of salivary gland stones (sialolithiasis), ultrasound shows echogenic structures that cast an acoustic shadow in the submandibular glands.[18]
- Thyroid and parathyroid disease
  - Pertinent findings: Ultrasound is useful in differentiating cysts from solid tumors.
  - Normal thyroid is hyperechoic to adjacent muscles and homogeneous, with diameter of the lobes <2 cm in anteroposterior (AP) and transverse views. Nodular hyperplasia reveal multiple internal septations, wall thickening, solid or partially solid mural nodules, or a combination of these findings.[2] Malignant lesions can appear solid and hypoechoic with microcalcifications. They often have lobulated margins.[18]
  - In Graves' disease, ultrasound will show gland enlargement, decreased echogenicity, occasional heterogeneity, and hypervascularity. Hashimoto's thyroiditis appears as enlarged and hypoechoic on ultrasound, with heterogeneous changes and increased vascularity.[7,18]

Chest/Breast

- Chest wall mass and breast cysts
  - Pertinent findings: Ultrasound enables differentiation of cysts from solid lesions and guides cyst aspirations and needle biopsies. Normal chest appears as a solid, hypoechoic collection of tissue. Neoplastic involvement of the ribs is generally visible, if present.[18]
- Pleural disease
  - Pertinent findings: Used in the presence of pleural effusion to perform thoracentesis. Pleural fluid as small as 3 mL is detectable with ultrasound.[18]

Abdomen

- Aorta and large abdominal vessels
  - Pertinent findings: Aneurysms, clots, and tumors
- Flank pain and hematuria
  - Pertinent findings: In complicated urinary tract infection involving abscess, ultrasound will show complex fluid collections or complex cystic masses (abscess). In the presence of large hematuria with minimal pain, renal cell carcinoma will appear as hypoechoic structures compared to normal adjacent renal parenchyma on sonography. Renal stones will appear as hyperechoic structures with posterior shadowing.[18]

- Hepatobiliary disease
  - Pertinent findings: In acute cholecystitis, gallstones, wall thickening, enlargement, and pericholecystic fluid will be visible. Murphy sign is commonly present. Gallstones appear as mobile, echogenic, intraluminal structures that cast shadows due to sound beam absorption by stones.
  - In cirrhosis, a shrunken liver with nodular contours and adjacent ascites may be visible. In hepatic steatosis, findings include increased echogenicity of the liver.[18]
- Pancreatitis diseases
  - Pertinent findings: Ultrasound is used to assess for tumors, cysts, and inflammatory processes. In chronic pancreatitis, calcifications that appear as multifocal, punctate, and hyperechoic foci may be visible on ultrasound. Pancreatic carcinoma appears as hypoechoic masses. Simultaneous dilation of the common bile duct and the pancreatic duct should always prompt a consideration of pancreatic cancer.[18]
- Portal hypertension
  - Pertinent findings: Slowed portal vein flow too slow to be detected by Doppler ultrasound or slows to undetectable varying with respirations[18]
- Traumatic abdominal injury (FAST Scan)
  - Pertinent findings: Focused Assessment with Sonography for Trauma (FAST) is a rapid bedside ultrasound examination that allows a timely screening and diagnosis in patients with blunt abdominal trauma (BAT). It involves evaluation of the hepatorenal recess, (Morrison's pouch), perisplenic space, pericardium, and the pelvis. It is possible to detect intraperitoneal and pericardial free fluid.[20]
  - Liver injury will appear as hyperechoic. Localized fluid around the spleen in the presence of traumatic injury may indicate splenic laceration.[7,12,18]

Pelvis

- Gynecologic and obstetric ultrasound is done to assess hematuria, urinary tract, bladder, uterus, and ovaries, and to monitor embryonic development.
  - Pertinent findings: Hydronephrosis and calcifications in the urinary system are noted if kidney stones are present. If urothelial tumors are present, small focal wall thickening, possibly with blood flow, will be demonstrated on Doppler evaluation.[18]
  - Ovarian cysts appear as anechoic areas with a thin or imperceptible wall, nodule, or internal echoes and exhibit posterior enhancement.[2] Hemorrhagic cysts demonstrate reticular pattern or fine, linear echoes and strands inside the cyst with internal echoes and posterior enhancement. Dermoid cysts appear as highly echogenic areas with posterior sound attenuation. Calcifications are commonly seen.[18]
- Obstetric
  - Pertinent findings: First trimester findings may include yolk sac, with anechoic lesion with central hyperechoic wall. Cardiac activity will

become visible at 5 to 7 mm size. Structures seen in the first trimester include the fetal bladder, stomach, choroid plexus, four extremities, and the abdominal cord insertion. During second and third trimester evaluations, fetal cardiac activity, fetal number, and presentation should be documented. By the third trimester, most fetal anatomic structures should be visible.[18]

- Ovarian torsion
  - Pertinent findings: Unilateral ovarian enlargement, with heterogeneous edema, hemorrhage, ischemia, or necrosis. Doppler demonstration of blood flow in an ovary does not exclude torsion.[18]
- Polycystic ovarian syndrome
  - Pertinent findings: Ovarian volume over 10 mL and identification of 12 or more follicles measuring between 2 and 9 mm[18]
- Male reproductive organ sonogram
  - Epididymitis/epididymo-orchitis
  - Pertinent findings: Enlargement and decreased echogenicity of the epididymis. Color Doppler imaging may detect inflammatory hyperemia and increased epididymal vascularity.[18]
- Scrotal mass
  - Pertinent findings: Hydroceles occur in the anterior aspect of the scrotum and displace the testes posteriorly. Spermatoceles (most common) appear as cystic lesions in the head of the epididymis and are filled with spermatozoa-containing fluid. Low echoes are seen in the lumen. Varicoceles appear as cystic masses most commonly on the left, and appear as numerous, dilated, tortuous, tubular channels in the peritesticular tissues.[18]
- Testicular pain
  - Pertinent findings: The left testis will most commonly torse in a counterclockwise direction, while the right testis will torse in the clockwise direction. The torsion knot will appear as a solid, heterogeneous mass adjacent to the testis. The echogenicity of the testis may be normal, decreased, or increased and may be homogenous or heterogeneous. Color Doppler will demonstrate asymmetric flow or absence of flow to the testis.[18]

Musculoskeletal

- Arterial and venous blood flow
  - Pertinent findings: Ultrasound helps in detecting deep venous thrombosis.
- Arthritis or crystal deposition
  - Pertinent findings: Crystal deposition will appear hyperechoic on the surface of cartilage. Osteoarthritis appears as well-defined bone excrescence at a margin of an involved joint. An effusion may be present. Rheumatoid arthritis will demonstrate bone cortex abnormalities. Rheumatoid nodules typically appear as hypoechoic nodules.[10,18]
- Infection
  - Pertinent findings: Changes associated with abscess include a well-defined, hypoechoic heterogeneous fluid collection with posterior through-transmission and hyperemia on Doppler. Changes associated

with cellulitis include hyperechoic and thickened subcutaneous tissue. Later, hypoechoic or anechoic branching channels are visualized, with distortion of soft tissues and possible increased vascular flow.[10,18]

- Soft tissue mass and foreign body
  - ○ Pertinent findings: Ganglion cysts appear as hypoechoic or anechoic multilocular noncompressible cysts. Lipomas appear as hypoechoic lesions within the soft-tissue mass. They are isoechoic to the surrounding subcutaneous fat tissue.[10,18]
  - ○ All foreign bodies are hyperechoic.[10,18]

Other frequently requested diagnostic studies and tests are listed in Table 3.3.

TABLE 3.3 Other Frequently Requested Diagnostic Studies in Family Medicine

Diagnostic Study	Indication
DEXA scan	At least once after age 65 in women. Measure bone mineral density, osteopenia, and osteoporosis and assess fracture risk. The T-score refers to the number of SD for the patient compared with normal young adults. Osteopenia is 1.0–2.0 SD below normal. Osteoporosis is ≥2.5 SD below normal
PCR	Technique in molecular genetics that is used to exponentially amplify a few copies of DNA segment to generate millions of copies of that target DNA sequence. PCR is often used to diagnose infections and mutations.
Potassium hydroxide prep (KOH)	Used to diagnose fungal infections of the skin and nails. Positive findings: Microscopic examination will show hyphae and grapelike clumps of thick-walled spores.
Pulmonary function tests	Evaluate pulmonary dysfunction caused by obstruction or restrictive diseases. Indications include dyspnea, staging of asthma and COPD, periodic evaluation of certain occupational workers, and monitoring disease progression after therapeutic interventions. Commonly used measurements are FVC (maximum amount of air in liters that can be exhaled forcibly and completely after a maximal inspiration); FEV_1; and FEV_1/FVC. An obstructive disease process, such as COPD, is implied by a low FEV_1/FVC ratio (<70%)
Tuberculosis blood test (Quanti-FERON Gold)	Blood test used for diagnosing *Mycobacterium tuberculosis*. It is more specific than PPD skin testing, and its accuracy is not affected by prior BCG vaccination.
Tuberculosis skin test	Skin test for *Mycobacterium tuberculosis* (TB) utilized for screening and diagnosing latent TB. Result is positive if induration ≥15 mm. For high-risk populations (e.g., patients experiencing homelessness, healthcare workers, prisoners), 10 mm induration is considered positive. For immunocompromised patients (e.g., patients with HIV/AIDS), 5 mm induration is considered positive

COPD, chronic obstructive pulmonary disease; BCG, bacille Calmette–Guérin; DEXA, dual-energy x-ray absorptiometry; FEV_1/FVC, ratio of a timed forced expiratory volume to the forced vital capacity; FEV_1, forced expiratory volume in one second; FVC, forced vital capacity; PPD, purified protein derivative; SD, standard deviations; TB, tuberculosis.

ADDITIONAL RESOURCES

1. American Board of Internal Medicine Laboratory Test Reference Ranges–August 2018. https://www.abim.org/~/media/ABIM%20Public/Files/pdf/exam/laboratory-reference-ranges.pdf.
2. Fischbach FT, Dunning MB. *A Manual of Laboratory and Diagnostic Tests*. Philadelphia, PA: Lippincott Williams & Wilkins; 2009.
3. Sloane PD. *Essentials of Family Medicine*. Philadelphia, PA: Lippincott Williams & Wilkins; 2008.
4. Johnson JD, Theurer WM. A stepwise approach to the interpretation of pulmonary function tests. *Am Fam Physician*. 2014;89(5):359–366.

REFERENCES

1. American College of Radiology. ACR appropriateness criteria. http://www.acr.org/Quality-Safety/Appropriateness-Criteria/Diagnostic. Accessed September 2, 2018.
2. Crownover B, Bepko J. Appropriate and safe use of diagnostic imaging. *Am Fam Physicians*. April 1, 2013;87(7):494–501.
3. Marks MP, Holmgren EB, Fox AJ, et al. Evaluation of early computed tomographic findings in acute ischemic stroke. *stroke*. 1999;30(2):389–392. doi:10.1161/01.STR.30.2.389
4. Heit JJ, Iv M, Wintermark M. Imaging of intracranial hemorrhage. *J stroke*. 2017;19(1):11. doi:10.5853/jos.2016.00563
5. Kim JJ, Gean AD. Imaging for the diagnosis and management of traumatic brain injury. *Neurotherapeutics*. 2011;8(1):39–53. doi:10.1007/s13311-010-0003-3
6. Uzelac A, Davis RW. *Blueprints Radiology*. Philadelphia, PA: Lippincott Williams & Wilkins; 2006.
7. Chen M, Pope T, Ott D. *Basic Radiology*. 2nd ed. New York, NY: McGraw-Hill; 2011. http://accessmedicine.mhmedical.com/content.aspx?bookid=360&sectionid=39669003. Accessed September 4, 2018.
8. Kerwin WS, Hatsukami T, Yuan C, Zhao XQ. MRI of carotid atherosclerosis. *AJR Am J Roentgenol*. 2013;200(3):W304–W313. doi:10.2214/AJR.12.8665
9. Shin J, Suh D, Choi C, et al. Vertebral artery dissection: spectrum of imaging findings with emphasis on angiography and correlation with clinical presentation. *RadioGraphics*. November 1, 2000;20(6):1687–1696. doi:10.1148/radiographics.20.6.g00nv081687
10. Manaster B, May D, Disler D. *Musculoskeletal Imaging*. 4th ed. Philadelphia, PA: Elsevier; 2013.
11. Paulson E, Coursey C. CT protocols for acute appendicitis: time for change. *AJR Am J Roentgenol*. 2009;193(5):1268–1271. doi:10.2214/AJR.09.3313
12. Shanmuganathan K, Mirvis SE, Chiu WC, et al. Triple-contrast helical CT in penetrating torso trauma: a prospective study to determine peritoneal violation and the need for laporotomy. *AJR Am J Roentgenol*. 2001;177(6):1247–1256. doi:10.2214/ajr.177.6.1771247
13. Abraham S, Rivero H, Erlikh I, et al. Surgical and nonsurgical management of gallstones. *Am Fam Physician*. May 15, 2014;89(10):795–802.
14. DeStigter KK, Keating DP. Imaging update: acute colonic diverticulitis. *Clin Colon Rectal Surg*. 2009;22(3):147. doi:10.1055/s-0029-1236158
15. Williams JC, Carr CM, Eckel LJ, et al. Utility of noncontrast magnetic resonance imaging for detection of recurrent vestibular schwannoma. *Otol Neurotol*. 2018;39(3):372–377. doi:10.1097/MAO.0000000000001698

16. Jamshed N, Dubin J, Eldadah Z. Emergency management of palpitations in the elderly: epidemiology, diagnostic approaches, and therapeutic options. *Clin Geriatr Med.* 2013;29:205–230. doi:10.1016/j.cger.2012.10.003
17. Maxwell R. *Maxwell Quick Medical Reference.* Grass Valley, CA: Maxwell Publishing Company; 2011.
18. Hertzberg B, Middleton W. *The Requisites of Ultrasound.* 3rd ed. Philadelphia, PA: Elsevier; 2016.
19. Haynes J, Arnold K, Aguirre-Oskins C, et al. Evaluation of neck masses in adults. AAFP.org. *Am Fam Physician.* May 15, 2015;91(10):698–706.
20. Scalea TM, Rodriguez A, Chiu WC, et al. Focused assessment with sonography for trauma (FAST): results from an international consensus conference. *J Trauma Acute Care Surg.* 1999;46(3):466–472. doi:10.1097/00005373-199903000-00022

4

Patient Education and Counseling in Family Medicine

AGE APPROPRIATE SCREENINGS

Office visits for health promotion and disease prevention, also known as "well visits" or "health maintenance" visits, are a large part of what a family medicine PA does on a daily basis. These visits allow an opportunity for patients and families to focus on their overall health, ask questions, and hear advice on lifestyle modifications and recommendations for preventive screenings. These visits occur much more frequently in infancy and childhood than they do in adulthood. Regardless of the reason for the patient's visit, whether it be for health maintenance, an acute problem, or management of a chronic condition, you should always check the patient's chart to see if they are up-to-date on preventive screenings and immunizations.

For infants and children, focus on the following aspects of care: disease detection, disease prevention, health promotion, and anticipatory guidance.[1] Developmental and disease surveillance should occur at every visit, with specific dedicated screenings at certain visits. Much of this is accomplished during the history and physical examination portions of the visit. Primary and secondary disease prevention measures should be discussed and recommended.[1] Health promotion focuses on wellness and evaluating social determinants of health.[1] All visits should conclude with anticipatory guidance. Anticipatory guidance gives advice to families regarding upcoming development, changes, and potential challenges. It should be timely, appropriate, and relevant.[1]

For adults, focus on health promotion and disease prevention. Specific attention should be directed toward recommended screening instruments and tests as well as ways to reduce risk factors for the development of chronic disease. Immunizations should not be forgotten in this population. A detailed history to include review of past medical/surgical history, social history, and family history is important as is a thorough physical examination.

Well-child exams are recommended at the following ages during infancy: initial newborn exam, 3 to 5 days, 1 month, 2 months, 4 months, 6 months, 9 months.[2] During early childhood, visits should occur at 12 months, 15 months, 18 months, 24 months, 30 months, 3 years, 4 years.[2] Visits occur annually from ages 5 to 21 years.[2]

In addition to the history, vital sign measurement, physical examination, developmental surveillance, psychosocial/behavioral assessment, and anticipatory guidance that occurs at well visits, the following additional screenings are recommended by the American Academy of Pediatrics:

INFANCY (BIRTH TO 9 MONTHS)

- *Hearing screening*: To be performed as a newborn and this should be verified by the provider by 2 months of age[2]
- *Developmental screening*: To be performed at the 9-month visit to assess vision, hearing, motor skills, and early communication skills[3]
- *Maternal depression screening*: To be performed by the 1-month visit and at the 2-, 4-, and 6-month visits
- *Newborn blood testing*: Confirm testing was complete, and review results at the time of initial newborn exam
- *Oral health risk assessment*: At the 6- and 9-month visit

EARLY CHILDHOOD (12 MONTHS TO 4 YEARS)

- *Body mass index (BMI) screening*: Begins at 24 months of age[2]
- *Blood pressure screening*: Routinely begins at 3 years of age
- *Vision screening*: At the 3-year and 4-year visits
- *Hearing screening*: At the 4-year visit
- *Developmental screening*: At the 18- and 30-month visits
- *Autism Spectrum Disorder screening*: At the 18- and 24-month visits

> **CLINICAL PEARL:** The Modified Checklist for Autism in Toddlers (M-CHAT) is a commonly used, validated instrument used to screen for autism spectrum disorders.

- *Anemia screening*: To be performed at the 12-month visit
- *Lead risk assessment*: To be performed at the 12- and 24-month visits. Specific questions include, Does the child live in or regularly visit a building built before 1950? Does the child live in or regularly visit a building built before 1978 that is being renovated or has recently been renovated? Does the child have a sibling or peer who has/had lead poisoning?[4]
- *Fluoride varnish*: Consider application of fluoride varnish once teeth are present; this may be reapplied every 3 to 6 months

MIDDLE CHILDHOOD (5–10 YEARS)

- *Vision screening*: 5-, 6-, 8-, and 10-year visits[2]
- *Hearing screening*: 5-, 6-, 8-, and 10-year visits

ADOLESCENCE (11–21 YEARS)

- *Vision screening*: 12- and 15-year visits[2]
- *Hearing screening*: Once between 11 and 14 years, once between 15 and 17 years, and once between 18 and 21 years
- *Tobacco, alcohol, drug use assessment*: Perform risk assessment at all adolescent visits, screen if risk dictates
- *Depression screening*: Begin at 12-year visit and repeat annually. The Patient Health Questionnaire (PHQ)-2 or other validated tools are recommended
- *Dyslipidemia*: Assess risk and consider screening between the ages of 17 and 21 years
- *HIV*: Screen between 15 and 18 years of age and repeat annually if at risk

ADULTHOOD (22 YEARS AND OLDER)

- *Alcohol use disorders*: Several validated instruments exist for screening for the presence of an alcohol use disorder. The Alcohol Use Disorders Identification Test (AUDIT) has been well studied. It consists of 10 multiple choice questions regarding the amount of alcohol consumed and behaviors related to alcohol use. The CAGE screening questions are a set of four questions, which can be easily memorized and asked by the clinician.
- *Tobacco use*: All adults should be asked about tobacco use at every visit. Even brief interventions in the clinical setting can be effective in aiding patients with tobacco cessation. Be aware of commonly used behavioral and pharmacological interventions to assist patients who wish to quit using tobacco.
- *Depression*: The PHQ-9 is an appropriate tool to use for depression screening. Annual screening is recommended.

REFERENCES

1. Hagan JF Jr, Shaw JS, Duncan PM. *United States. Health Resources and Services Administration, United States. Department of Health and Human Services, United States. Maternal and Child Health Bureau. Bright Futures: Guidelines for Health Supervision of Infants, Children, and Adolescents.* 4th ed. Elk Grove Village: American Academy of Pediatrics; 2017.
2. https://www.aap.org/en-us/Documents/periodicity_schedule.pdf. Updated February 2017. Accessed September 2018.
3. Council on Children With Disabilities, Section on Developmental Behavioral Pediatrics, Bright Futures Steering Committee, Medical Home Initiatives for Children With Special Needs Project Advisory Committee. Identifying infants and young children with developmental disorders in the medical home: an algorithm for developmental surveillance and screening. *Pediatrics.* 2006;118:405.
4. Committee on Environmental Health. Screening for elevated blood lead levels. *Pediatrics.* 1998;101(6):1072–1078.

IMMUNIZATIONS

The evidence is clear that vaccines reduce the risk of certain diseases and promote public health and wellness. Family medicine physician assistants (PAs) are integral to the promotion of adherence to immunization recommendations. Most patients will consent to vaccination, but some will not. Others are unsure of how they feel about vaccines. It is vital for PAs to feel comfortable discussing the role of vaccination, the recommended schedule, and any concerns about vaccine safety their patients or families may have. The Centers for Disease Control and Prevention (CDC) have a variety of resources available to clinicians to help them build this skill.[1]

It is important to note, the CDC's recommended vaccine schedule may change yearly. It is always easily accessible through its website or smartphone app. The immunization schedules provide details on when to administer each dose of the vaccine and what to do if a dose is missed or if a patient is behind schedule on immunizations and needs to catch up. Providers can also access current vaccine information statement (VIS) handouts for patients. These documents are specific to each vaccine and are available in several languages. They explain the reason each vaccine is recommended, the general dosing schedule, contraindications to the vaccine, possible adverse effects and recommended actions, and information on the National Vaccine Injury Compensation Program (VCIP).

CHILDREN AND ADOLESCENTS

Recommended vaccinations for children and adolescents are noted in Table 4.1.

ADULTS

Recommended routine vaccinations for adults are noted in Table 4.2.

REFERENCES

1. https://www.cdc.gov/vaccines/hcp/patient-ed/educating-patients.html. Updated August 2, 2016. Accessed September 2018.
2. https://www.cdc.gov/vaccines/schedules/downloads/child/0-18yrs-child-combined-schedule.pdf. Updated May 14, 2018. Accessed September 2018.
3. Recommended immunization schedule for adults aged 19 years or older, United States, 2018. www.cdc.gov. https://www.cdc.gov/vaccines/schedules/downloads/adult/adult-combined-schedule.pdf. Updated April 24, 2018. Accessed September 2018.
4. Grohskopf LA, Sokolow LZ, Broder KR, et al. Prevention and control of seasonal influenza with vaccines: recommendations of the advisory committee on immunization practices—United States, 2018–19 Influenza Season. *MMWR Recomm Rep*. 2018;67(No. RR-3):1–20. doi:10.15585/mmwr.rr6703a1
5. Liang JL, Tiwari T, Moro P, et al. Prevention of pertussis, tetanus, and diphtheria with vaccines in the United States: recommendations of the advisory committee on immunization practices (ACIP. *MMWR Recomm Rep*. 2018;67(No. RR-2):1–44. doi:10.15585/mmwr.rr6702a1
6. Dooling KL, Guo A, Patel M, et al. Recommendations of the advisory committee on immunization practices for use of herpes zoster vaccines. *MMWR Morb Mortal Wkly Rep*. 2018;67:103–108. doi:10.15585/mmwr.mm6703a5

TABLE 4.1 Recommended Routine Vaccines for Children and Adolescents

Vaccine Name	Vaccine Abbreviation	Number of Doses	Recommended Ages for Routine Dosing	Notes
Hepatitis B	Hepatitis B	3 doses	Birth 1–2 months 6–18 months	Birth dosing schedule changes and the addition of HBIG may be indicated if mother tests positive for hepatitis B
Rotavirus	RV1	2 doses	2 months 4 months	This vaccine is an oral suspension, not an injection
	RV5	3 doses	2 months 4 months 6 months	Either RV1 or RV5 may be administered, but not both
Diphtheria, tetanus, and acellular pertussis	DTaP	5 doses	2 months 4 months 6 months 15–18 months 4–6 years	Be sure not to confuse this vaccine with the tetanus, diphtheria, and acellular pertussis vaccine (Tdap). The Tdap vaccine is indicated for children >7 years and adults
Haemophilus influenzae type b	HiB (PRP-T)	4 doses	2 months 4 months 6 months 12–15 months	Administer either formulation of this vaccine, not both HiB (PRP-T) is sold under the brand names ActHIB and Hibrix
	HiB (PRP-OMP)	3 doses	2 months 4 months 12–15 months	Hib (PRP-OMP) is sold under the brand name PedvaxHIB
Pneumococcal conjugate	PCV13	4 doses	2 months 4 months 6 months 12–15 months	

(continued)

TABLE 4.1 Recommended Routine Vaccines for Children and Adolescents (*continued*)

Vaccine Name	Vaccine Abbreviation	Number of Doses	Recommended Ages for Routine Dosing	Notes
Poliovirus vaccine (inactivated)	IPV	4 doses	2 months 4 months 6–18 months 4–6 years	Not recommended for people 18 years and older
Influenza vaccine (inactivated)	IIV	In a child aged 6 months to 8 years who did not receive at least 2 doses of the previous year's flu vaccine before July 1 of the current year: 2 doses Children 9 years and older: 1 dose	Immunization begins at 6 months of age and is recommended annually	The LAIV recommendations typically vary by year
Measles, mumps, and rubella	MMR	2 doses	12–15 months 4–6 years	There is no evidence to suggest this vaccine causes autism This is a live, attenuated vaccine
Varicella	VAR	2 doses	12–15 months 4–6 years	This is a live, attenuated vaccine
Hepatitis A	Hepatitis A	2 doses	Give between the first and second birthdays Separate doses by 6–18 months	
Meningococcal serogroups A, C, W, Y	MenACWY-D MenACWY-CRM	2 doses	11–12 years 16 years	MenACWY-D is sold under the brand name Menactra MenACWY-CRM is sold under the brand name Menveo

Tetanus, diphtheria, and acellular pertussis	Tdap	1 dose	11–12 years	Be sure not to confuse this vaccine with the diphtheria, tetanus, and acellular pertussis vaccine (DTaP) For pregnant adolescents, one dose of this vaccine should be administered between 27 and 36 weeks' gestation.
Human papillomavirus	HPV	Patients ages 9–14 years at initiation of series: 2 doses Patients ages 15 years or older at initiation of series: 3 doses	Initiate at 11–12 years for most patients	Begin the series at age 9 years for patients with a history of sexual abuse The 3-dose series is recommended for immuno-compromised patients, including those with HIV

HBIG, Hepatitis B immune globulin; LAIV, live attenuated influenza vaccine.

Source: https://www.cdc.gov/vaccines/schedules/downloads /child/0-18yrs-child-combined-schedule-pdf. Updated May 14, 2018. Accessed September 2018.[2]

TABLE 4.2 Recommended Routine Vaccinations for Adults

Influenza immunization information:[3,4] In the United States, patients are at highest risk for contracting influenza in late fall through early spring. Certain populations, such as those who are in the extremes of age, those who have chronic medical conditions, and women who are pregnant, are at greatest risk for increased morbidity and mortality from influenza. People should be immunized against influenza as soon as the vaccine for that year becomes available, and especially by the end of October of each year. A high-dose influenza vaccine exists for older adults and should be considered for those ≥65 years and older. Individuals with egg allergies may receive the influenza vaccine, but providers administering the vaccine should only do so if they are able to recognize and manage severe allergic reactions. Some available formulations of the influenza vaccine are not prepared using embryonated eggs.

Vaccine Name	Vaccine Abbreviation	Number of Doses	Recommended Routine Dosing	Notes
Influenza	IIV	1 dose, annually	Annually	Also recommended for pregnant women

Tetanus, diphtheria, and pertussis immunization information:[5] *Pertussis* is transmitted through respiratory droplets and carries an increased risk of morbidity in all age groups, but especially in those patients <12 months of age who also have an increased risk of mortality. Patients <2 months of age are at highest risk of death. Infants have not yet received vaccinations to protect against pertussis, and they are at risk of contracting the illness from those around them who are not fully immunized. There has been an increase in the number of cases of pertussis in recent years. *Tetanus* bacteria (*Clostridium tetani*) are found in soil and animal waste; they generally enter the human body through an opening in the skin or mucous membranes. Tetanus toxin causes spasm of skeletal muscles and can have long-term sequelae. *Diphtheria* infections result in thick, gray, pseudomembranes that form in the larynx and can compromise the airway. Neurologic and cardiac complications can also be seen with diphtheria.

Vaccine Name	Vaccine Abbreviation	Number of Doses	Recommended Routine Dosing	Notes
Tetanus, diphtheria, and pertussis	Tdap	1 dose	For those who have not received a dose of Tdap in childhood, administer 1 dose Tetanus and diphtheria toxoids (Td) booster should be administered every 10 years	One dose recommended between 27 and 36 weeks' gestation during each pregnancy

Zoster immunization information:[6] Zoster, commonly known as shingles, manifests as a painful, blistering rash caused by reactivation of the varicella zoster virus. The incidence of zoster increases with age. Patients who contract zoster are at risk for developing a condition called postherpetic neuralgia, which is pain that persists for at least 90 days after the zoster rash has resolved. The incidence of postherpetic neuralgia also increases with age.

Vaccine Name	Vaccine Abbreviation	Number of Doses	Recommended Routine Dosing	Notes
Zoster	RZV (*preferred zoster vaccine*)	2 doses	Give 2 doses, 2–6 months apart to patients >50 years old Give 2 doses, 2–6 months apart to patients who previously received ZVL; give at least 2 months after ZVL	Give this vaccine regardless of whether or not a patient has had zoster in the past, and regardless of whether they have received the ZVL vaccine in the past More efficacious than ZVL
	ZVL	1 dose	Indicated for those ≥60 years old	Contraindicated in pregnant women and patients with severe immunodeficiency

Human papillomavirus immunization:[7] The HPV vaccine helps prevent infections caused by HPV, as well as other HPV-associated cancers and diseases. The following cancers can be caused by HPV: cervical, vaginal, penile, oropharyngeal, and anal. This vaccine is recommended to be administered during adolescence, but is indicated through 26 years of age. If initiating the series at the age of 15 years or older, the 3-dose series is recommended.

Vaccine Name	Vaccine Abbreviation	Number of Doses	Recommended Routine Dosing	Notes
Human papillomavirus	HPV	A 3-dose schedule is recommended for boys and girls who are 11 or 12 years old. The second dose should be given 1 to 2 months after the first dose and the third dose 6 months after the first dose.	May administer to women up to age 26 years, and men up to age 21 years. Men and women may be vaccinated up to 45 years based on clinical judgment	Not recommended during pregnancy Recommended for adults who are immunocompromised Recommended for men who have sex with men

(continued)

TABLE 4.2 Recommended Routine Vaccinations for Adults (*continued*)

Pneumococcal vaccine information: This vaccine helps prevent against serious infections such as meningitis, pneumonia, and bacteremia caused by *Streptococcal pneumonia.*[8] The vaccine is recommended in children and adults.

Indications for the administration of PCV13 and PPSV23 in adults:[9] Immunocompetent adults ≥65 years old should receive both the PCV13 vaccine and the PPSV23 vaccine. The PCV13 vaccine should be given first. The PPSV23 should be given 12 months later. The two vaccines should not be administered together. The intervals between these vaccines vary for those with cochlear implants, functional or anatomic asplenia, cerebrospinal fluid leaks, or those who are immunocompromised; refer to the CDC's website for specific intervals for these higher risk patients.

One dose of PPSV23 should be administered to patients ages 19–64 years who have the following conditions: chronic heart disease (not just hypertension), chronic lung disease, chronic liver disease, alcoholism, diabetes mellitus, those who are cigarette smokers.[3]

Vaccine Name	Vaccine Abbreviation	Number of Doses	Recommended Routine Dosing	Notes
Pneumococcal conjugate	PCV 13	1 dose	Immunocompetent adults ≥65 years of age	Recommended to administer PCV13 at least 1 year *before* PPSV23
Pneumococcal polysaccharide	PPSV23	1 dose	Immunocompetent adults ≥65 year of age, at least 1 year *after* administration of PCV13	If administered and the patient had not received PCV13, give a dose of PCV13 at least 1 year after PPSV23

Hepatitis B immunization:[10] Although now part of the childhood immunization schedule, the hepatitis B vaccine has not always been. Many adults, unless they work in healthcare, may be unimmunized. Hepatitis B is spread through sexual contact or blood, and increases a person's risk for cirrhosis and liver cancer. The vaccine is recommended for adults who are at risk for contracting hepatitis B as well as those who request the vaccine regardless of whether or not they have risk factors.

Vaccine Name	Vaccine Abbreviation	Number of Doses	Recommended Routine Dosing	Notes
Hepatitis B	Hep B	3 doses	0, 1, 6 months	There are groups of patients for whom the hepatitis B vaccine should be recommended. They include healthcare workers, sexual exposure risk, those receiving dialysis, injection drug users, and those with chronic liver disease, HIV infection, or diabetes mellitus

ZVL, live zoster vaccine.

Source: Recommended immunization schedule for adults aged 19 years or older, United States, 2018. www.cdc.gov. https://www.cdc.gov/vaccines/schedules/downloads/adult/adult-combined-schedule.pdf. Updated April 24, 2018. Accessed September 2018.

7. Meites E, Kempe A, Markowitz LE. Use of a 2-dose schedule for human papillomavirus vaccination — updated recommendations of the advisory committee on immunization practices. *MMWR Morb Mortal Wkly Rep.* 2016;65:1405–1408. doi:10.15585/mmwr.mm6549a5

8. Tomczyk S, Bennett N, Stoecker C, et al. Use of 13-valent pneumococcal conjugate vaccine and 23-valent pneumococcal polysaccharide vaccine among adults aged ≥65 years: recommendations of the advisory committee on immunization practices (ACIP). *MMWR Morb Mortal Wkly Rep.* 2014;63:822–825.

9. Kobayashi M, Bennett N, Gierke R, et al. Intervals between PCV13 and PPSV23 vaccines: recommendations of the advisory committee on immunization practices (ACIP). *MMWR Morb Mortal Wkly Rep.* 2015;64:944–947.

10. Schillie S, Vellozzi C, Reingold A, et al. Prevention of hepatitis B virus infection in the United States: recommendations of the advisory committee on immunization practices. *MMWR Recomm Rep.* 2018;67(No. RR-1):1–31. doi:10.15585/mmwr.rr6701a1

PREVENTIVE MEDICINE GUIDELINES

Preventive medicine guidelines for common disorders are listed in Tables 4.3 through 4.12.

TABLE 4.3 Preventive Medicine Guidelines: Abdominal Aortic Aneurysm

Disorder: Abdominal Aortic Aneurysm	
Narrative and Rationale: AAA are more common in adults >50 years of age. Although they are most often asymptomatic, rupture has a high mortality rate. Cigarette smoking increases the risk of developing an AAA.	
Recommendation(s)	**Level of Evidence**
One-time screening, using ultrasound, for men ages 65–75 years who have ever smoked	B
For men ages 65–75 who have never smoked, clinician judgment should be used to determine who to screen	C
For women ages 65–75 who have ever smoked, evidence is insufficient to recommend screening.	I
For women who have never smoked, routing screening is not recommended	D

AAA, abdominal aortic aneurysms.

Source: https://www.uspreventiveservicestaskforce.org/Page/Document/RecommendationStatementFinal/abdominal-aortic-aneurysm-screening. Accessed September 2018.

TABLE 4.4 Preventive Medicine Guidelines: Breast Cancer

Disorder: Breast Cancer
Narrative and Rationale: Appropriate breast screening in the average risk patient strives to emphasize the importance of screening mammogram to detect an early breast carcinoma while reducing mortality of breast cancer. The current approach is patient-provider shared decision-making in starting and ending screening.

(continued)

TABLE 4.4 Preventive Medicine Guidelines: Breast Cancer (*continued*)

Recommendation(s)	Level of Evidence
40–49 years of age: Initiate screening annually or biennially. USPSTF states screening mammogram in this age group should be individual-ized/shared decision	C
50–75 years of age: Annual or biennial per the ACOG; the USPSTF states biennial	B
>75 years of age: Based on shared decision-making, state both the ACOG and the USPSTF	A

ACOG, American College of Obstetricians and Gynecologists; USPSTF, U.S. Preventive Services Task Force.
Source: www.acog.org, Practice Bulletin No. 179, July 2017, Table 1. Accessed September 2018.

TABLE 4.5 Preventive Medicine Guidelines: Cervical Cancer

Disorder: Cervical Cancer

Narrative and Rationale: The goal of appropriate cervical cancer screening is to reduce overmanagement of precursor cervical lesions that will regress or resolve over a short period of time. The use of HPV testing in age-appropriate patients guides the screening intervals and management.

Recommendation(s)	Level of Evidence
21 years of age: Pap starts, regardless of first coitus or high-risk behavior	A
21–29 years of age: Pap every 3 years, Pap only, HPV cotesting should not be done <30 years of age	A
30–65 years of age: Pap every 3 years without HPV cotesting or every 5 years with HPV cotesting	A
>65 years of age: No further screening with negative prior screening and negative history of CIN 2 or higher cervical dysplasia if patient is up-to-date	A
>65 years of age: With history of CIN 2, CIN 3, or AIS continue screening for 20 years after diagnosis	B
Hysterectomy: No screening indicated	A

CIN, cervical intraepithelial neoplasia; HPV, human papilloma virus.
Source: www.cdc.gov/cancer/cervical/pdf/guidelines.pdf, Accessed September 2018.
www.acog.org, 2016 cervical screening, Accessed September 2018.

TABLE 4.6 Preventive Medicine Guidelines: Colorectal Cancer

Disorder: Colorectal Cancer

Narrative and Rationale: Colorectal cancer is a leading cause of death and is seen more commonly in older adults. Early detection of colorectal cancer, before the age of 75, is beneficial. Screening tests include stool-based testing such as the FITs; flexible sigmoidoscopy; and colonoscopy. Generally, FIT testing should be repeated annually, and sigmoidoscopy/colonoscopy every 10 years.

(continued)

TABLE **4.6** Preventive Medicine Guidelines: Colorectal Cancer (*continued*)

Recommendation(s)	Level of Evidence
Screening should begin at age **50 years** and continue until age **75 years**	A
For those adults between the ages of **75 and 85 years**, screening decisions should be **individualized**. Consider screening especially in those who have not been screened before, those who could tolerate treatment for colorectal cancer, and those who do not have a significantly limited life expectancy.	C

FIT, fecal immunochemical tests.

Source: https://www.uspreventiveservicestaskforce.org/Page/Document/RecommendationStatementFinal/colorectal-cancer-screening2. Accessed September 2018.

TABLE **4.7** Preventive Medicine Guidelines: Diabetes Mellitus, Type 2

Disorder: Diabetes Mellitus, Type 2	
Narrative and Rationale: Diabetes is a risk factor for cardiovascular disease as well as increased risk of the development of renal and ophthalmologic disease. Often patients are completely asymptomatic in the early stages of the disease. For people with abnormal glucose levels who do not yet meet the diagnostic criteria for diabetes, intensive lifestyle modifications can reduce risk.	
Recommendation(s)	**Level of Evidence**
Asymptomatic **overweight** or **obese** adults between the ages of **40 and 70** years should be screened for blood glucose levels. If abnormal, intensive behavioral interventions regarding nutrition and physical activity are recommended.	B
Consider screening earlier than the age of 40 if patients have a **family history** of diabetes mellitus, had **gestational diabetes,** or belong to **high-risk racial/ethnic groups** such as African Americans, American Indians, Alaskan Natives, Asian Americans, Hispanics or Latinos, Native Hawaiians, or Pacific Islanders.	

Source: https://www.uspreventiveservicestaskforce.org/Page/Document/RecommendationStatementFinal/screening-for-abnormal-blood-glucose-and-type-2-diabetes. Accessed September 2018.

TABLE **4.8** Preventive Medicine Guidelines: Preventing Falls

Disorder: Falls Prevention (In Community-Dwelling Adults)	
Narrative and Rationale: Among elderly persons, falls are a leading cause of morbidity and mortality. Fall prevention focuses on identifying those who are at risk for falls and mitigating that risk. A history of falls is a strong predictor of future falls.	
Recommendation(s)	**Level of Evidence**
Exercise interventions are recommended to prevent falls in adults **≥65 years old.** These generally include exercises to improve gait, balance, and flexibility.	B

(*continued*)

TABLE 4.8 Preventive Medicine Guidelines: Preventing Falls (*continued*)

Clinical judgment should be used when recommending **multifactorial interventions** to prevent falls. Interventions may include assessment of risk factors, environment, cognition, and psychological health, and are often performed by an interdisciplinary team.	C
Vitamin D supplementation to prevent falls is **not recommended.**	D

Source: https://www.uspreventiveservicestaskforce.org/Page/Document/RecommendationStatementFinal/falls-prevention-in-older-adults-interventions1. Accessed September 2018.

TABLE 4.9 Preventive Medicine Guidelines: Hepatitis C

Disorder: Hepatitis C

Narrative and Rationale: Hepatitis C is the most common blood-borne pathogen in the United States. It is a common cause of chronic liver disease and an increasingly common cause of hepatocellular carcinoma. The most significant risk factor is injection drug use. Treatment of hepatitis C is very effective.

Recommendation(s)	Level of Evidence
A **one-time** screening for hepatitis C should be offered to all **adults** born between the years **1945 and 1965.**	B

Source: https://www.uspreventiveservicestaskforce.org/Page/Document/RecommendationStatementFinal/hepatitis-c-screening. Accessed September 2018.

TABLE 4.10 Preventive Medicine Guidelines: Hyperlipidemia

Disorder: Hyperlipidemia

Narrative and Rationale: Lipid screening is one component of global cardiovascular risk assessment. Guidelines will vary. Detection and treatment of elevated lipids reduces a patient's risk of developing cardiovascular disease.

Recommendation(s)	Level of Evidence
Adults with **diabetes** should be screened **annually.**	B
Men aged 20–45 years and **women aged 20–55** years should be screened at **age 20** and every **5 years** thereafter.	C
Men aged 45–65 years and **women aged 55–65 years without risk factors** for atherosclerotic cardiovascular disease should be screened **at least once every 1–2 years** and more frequently if risk factors are present.	A
Adults >**65 years** old with **0–1 risk factors** should be screened **annually.**	A
The **clinician's judgment**, and **individual patient circumstances**, should guide the frequency of lipid testing.	C

Source: Jellinger PS. American Association of Clinical Endocrinologists/American College of Endocrinology Management of Dyslipidemia and Prevention of Cardiovascular Disease Clinical Practice Guidelines. *Diabetes Spectr.* 2018;31:234–245.[1]

TABLE 4.11 Preventive Medicine Guidelines: Hypertension

Disorder: Hypertension	
Narrative and Rationale: Although it is a common condition, hypertension is often asymptomatic and patients may have the disease for a long period of time before it is diagnosed and treated. Hypertension increases a patient's risk of heart failure, stroke, heart attack, and kidney disease. Care should be taken to use proper technique to measure blood pressure and to confirm abnormal readings with multiple measurements over time.	
Recommendation(s)	**Level of Evidence**
Patients **18 years of age** and older should be screened for hypertension. Before beginning treatment, **abnormal readings should be confirmed** outside of the clinical setting.	A

Source: https://www.uspreventiveservicestaskforce.org/Page/Document/RecommendationStatementFinal/
high-blood-pressure-in-adults-screening. Accessed September 2018.

TABLE 4.12 Preventive Medicine Guidelines: Prostate Cancer

Disorder: Prostate Cancer	
Narrative and Rationale: Prostate cancer is common and will affect approximately 11% of men in their lifetime. It is often slow-growing and asymptomatic, and a larger number of men will be diagnosed upon autopsy after death from other causes. Prostate cancer can also be aggressive, causing death. African American men are at increased risk for prostate cancer. The PSA test is a blood test used to screen for prostate cancer; however, elevated PSA levels can also be seen for other reasons, such as a benign prostatic hyperplasia.	
Recommendation(s):	**Level of Evidence**
PSA screening is an **individualized** decision for **men ages 55–69 years**. The decision should be made after discussion with a clinician considering overall risk and the potential for false-positive results that can lead to additional testing as well as overdiagnosis and overtreatment of prostate cancer, if detected.	C
PSA testing is not recommended for men ≥70 years old	D

PSA, prostate-specific antigen.
Source: https://www.uspreventiveservicestaskforce.org/Page/Document/RecommendationStatementFinal/
prostate-cancer-screening1. Accessed September 2018.

REFERENCE

1. Jellinger PS. American Association of clinical endocrinologists/American college of endocrinology management of dyslipidemia and prevention of cardiovascular disease clinical practice guidelines. *Diabetes Spectr.* 2018;31:234–245. doi:10.2337/ds18-0009

SELECTED PATIENT EDUCATION TOPICS PERTINENT TO FAMILY MEDICINE

Selected patient education topics are listed in Tables 4.13 and 4.14.

TABLE 4.13 Contraception and Family Planning

Method	Indications	Contraindications	Notes
Combination estrogen and progestin pills (COC)	Prevent pregnancy	Tobacco use >15 cigarettes/day and >35 years old HTN >160/100 VTE or thrombogenic factors (factor V, MTHFR) Migraine with aura >35 years old Breast cancer Cirrhosis of liver	Daily oral administration, compliance is required to achieve optimal effectiveness. Can be used until menopause is reached in non-smoking healthy women
Combination estrogen and progestin dermal patch	Same as oral contraceptive pills	Same as oral contraceptive pills	Weekly dermal administration, placed on the skin of abdomen, upper arm, or buttock; may cause adhesive sensitivity. Compliance = effectiveness
Combination estrogen and progestin vaginal ring	Same as oral contraceptive pills	Same as oral contraceptive pills	Monthly vaginal insertion 3 weeks on 1, week off; best used in patients that have systemic side effects from the pill
POP-Norethindrone 0.35 mg	Prevent pregnancy where estrogen is contraindicated, estrogen is not desired, or in breastfeeding patients	Known or suspected pregnancy Known or suspected breast cancer Undiagnosed abnormal uterine bleeding Liver tumors and liver disease	Daily administration, 28 pills/pack—no placebo week Unpredictable bleeding is common Compliance is crucial: same time every day due to short half-life of POP
Progestin only IM- DMPA injection	Prevention of pregnancy, long acting	Planning pregnancy within the year Long-term use of corticosteroid therapy with history of nontraumatic bone fracture Use of aminoglutethimide (Cushing's syndrome)—decreases the metabolism of progestins Known or suspected pregnancy Known or suspected breast cancer Undiagnosed abnormal uterine bleeding Liver tumors and liver disease	Injectable—IM administration every 12 weeks. Irregular vaginal bleeding to be expected until amenorrhea is reached. Bone loss is noted in DMPA use; it is reversible with discontinuation Calcium and vitamin D supplementation is recommended with use Return to fertility can be delayed up to 18 months

LARC: IUD—progestin only (levonorgestrel) and nonhormonal (TCu380A) Dermal implant- progestin only (etonogestrel)	Long-term reversible contraception Desire for estrogen free or hormonal free **IUD: Progestin (LNg): 5- and 3-year options** **Copper (nonhormonal): 10 years** **Dermal implant: Etonogestrel (68 mg) single rod**	**IUD:** Distortion of uterine cavity Current pelvic infection Known or suspected pregnancy Undiagnosed abnormal vaginal bleeding Breast cancer—LNg Liver disease—LNg Wilson's disease or copper allergy—in TCu380A **Dermal implant:** Current or past history of thrombosis/thromboembolic event Hypersensitivity to rod component	**IUD: intrauterine device:** LNg IUD 3 doses (52 mg, 19.5 mg are 5-year options, and 13.5 mg is a 3-year option) LNg IUD is recommended as first-line contraception in the adolescent population Misoprostol 200 mcg indicated 4–6 hours prior to insertion of either IUD in nulliparous women to aid in the dilation and ease of insertion **Dermal implant:** subdermal single 40 × 2 mm semirigid plastic rod, 68 mg
Barrier methods: Condoms (male and female) Diaphragm Vaginal sponge, spermicide Cervical cap NFP	Prevention of pregnancy in patients that desire nonhormonal options, as needed contraception, not comfortable with insertion of devices	Improper use of condom	Education of the proper use is critical; access and availability of condoms, vaginal sponge, and spermicide may limit use. Cooperative partner in NFP, education regarding NFP by medical provider, understanding signs/symptoms of ovulation
Sterilization—male and female	Permanent, surgical		Bilateral tubal ligation for females Vasectomy for males

COC, combined oral contraceptives; DMPA, depot medroxyprogesterone acetate; HTN, hypertension; IM, intramuscular; LARC, long-acting reversible contraception; MTHFR, methylenetetrahydrofolate reductase; NFP, natural family planning; POP, progestin only pills; VTE, Venous thromboembolism.

TABLE **4.14** Recommended Screenings for Pregnancy

Gestation	Indicated Testing/Screenings	Notes
Initial visit preferred 6–12 weeks	CBC with diff, RPR, rubella, HepBsAg, type and screen, urinalysis, urine culture, HIV, cervical cultures (GC/chlamydia), cystic fibrosis carrier screening	The following tests if indicated by risk factors: hepatitis C, toxoplasmosis, CMV, varicella, TSH, TB, hemoglobin electrophoresis– sickle cell, thalassemia, or other hemoglobinopathies, Tay-sachs and Canavan for those of Eastern European Jewish ancestry, early glucola screening for prior gestational diabetics
2nd trimester	**18–20 weeks:** Anatomical ultrasound **24–26 weeks:** Hgb, platelets, antibody screen, 1-hour glucola (oral glucose tolerance test), 3-hour glucola if indicated	If antibody screen negative in Rh negative patient, Rho(D) immune globulin to be given at 28 weeks. If positive antibody, refer to high-risk maternal services. Failed 1-hour glucola >135 proceed to 3-hour glucola
3rd trimester screening	Vaginal screening at 35–37 weeks for **group B strep** and repeat hgb. In high-risk patients repeat GC/chlamydia, HIV, and RPR	
Genetic testing	**FTS** done between 10 and 13.6 weeks **NIPT**-cfDNA test: Done at any time after 10 weeks testing for trisomy 21, trisomy 18, trisomy 13, and sex aneuploidy **Quad Screen:** 15–22.6 weeks, screening for trisomy 21, trisomy 18, and ONTD **MSAFP:** Done between 15 and 20 weeks for ONTD	FTS: Combination of an ultrasound that measures the NT of the fetus and maternal serum screening. If more invasive testing is indicated, amniocentesis and CVS

CBC, complete blood count; cfDNA, cell free DNA; CMV, cytomegalovirus; CVS, chorionic villi sampling; FTS, first trimester screen; MSAFP, maternal serum alpha fetoprotein; NIPT, noninvasive prenatal test; NT, nuchal translucency; ONTD, open neural tube defects; RPR, rapid plasma reagin; TB, tuberculosis; TSH, thyroid-stimulating hormone.

Source: ACOG Practice Bulletin No 163. May 2016. Accessed September 2018; ACOG Routine testing during pregnancy. September, 2017. https://www.acog.org/Patients/FAQs/Routine-Tests-During-Pregnancy? September 2017. Accessed September 2018.

ELECTRONIC RESOURCES

CDC Immunization schedule for children and adolescents 2018:

> https://www.cdc.gov/vaccines/schedules/downloads/child/0-18yrs-child
> -combined-schedule.pdf

CDC Immunization schedule for adults 2018:

> https://www.cdc.gov/vaccines/schedules/downloads/adult/adult
> -combined-schedule.pdf

Vaccine Information Statement Handouts:

> https://www.cdc.gov/vaccines/hcp/vis/current-vis.html

5

Urgent Management in Family Medicine

CHEST PAIN

INTRODUCTION

Chest pain may be caused by disorders that involve the chest wall, intrathoracic and abdominal structures, as well as psychophysiological sources. The incidence of severe heart disease in patients presenting with chest pain is highly dependent on the care setting. Five percent of ED visits and up to 40% of admissions are because of chest pain; however, <15% of these patients are diagnosed with acute coronary syndrome (ACS).[1] Many of these patients may first present to the family medicine clinic.

The most common causes of acute, severe chest pain are myocardial ischemia, pericarditis, aortic dissection, and pulmonary embolism (PE), compared to the most common causes of chronic, recurrent chest pain, which are angina, esophageal reflux, or musculoskeletal pain.[2]

> **CLINICAL PEARL:** Coronary artery disease (CAD) is most likely to be underdiagnosed in the female patient population <60 years old and in African Americans.

Clinical Presentation

> **CLINICAL PEARL:** Must-not-miss causes of chest pain include the following:
>
> **1.** ACS
> **2.** Aortic dissection
> **3.** Pneumothorax
> **4.** Esophageal rupture
> **5.** Pulmonary emboli

History

Taking the patient's history should determine if the pain is acute or chronic and elicit the onset, quality, radiation of the pain, and associated symptoms. The initial goal of the history is to determine if the patient is experiencing a life-threatening event such as ACS, PE, or aortic aneurysm/dissection so that treatment can be initiated immediately. Framing the differential diagnosis as cardiac, pulmonary, or gastrointestinal is helpful. The physical exam should focus on eliciting signs of hemodynamic compromise.

Symptoms suggestive of a cardiovascular cause of chest pain:

- Chest discomfort pain described as substernal pressure, radiation to neck, jaw, arm
- Discomfort/pain aggravated by exertion, relieved with nitroglycerin or rest within 10 minutes
- Pain/discomfort is sudden onset, tearing, or knifelike
- Pain relieved with sitting up or leaning forward
- Pain associated with shortness of breath, nausea, vomiting
- Neurologic deficits

Symptoms suggestive of a gastrointestinal cause of chest pain:

- Sharp pain radiating to trapezius
- Pain/discomfort radiating anterior to posterior mid scapula, epigastric region, or right upper quadrant (RUQ)
- Recent concerns of active, intermittent bleeding
- Substernal burning, aggravated with meals or recumbent position relieved with antacids
- Pain worsened by swallowing, relieved with nitroglycerin or calcium channel blocker
- Difficulty swallowing

Symptoms suggestive of a musculoskeletal cause of chest pain:

- Pain that is aggravated by breathing
- Sharp pain aggravated by deep inspiration
- Pain worse with movement, breathing, or coughing

Symptoms suggestive of a pulmonary cause of chest pain:

- Pain that is aggravated by breathing that is relieved with sitting up or leaning forward

- Sharp pain aggravated by deep inspiration
- Pain that is unilateral, sudden in onset, sharp, and pleuritic

Pertinent past medical history to obtain that may narrow the differential diagnosis:

- Diabetes mellitus (DM), personal or family history of CAD: Cardiovascular
- Peripheral vascular disease: Cardiovascular
- Hypertension: Cardiovascular
- Peptic ulcer disease: Gastrointestinal
- History of hypercoagulable state: Pulmonary, gastrointestinal

Allergies:

- Specifically to medications that may be required for treatment. Examples include aspirin, heparin, intravenous (IV) contrast dye, thienopyridines

Medications:

- Recent use of phosphodiesterase inhibitors: Sildenafil, tadalafil, or varde-nafil

> **CLINICAL PEARL:** Twelve percent of patients presenting to the ED with acute myocardial infarction (AMI) have no cardiac risk factors.[3]

Physical Examination

Evaluate for:

- Vitals: hyper/hypotension, disparate blood pressure (BP) right/left arms, low pulse pressure, tachycardia, abnormal rhythm, hypoxemia, fever
- Neck: Jugular venous distension (JVD), nodular thyroid
- Chest: Diminished breath sounds, crackles, pleural rub, egophony, wheezes
- Heart: Rate, rhythm, pericardial friction rub, murmurs of valvular regur-gitation, stenosis, atrial septal defect (ASD), S_3, S_4
- Abdominal: Epigastric, upper quadrant, periumbilical tenderness
- Extremities: Presence of edema, evaluate pulses
- Neuro: Identify sensory motor, focal abnormalities
- Musculoskeletal: Costochondral tenderness to palpation

> **CLINICAL PEARL:** The presence of pain upon palpation reduces the chance of a cardiovascular cause of the chest pain.

> **CLINICAL PEARL:** The likelihood of myocardial infarction (MI) is higher in the presence of pain radiating to both arms, hypotension, S_3 gallop on physical examination, or diaphoresis.

Specific clinical findings that can help narrow the differential diagnosis are outlined in Tables 5.1 through 5.4.

TABLE 5.1 Suspected Cardiovascular Cause of Chest Pain

Disorder	Typical Characteristics
Angina	Substernal pressure, neck, jaw, arm, duration <30 minutes Associated with dyspnea, diaphoresis, nausea, vomiting Aggravated with exertion, relieved with NTG or rest within 10 minutes
Myocardial infarction	Greater intensity of above symptoms Duration >30 minutes
Pericarditis	Aggravated by breathing, relieved with sitting up or leaning forward Pericardial friction rub
Aortic dissection	Sudden onset, tearing/knifelike pain located anteroposterior, mid scapular Asymmetric BP, pulses New murmur of aortic insufficiency Neurological deficits

BP, blood pressure; NTG, Nitroglycerin.

TABLE 5.2 Suspected Pulmonary Cause of Chest Pain

Disorder	Typical Characteristics
Pneumonia	Pleuritic pain, dyspnea Fever, cough, sputum production, tachypnea Decreased breath sounds and dullness to percussion
Pleuritis	Sharp pain aggravated by deep inspiration, unaffected by movement or palpation When pleuritic inflammation occurs near the diaphragm, pain can be referred to the neck or shoulder Pleural friction rub
Pneumothorax	Sudden onset of pain, sharp, pleuritic Unilateral decreased, hyperresonant breath sounds
Pulmonary embolus	Pleuritic chest pain, sudden onset Tachypnea, tachycardia
Pulmonary hypertension	Dyspnea, exertional chest pressure Hypoxemia Increased P2 component on cardiac auscultation Right ventricular heave

TABLE 5.3 Suspected Gastrointestinal Cause of Chest Pain

Disorder	Typical Characteristics
GERD	Substernal burning, acid taste Dysphagia Aggravated with meals, recumbent position Relieved with antacids

(continued)

TABLE 5.3 Suspected Gastrointestinal Cause of Chest Pain (*continued*)

Disorder	Typical Characteristics
Esophageal spasm	Intense substernal pain Worsened by swallowing, relieved with NTG, CCB
Mallory–Weiss tear, esophageal rupture	Vomiting followed by sudden chest pain
Peptic ulcer disease	Epigastric, associated with meals Hematemesis, melena
Biliary disease	RUQ pain, nausea, vomiting
Pancreatitis	Epigastric, back discomfort

CCB, calcium channel blocker; GERD, gastroesophageal reflux disease; NTG, nitroglycerin; RUQ, right upper quadrant.

TABLE 5.4 Cause of Chest Pain: Other

Disorder	Typical Characteristics
Costochondritis	Localized, sharp, or dull pain Worse with movement, breathing, cough, palpation
Cervical disk disease	Aggravated by movement, lasting for hours, neuropathy
Herpes zoster	Severe unilateral pain, rash in dermatomal distribution
Anxiety	Tightness in the chest

Diagnosis

The *HEART Score* and *Thrombolysis in Myocardial Infarction* (TIMI) score are two systems that can be used to risk stratify the patient with suspected cardiovascular cause of chest pain. These are compared in Table 5.5.

In ruling out pulmonary emboli, the *Wells Score* (Table 5.6) is the most commonly used and best validated prediction rule used in determining the pretest probability of pulmonary emboli. A score >6.0 is associated with a high probability of a PE.

TABLE 5.5 Comparison of the HEART Score and Thrombolysis in Myocardial Infarction Score

HEART Score[3–8]	TIMI[1]
Parameters	**Parameters (1 point each)**
Patient history	Patient age ≥65
EKG findings	≥3 CAD risk factors: hypertension, hyper-
Patient age	cholesterolemia, diabetes, family history of
Known risk factors	CAD, or current smoker
Initial troponin levels	Known CAD (stenosis ≥50%)
	ASA use in past 7 days
	Severe angina (≥2 episodes in 24 hours)
	EKG ST changes ≥0.5 mm
	Positive cardiac marker

(*continued*)

TABLE 5.5 Comparison of the HEART Score and Thrombolysis in Myocardial Infarction Score (*continued*)

HEART Score[3–8]	TIMI[1]
Interpretation	Interpretation
The likelihood of MI is higher if there is pain radiating to both arms, hypotension, an S_3 gallop on physical examination, or diaphoresis.	Patients with a score <2 are considered low risk and have a 5% risk of cardiac event.
A normal level of troponin T or troponin I between 6 and 72 hours after the onset of chest pain is strong evidence against MI and acute coronary syndrome, particularly if the EKG is normal or near normal.[9,10]	Patients with a score of 4.0 to 5.0 have a 20% to 26% risk of a cardiac event.
Other factors predicting MI include age < 60 years, male sex, and prior MI.[11]	Patients with a score of ≥6 have a 41% risk of a cardiac event.

CAD, coronary artery disease; MI, myocardial infarction; TIMI, thrombolysis in myocardial infarction.

TABLE 5.6 Wells Scoring

Features	Score
Tachycardia >100	1.5
Immobilization (bed rest for 3 or more days)	1.5
Previous diagnosis of PE or DVT, or surgery within the past 4 weeks	1.5
Hemoptysis	1
Cancer/malignancy (in treatment, treatment in last 6 months, or palliative treatment)	1
Clinical signs and symptoms consistent with a DVT	3
PE is no.1 diagnosis OR equally likely (an alternative diagnosis is less likely than PE)	3

DVT, deep vein thrombosis; PE, pulmonary embolism.

Specific testing should be ordered based on the suspected diagnosis and may include the following:

- D-dimer assay in suspected PE can help determine whether further evaluation with helical CT, ventilation-perfusion scan, or venous ultrasound is needed.[4]
- 12-ead EKG within 10 minutes of presentation, findings suggestive of ischemia include the following:[5]
  - ○ Transient ST segment changes 0.05 mV (0.5 mm) or greater
  - ○ T-wave inversions 0.2 mV (2 mm) or greater
  - ○ ST elevation MI can be diagnosed with ST segment elevation in two contiguous leads on electrocardiography

- Cardiac troponin levels are to be obtained at presentation, 3 and 6 hours after the patient's symptoms began.[6–8]
  - Troponin values above the 99th percentile of the upper limit of normal (ULN; laboratory specific) are required to diagnose myocardial necrosis.
  - An increase or decrease of at least 20% from the initial lab is required for the diagnosis of acute myocardial necrosis.[5]
  - A normal level of troponin T or troponin I between 6 and 72 hours after the onset of chest pain is strong evidence against MI and ACS, particularly if the EKG is normal or near normal.
- Echocardiography may be considered when an acute ischemic event has not occurred. This test can help to identify other cardiac causes of chest pain, such as cardiac tamponade, severe valvular disease, and hypertrophic cardiomyopathy. Lack of regional wall motion abnormalities carries a high negative predictive value for ischemia.
- Chest x-ray (CXR) identifies pulmonary edema, cardiomegaly, widened mediastinum, pneumonia, effusion, and pneumothorax.
  - Aortic dissection: CXR revealing widened mediastinum
    - Pneumothorax: CXR lung collapse, tracheal deviation requiring chest tube placement for reexpansion
  - Pneumonia: Infiltrates, consolidation
- CT scan of the chest:
  - Aortic dissection: Can detect a false lumen. This condition can also be seen on MRI.
  - Esophageal rupture: CT is the test of choice and will show an ipsilateral pleural effusion with free air in the mediastinum and thorax. This condition requires surgical exploration, primary suture repair, thoracomediastinal lavage, and drainage.
- Esophagogastroduodenoscopy (EGD): Evaluate for gastroesophageal reflux disease (GERD), Mallory–Weiss tear, peptic ulcer disease
- Barium swallow: Can identify esophageal spasm
- RUQ ultrasound: Can rule out biliary disease

Management

The primary responsibility of the family medicine PA is to efficiently recognize conditions that require urgent care, stabilize the patient, and determine the need for hospital admission. You must recognize clinical presentations suggestive of an unstable condition. Many of the conditions discussed above will require care in the ED, and the management is dependent on the primary diagnosis. If it is determined that hospital admission is not required, proceed with specific management details as found in Chapter 2, Common Disease Entities in Family Medicine.

REFERENCES

1. Mistry NF, Vesely MR. Acute coronary syndromes. *Cardiol Clin.* November 1, 2012;30(4):617–627. doi:10.1016/j.ccl.2012.07.010
2. Than M, Flaws D, Sanders S, et al. Development and validation of the emergency department assessment of chest pain score and 2 h accelerated diagnostic protocol. *Emerg Med Australas.* February 2014;26(1):34–44. doi:10.1111/1742-6723.12164

3. Berger JP, Buclin R, Haller E, et al. Right arm involvement and pain extension can help to differentiate coronary diseases from chest pain of other origin: a prospective emergency ward study of 278 consecutive patients admitted for chest pain. *J Intern Med.* 1990;227:165–172. doi:10.1111/j.1365-2796.1990.tb00138.x

4. Weaver WD, Eisenberg S, Martin JS, et al. Myocardial infarction triage and intervention project—phase I: patient characteristics and feasibility of prehospital initiation of thrombolytic therapy. *J Am Coll Cardiol.* 1990;15:925–931. doi:10.1016/0735-1097(90)90218-E

5. Barstow C, Rice M, McDivitt JD. Acute coronary syndrome: diagnostic evaluation. *Am Fam Physician.* 2017;95(3):170–177.

6. Pickering JW, Flaws D, Smith SW, et al. A risk assessment score and initial high sensitivity troponin combine to identify low risk of acute myocardial infarction in the emergency department. *Acad Emerg Med.* 2018;25(4):434–443. doi:10.1111/acem.13343

7. Ebell MH, Flewelling D, Flynn CA. A systematic review of troponin T and I for diagnosing acute myocardial infarction. *J Fam Pract.* 2000;49:550–556.

8. Ebell MH, White LL, Weismantel D. A systematic review of troponin T and I values as a prognostic tool for patients with chest pain. *J Fam Pract.* 2000;49:746–753.

9. Tierney WM, Fitzgerald J, McHenry R, et al. Physicians' estimates of the probability of myocardial infarction in emergency room patients with chest pain. *Med Decis Making.* 1986;6:12–17. doi:10.1177/0272989X8600600103

10. Solomon CG, Lee TH, Cook EF, et al. Comparison of clinical presentation of acute myocardial infarction in patients older than 65 years of age to younger patients: the multicenter chest pain study experience. *Am J Cardiol.* 1989;63:772–776. doi:10.1016/0002-9149(89)90040-4

11. Panju AA, Hemmelgarn BR, Guyatt GH, et al. The rational clinical examination. Is this patient having a myocardial infarction? *JAMA.* 1998;280:1256–1263. doi:10.1001/jama.280.14.1256

ELECTRONIC RESOURCES

https://www.mdcalc.com/

https://s.aafp.org/

https://www.nhlbi.nih.gov/files/docs/research/2012_ChartBook.pdf

GLUCOSE EMERGENCIES: DIABETIC KETOACIDOSIS AND HYPERGLYCEMIC HYPEROSMOLAR STATE

INTRODUCTION

Diabetic ketoacidosis (DKA), hyperglycemic hyperosmolar state (HHS), and hypoglycemia are three serious complications of DM requiring early recognition, diagnosis, and treatment. Mortality in patients with HHS is 10 times higher than in adults and children diagnosed with DKA. In the United States, approximately 145,000 cases of DKA occur each year. DKA can be a common presentation for an initial diagnosis of type I DM, and is a leading cause of mortality among children and young adults. Previous research finds that 29% of patients <20 years of age with type 1 diabetes and 10% with type 2 diabetes presented in DKA at diagnosis.[1] Prognosis in these patients correlates with the degree of dehydration, comorbidities, and advanced age (>60 years). HHS is less common; however, it is associated with a mortality of 20%.[2] Hypoglycemic episodes can occur in approximately one-third of patients who are being treated with subcutaneous insulin, and they are listed as an underlying cause in approximately 5% of total hospitalizations in the United States that are due to diabetes.[1]

Clinical Presentation

Historical and physical examination findings are presented in Table 5.7.

TABLE 5.7 Comparison Patient History: Diabetic Ketoacidosis Versus Hyperglycemic Hyperosmolar State

Historical Findings

DKA	HHS
Type I DM	Type 2 DM
Presents within days of developing symptoms	Several weeks' history of polyuria, weight loss, decreased oral intake
Younger age at presentation, female	Advanced age
Nausea, vomiting, abdominal pain	May be precipitated by significant medical event such as MI, stroke, sepsis, alcohol misuse, hepatic failure, pancreatitis
Polyuria, polydipsia	
Weight loss	
Precipitated by infection, medication noncompliance, pregnancy, psychiatric disorders	Polyuria, polydipsia
Lower socioeconomic status	Altered mental state
Medications that may precipitate the event include glucocorticoids, atypical antipsychotics	Medications that may precipitate the event include corticosteroids, thiazides, and sympathomimetic agents
Family history of DM	

Physical Examination

Fluid deficit 3–5 L	Fluid deficit 9–10 L
Fever	Fever
Acetone breath	Tachycardia
Kussmaul's respirations	Hypotension
Tachycardia	Dry mucous membranes
Hypotension	
Dry mucous membranes	
Abdominal tenderness	

DKA, diabetic ketoacidosis; DM, diabetes mellitus; HHS, hyperglycemic hyperosmolar state; MI, myocardial infarction.

CLINICAL PEARL: Coexistence of DKA and HHS is reported in approximately one-third of cases.

Diagnosis

The diagnostic evaluation is presented in Table 5.8.

LABS

- Complete blood count (CBC): Leukocytosis
- Comprehensive metabolic panel (CMP): Elevated glucose, ketosis, potassium, and phosphate may be normal, sodium levels may be low, azotemia
- Abnormalities in serum osmolality
- Serum beta-hydroxybutyrate elevation
- Lipid panel: Hypertriglyceridemia
- Arterial blood gas: Metabolic acidosis, low CO_2 and HCO_3
- Cultures: When indicated

TABLE 5.8 Diagnostic Workup: Diabetic Ketoacidosis Versus Hyperglycemic Hyperosmolar State

DKA	HHS
Diagnosis	Diagnosis
Plasma glucose 250–600 mg/dL	Plasma glucose 600–1,200 mg/dL
Sodium 125–135 mEq/L	Sodium 135–145 mEq/L
Potassium normal to increased	Potassium normal
Phosphate normal, deceased	Normal
Serum osmolality 300–320 mmol/kg	Serum osmolality 330–380 mmol/kg
Serum bicarbonate <15 mEq/L	Normal
Creatinine mildly elevated	Moderately elevated
Plasma ketones marked elevation	Normal, mild elevation
pH ≤7.30, PCO_2 20–30 mmHg	pH ≥7.30 PCO_2 normal
Urine or blood acetoacetate (nitroprusside reaction) positive	Urine or blood acetoacetate (nitroprusside reaction) negative
Urine or blood beta-hydroxybutyrate, mmol/L >3	Urine or blood beta-hydroxybutyrate, mmol/L >3
Anion gap, mmol/L >10–12	Anion gap, mmol/L <12

DKA, diabetic ketoacidosis; HHS, hyperglycemic hyperosmolar state.

Management

The primary responsibility of the family medicine physician assistant (PA) is to recognize the presence of a glucose emergency, stabilize the patient, and determine the need for hospital admission. Management of these conditions does not typically occur in the outpatient setting. Treatment goals are to restore volume, stop ketogenesis, correct electrolyte imbalance, and restore serum glucose levels to ≤138 mg/dl.

DIABETIC KETOACIDOSIS

- IV fluids:
  - 0.9% NaCl (10–15 mL kg/h, 2–3 L) × 1 to 3 hours, then
  - 0.45% NaCl (150–300 mL/h) until BS ≤250 mg/dL, then
  - $D_5$0.45% NaCl

- Infusion of regular human insulin with bolus dose of 0.1 U/kg, followed by continuous IV infusion of 0.1 U/kg/h (5 to 10 U/h)
- Initial bolus subcutaneous dose of 0.2 to 0.3 U/kg; the administration of lispro or aspart (subcutaneous doses of 0.1 U/kg/h or 0.2 U/kg/2 h) in mild to moderate DKA
- Potassium supplementation 20 to 40 mEq of potassium per liter of fluids is routine to maintain normal levels with serum potassium levels <5 mEq
- Labs: Capillary blood sugar (BS) levels every 1 to 2 hours, electrolytes (K, bicarbonate phosphate) and anion gap every 4 × 24 hours

CLINICAL PEARL: The acidotic state forces potassium out of the cell, causing a relatively higher serum potassium level despite the total body deficit. Insulin administration will drive potassium into the cells, resulting in hypokalemia.

HYPERGLYCEMIC HYPEROSMOLAR STATE
- IV fluid deficits repleted over 48 hours with:
  - 0.9% NaCl (1–3 L) × 2 to 3 hours, then
  - 0.45% NaCl × 48 hours, then
  - D_5W when levels <250 mg/dL
- Insulin infusion: Regular human insulin with bolus dose of 0.1 U/kg, followed by continuous IV infusion of 0.1 U/kg/h (5–10 U/h)

GLUCOSE EMERGENCIES: HYPOGLYCEMIA

INTRODUCTION

Hypoglycemia is the most common life-threatening complication of diabetes management. Sudden nocturnal death is the cause of 6% of deaths in diabetic patients <40 years of age. It occurs more commonly in the younger patient population and in those with insulin therapy. Additional risk factors include male sex, duration of DM, tight glucose control, alcohol use, and the patient's lack of awareness of low blood sugar symptoms. The most common causes of hypoglycemia are missed meals, medication dosing error, increased physical activity, and medications such as beta-blockers, sulfonylureas, other insulin secretagogues, and possibly ACE inhibitors.

American Diabetes Association Workgroup on Hypoglycemia defines hypoglycemia as:[3,4]

- Severe hypoglycemia: Symptoms that require carbohydrate administration, resuscitative action
- Documented symptomatic hypoglycemia: Symptoms of low blood sugar with plasma glucose levels ≤70 mg/dL
- Probable symptomatic hypoglycemia: Symptoms of low blood sugar with no associated documentation of normal plasma glucose levels

- Relative hypoglycemia: Symptoms of low blood sugar in the patient with DM with plasma glucose levels ≥70 mg/dL

Clinical Presentation

HISTORICAL FINDINGS

- General: Anxiety, sweating, hunger, fatigue, pale
- Cardiac: Palpitations, elevated BP
- Neuro: Paresthesias, confusion, altered mental status

Physical Examination

- Elevated BP
- General: Anxious
- Skin: Pallor, diaphoretic
- Cardiac: Tachycardia
- Neuro: Altered mental status, tremors

Diagnosis

- Capillary blood glucose
- If cause is unknown, additional labs should include insulin, proinsulin, C-peptide, urine/plasma sulfonylurea, cortisol, ethanol

Management

- Medical therapy: Glucose tablets, juices, glucagon injection, dextrose infusion until blood glucose level >55 mg/dL
- Insulin preparations: Assess for alternative types of insulin, such as lispro, aspart, and insulin pumps to lessen risk of hypoglycemia
- Patient education stressing the importance of self-glucose monitoring and psychosocial support
- Review patient's medications: Avoid agents known to precipitate hypoglycemic attacks

REFERENCES

1. Kitabchi AE, Umpierrez GE, Miles JM, et al. Hyperglycemic crises in adult patients with diabetes. *Diabetes Care.* 2009;32:1335–1343. doi:10.2337/dc09-9032
2. Umpierrez G, Korytkowski M. Diabetic emergencies — ketoacidosis, hyperglycaemic hyperosmolar state and hypoglycaemia. *Nat Rev Endocrinol.* April 2016;12:222–232. doi:10.1038/nrendo.2016.15
3. Workgroup on Hypoglycemia, American Diabetes Association. Defining and reporting hypoglycemia in diabetes: a report from the American diabetes association workgroup on hypoglycemia. *Diabetes Care.* 2005;28:1245–1249. doi:10.2337/diacare.28.5.1245
4. Seaquist ER, Anderson J, Childs B, et al. Hypoglycemia and diabetes: a report of a workgroup of the American diabetes association and the endocrine society. *Diabetes Care.* 2013;36:1384–1395. doi:10.2337/dc12-2480

HYPERTENSIVE EMERGENCY

INTRODUCTION

Hypertensive emergencies are defined as systolic blood pressure (SBP) >180/120 mmHg associated with clinical or laboratory evidence of target organ damage.[1] Hypertensive emergencies require intensive care management with continuous hemodynamic monitoring. Examples of targeted end-organ damage include aneurysm dissection, intracranial hemorrhage, acute ischemic stroke, encephalopathy, acute myocardial ischemia, acute left ventricular dysfunction with pulmonary edema, visual changes, and acute renal failure.[2] It is also important to be able to determine how quickly the BP has risen when deciding on therapy. Patients who have chronic elevations in BP may be able to tolerate higher levels and there may be no need for ED management.

Systemic BP >180/120 mmHg without any evidence of end-organ damage is consistent with the diagnosis of hypertensive urgency. Patients diagnosed with hypertensive urgency can be managed by initiating or intensifying the existing oral antihypertensive regimen and following up within 24 to 48 hours. Approximately 1% of patients with hypertension will develop acute elevations in BP at some point during their lifetime. The incidence is higher in men, blacks, and the elderly. Additional risk factors include lack of a primary care provider, patient noncompliance, and illicit drug use. Lack of appropriate treatment for acute hypertension is associated with an increase in mortality.[1]

Clinical Presentation

Historical findings may include the following:

- ENT: Vision changes, epistaxis
- Cardiac: Chest pain, palpitations, dyspnea, pulmonary edema
- GI: Nausea
- GU: Decreased urinary output, bloody urine
- Neuro: Headache, lightheadedness, altered level of consciousness, focal deficits
- Medications: Review compliance with medications prescribed, ask about new medications (nonsteroidal anti-inflammatory drugs [NSAIDS], weight loss medications, herbal supplements, sympathomimetics, steroids, cold medications)
- Past medical history: CAD, heart failure (HF), kidney disease, peripheral vascular disease, DM, sleep apnea
- Family history: Hypertension
- Social history: Smoking, alcohol, and illicit drugs

Physical Examination

Evaluate for:

- BP measurements: Take a minimum of two readings, averaged to confirm, then allow patient to rest about 30 minutes before repeating. Obtain postural BP in the elderly patient

- Eyes: Retinopathy with arteriolar changes, hemorrhages, exudates, papilledema (sign of hypertensive emergency), visual field defects
- Neck: JVD
- Chest: Crackles, decreased breath sounds
- Cardiac: S_3, irregular rhythm, murmur, displaced point of maximal impulse (PMI)
- Abdomen: Renal, aortic bruits
- Extremities: Peripheral edema, diminished pulses
- Neuro: Focal sensory, motor deficits, altered level of consciousness

Diagnosis

LABS

- CBC: Microangiopathic anemia
- Serum creatinine with glomerular filtration rate (GFR): Decreased renal function
- Electrolytes: Na+, K, Ca: Metabolic abnormalities
- Urinalysis: Proteinuria, hematuria

IMAGING

- CXR: May show cardiomegaly and/or pulmonary edema
- Echocardiogram: Evaluate for left ventricular dysfunction or wall motion abnormalities suggestive of ischemia, as well as left ventricular hypertrophy

> **CLINICAL PEARL:** Clinical judgment should be used to determine which tests are useful, given the individual patient, risk factors, and objective findings.

- Electrocardiogram: May reveal arrhythmias, ischemia, ventricular dysfunction, or wall motion abnormalities. arrhythmias, ischemia

Management

Over 5% of hospitalized patients require IV therapy to manage their BP elevations.[1] The family medicine PA will not be responsible for administering IV meds, but you should know when to pursue inpatient management. In the setting of a hypertensive emergency, management includes the following:

1. Admission to an intensive care unit; too rapid of a reduction in BP can result in reduced organ perfusion leading to ischemia and infarction
2. Continuous monitoring of BP and target organ damage
3. Patients with critical conditions such as aortic dissection; eclampsia systolic BP should have a target BP of <120 to 140 mmHg within the first hour. Refer to Table 5.9 for treatment options.
4. All other patients should have systolic BP lowered by 25% within the first hour. These treatment options are outlined in Table 5.9.
5. Target systemic pressures to 160/100 mmHg during hours 2 to 7
6. Target normalization of systemic BP over the next 24 to 48 hours[2]
7. Additional antihypertensive agents for oral use are listed in Tables 5.9 and 5.10.

TABLE 5.9 Treatment Options for Rapid Blood Pressure Reduction

Drug	Class	Dose	Target Organ	Contraindications and Indications
Enalapril	ACE inhibitor	Initial 1.25 mg over 5 minutes Titrated—5 mg q6h		Contraindicated in acute myocardial ischemia, bilateral renal artery stenosis
Fenoldopam	Dopamine receptor selective agonist	Initial 0.1–0.3 mcg/kg/min; max dose 1.6 mcg/kg/min	Acute pulmonary edema, encephalopathy, aortic dissection, acute renal failure	Contraindicated with glaucoma, sulfite allergy
Phentolamine	Adrenergic blocker, alpha antagonist	IV bolus dose 5 mg		Indicated with catecholamine excess (pheochromocytoma, cocaine toxicity, amphetamine overdose)
Esmolol	Adrenergic blocker, beta antagonist	500–1,000 mcg/kg/min over 1 minute, 50-mcg/kg/min infusion	ACS, aortic dissection	Contraindicated in bradycardia, decompensated CHF; high doses may affect lung function
Labetalol	Adrenergic blocker, alpha and betaantagonists	0.3- to 1.0-mg/kg dose slow IV injection or 0.4- to 1.0-mg/kg/h IV infusion (max 3 mg/kg/h)	ACS, encephalopathy, aortic dissection, eclampsia	Contraindicated in pulmonary disease and second/ third degree heart block
Hydralazine	Direct vasodilator	Initial 10 mg via slow IV infusion, q4–6h prn	Eclampsia	Not recommended as first-line therapy, response can be unpredictable
Sodium nitroprusside Nitroglycerin	Nitric oxide dependent vasodilators	0.3–0.5 mcg/kg/min (max 10 mcg/kg/min) Initial 5 mcg/min	Acute pulmonary edema, aortic dissection ACS	Intra-arterial BP monitoring required, risk of cyanide toxicity Best for patients with ACS, acute pulmonary edema, Contraindicated in volume depleted patients
Clevidipine Nicardipine	Dihydropyridine calcium channel blockers	1–2 mg/h Initial 5 mg/h	Encephalopathy, aortic dissection, eclampsia, acute renal failure, cocaine overdose	Contraindicated with allergies to soy, eggs; maximum duration 72 hours Contraindicated with aortic stenosis

ACE, angiotensin-converting-enzyme inhibitor; ACS, acute coronary syndrome; CHF, congestive heart failure; IV, intravenous.

Source: Whelton PK, Carey RM, Aronow WS, et al. ACC/AHA/AAPA/ABC/ACPM/AGS/APhA/ASH/ASPC/NMA/PCNA. Guideline for the prevention, detection, evaluation, and management of high blood pressure in adults. *J Am Coll Cardiol.* 2017;71:e127–e248. doi:10.1016/j.jacc.2017.11.006

TABLE 5.10 Management of Severe Hypertension: Asymptomatic, No Evidence of Target Organ Damage

Class	Drug	Dose	Onset of Action
Alpha blocker	Prazosin	1–2 g twice daily	Hours
ACE inhibitor	Captopril Lisinopril	25 mg two to three times daily 20 mg daily	Hours
ARB	Telmisartan Losartan	40 mg daily 50–100 mg daily	
Beta-blocker	Labetalol	100 mg twice daily	Hours
Calcium channel blocker	Diltiazem Amlodipine	30 mg four times daily 5–10 mg daily	Hours
Central alpha-2 adrenergic agonist	Clonidine	0.1–0.2 mg twice daily	Hours

Source: Gauer, R. (2017). Severe asymptomatic hypertension: evaluation and treatment. *American Family Physician,* 95(8):492–500.

For patients with severe, resistant hypertension who do not require admission to the hospital, you should be aware of the optimal medications to use in the outpatient setting to achieve blood pressure control. Common drug classes with examples of each are listed in Table 5.10. Other drug options are available within each class as well.

CLINICAL PEARL: Oral therapy is discouraged for hypertensive emergencies.

REFERENCES

1. Whelton PK, Carey RM, Aronow WS, et al. ACC/AHA/AAPA/ABC/ACPM/AGS/APhA/ASH/ASPC/NMA/PCNA. Guideline for the prevention, detection, evaluation, and management of high blood pressure in adults. *J Am Coll Cardiol.* 2017;71:e127–e248. doi:10.1016/j.jacc.2017.11.006
2. Gauer R. Severe asymptomatic hypertension: evaluation and treatment. *Am Fam Physician.* 2017;95(8):492–500.

ELECTRONIC RESOURCES

https://www.ncbi.nlm.nih.gov/pmc/articles/PMC270718/pdf/cc2351.pdf

http://www.onlinejacc.org/content/accj/71/19/e127.full.pdf?_ga=2.58572202.1816725587.1532873862-625759609.1531531330

Nausea and Vomiting

Introduction

Acute gastroenteritis results in over one million primary care visits annually and 10% of hospital admissions per year. Gastrointestinal complaints are included in the list of the top 20 reasons for primary care visits, and nausea, vomiting, and diarrhea are the most common presenting complaints.[1] The three most common causes of acute nausea and vomiting are gastroenteritis, pregnancy, and migraines. To aid in the diagnosis as well as management of nausea and vomiting, it helps to understand the major feedback control systems and the most likely conditions associated with them. The following categories represent the most common etiologies:

- Infections: Norwalk or rotavirus, bacteria, and bacterial associated toxins, *Staphylococcus aureus*, *Clostridium*, *Shigella*, *Campylobacter*, hepatitis A or B, appendicitis, pyelonephritis
- Hepatobiliary, pancreatic: Pancreatitis, cholelithiasis
- Medications: NSAIDs, antibiotics, calcium channel blockers, opioids, estrogens
- Mechanical obstruction: Peptic ulcer with associated edema, malignancy, previous abdominal surgery
- Dysmotility: Gastroparesis, postviral illness, postvagotomy, irritable bowel syndrome
- Metabolic: DKA, pregnancy, uremia, thyroid disorders
- Vestibular disorders: Benign positional vertigo, Meniere's, labyrinthitis, migraines

Clinical Presentation

A comparison of clinical presentations with possible etiologies is seen in Table 5.11.

HISTORICAL FINDINGS
- General: Fever, fatigue, dehydration, weight loss, stressors
- Skin: Jaundice
- Ear, nose, and throat (ENT): Visual changes, headaches, dizziness, vertigo
- Gastrointestinal (GI): Early morning nausea and vomiting can be associated with alcohol use disorders, pregnancy, or metabolic disturbances. Vomiting shortly following a meal can be seen with gastroparesis, ulcers, or gastritis. Symptoms that occur hours following a meal can be secondary to an obstruction. Pain that is relieved by vomiting suggests obstruction. Abdominal pain that is not associated with meals is less likely to be peptic ulcer disease or cancer. Other factors less associated with these entities include the absence of dark or blood tinged stool, and no relationship to meals
- Genitourinary (GU): Urogenital review of systems is important, including last menstrual period
- Neuro: Autonomic insufficiency, including orthostasis, lack of sweating

TABLE 5.11 Clinical Presentation: Possible Causes of Nausea and Vomiting

Feature	Differential Diagnosis
Timing of nausea/vomiting	
Acute onset and associated *with abdominal pain*	Gastroenteritis, cholecystitis, pancreatitis, obstruction, peritonitis
Acute onset *without abdominal pain*	CNS bleed, ketoacidosis, MI, hepatitis, medications
Insidious onset	Reflux disease, peptic ulcer disease, gastroparesis, medications, metabolic disorders, pregnancy
Associated symptoms	
Diarrhea, headache, myalgias	Viral gastroenteritis
Vomiting	
Bilious	Small bowel obstruction
Coffee ground	Ulcers, gastritis
Undigested food, chime	Gastroparesis, gastric outlet obstruction
Projectile	Elevated intracranial pressure
AM, before breakfast	Alcohol, elevated intracranial pressure, uremia
During or soon after meals	Anorexia, bulimia
Occurs >1 hour pc	Gastroparesis, gastric outlet obstruction
Habitual postprandial, continuous	Major depression
Fecal matter, foul odor	Obstruction
Diarrhea	
No fever, chills	Noninfectious
Large volume, watery stools, fever, chills, nausea, vomiting, and abdominal cramping	Gastroenteritis
	Colitis (infectious, inflammatory)
Fever, tenesmus, mucous, and bloody stools	

CNS, central nervous system; MI, myocardial infarction.

- Medications: Digoxin, calcium channel blockers
- Past medical history: Functional bowel disorder, diabetes
- Social history: Toxin exposure, ill contacts, contaminated foods
- Surgical history: Specifically focusing on abdominal surgeries

CLINICAL PEARL: Pertinent findings include timing, relationship to meals, associated symptoms, and characteristics of vomitus. Absence of headaches, severe abdominal pain, recent medication changes, and bleeding narrows the differential.

CLINICAL PEARL: Critical to the history is the presence of abdominal pain, significant headache, or recent initiation of certain medications, which may be associated with a more concerning etiology. When not present, the most likely cause remains an acute gastroenteritis.

Physical Examination

Evaluate for:

- General: Fever, tachycardia, hypotension, and orthostasis
- Skin: Pale, dry, jaundiced skin
- ENT: Papilledema, retinopathy, nystagmus, oral cavity dry mucosa, poor dentition
- Neck: Stiffness, adenopathy
- Abdomen: Distention, visible peristalsis, abnormal bowel sounds, peritoneal signs, organomegaly, celebravascukar accident (CVA) tenderness, increase in pain with tensing of abdominal muscles
- Rectal: Stool color, mucous, blood
- Neuro: Nystagmus, ataxia, asterixis
- Extremities: Edema

CLINICAL PEARL: The pertinent historical findings of timing, associated symptoms, alleviating factors, and aggravating factors are often enough to identify the cause.

Diagnosis

LABS

- CBC: Evaluate for anemia, leukocytosis
- Comprehensive metabolic panel: Evaluate hydration status, abnormal electrolytes (associated with metabolic disorders, psychogenic causes), prerenal azotemia
- Hepatic panel: Look for aminotransferase elevation suggestive of inflammation of hepatocytes; alkaline phosphatase and bilirubin elevations are suggestive of cholestatic obstructive pattern
- Hepatitis A virus (HAV), hepatitis B virus (HBV) antibodies
- C-reactive protein: Active inflammation
- Amylase and lipase: Pancreatitis
- Thyroid-stimulating hormone: Hyper/hypothyroidism
- Stool studies: Ova parasites, cultures
- Urinalysis: Infection
- Urine pregnancy testing

IMAGING

- Gastric emptying study: Gastroparesis
- Abdominal radiography: Obstruction
- Ultrasonography: Cholecystitis/lithiasis
- CT with contrast: Pancreatitis, inflammatory bowel disease, localizing obstruction
- CT: Intracranial lesions, elevated intracranial pressure
- Magnetic resonance cholangiopancreatography (MRCP): Pancreatic ductal obstruction
- Endoscopy: GERD, peptic ulcer disease (PUD)

Management

Treatment options will depend upon the definitive diagnosis. The decision to admit the patient will depend upon objective evidence of volume depletion, orthostatic changes, patient age, ability to maintain adequate hydration, or the presence of a surgical abdomen, central nervous system (CNS) lesion, or metabolic emergency. Treatment options based on symptoms and the underlying pathophysiology are outlined in Table 5.12 and Table 5.13.

TABLE 5.12 Nausea Treatment Based on Cause

Condition	Neuro-transmitter Pathways	Chemical Mediators	Treatment Options
Medications, metabolic disorders, gastroenteritis	Visceral stimulation	Dopamine and serotonin	Serotonin antagonists and dopamine antagonists, e.g., metoclopramide, promethazine, prochlorperazine
Motion sickness, vestibular diseases	Vestibular and CNS activation	Histamine and acetylcholine	Antihistamines and anticholinergics, e.g., meclizine, scopolamine, dimenhydrinate
Gastroparesis	Chemoreceptor trigger zone activation	Dopamine and serotonin	Serotonin antagonists and dopamine antagonists, e.g., metoclopramide, promethazine, prochlorperazine
Chemotherapy, severe gastroenteritis	Chemoreceptor trigger zone activation	Dopamine and serotonin	Selective serotonin receptor (5-HT_3) antagonists; substance P receptor inhibitors—dexamethasone

CNS, central nervous system.

TABLE 5.13 Medications Specific to Clinical Conditions

Condition	Treatment
Pregnancy	Doxylamine, pyridoxine
Migraine	Metoclopramide + aspirin Prochlorperazine Chlorpromazine Promethazine Triptans
Gastroenteritis	Ondansetron
Functional	Ginger (affects 5-HT3 and cholinergic receptors) Low-dose tricyclic antidepressants

CLINICAL PEARL: Serotonin antagonists have largely replaced the dopamine antagonists because of their side effects. Use caution when using serotonin antagonists in patients with prolonged QT intervals as these drugs may also prolong the QT interval.

> **CLINICAL PEARL:** Serotonin antagonists are most effective in treating gastroenteritis.

> **CLINICAL PEARL:** Because of the significant extrapyramidal effects associated with metoclopramide, it should not be used in the elderly and patients receiving antipsychotics and other dopamine antagonists.

REFERENCES

1. Anderson WD 3rd, Strayer SM. Evaluation of nausea and vomiting [published corrections appear in Am Fam Physician. 2013,88(11):728 and Am Fam Physician. 2014,89(3):152]. *Am Fam Physician.* 2013;88(6):371–379.

6

Common Procedures in Family Medicine

CERUMEN OR FOREIGN BODY REMOVAL

Indication

The goal is to remove cerumen or a foreign body from the ear canal of symptomatic patients with a minimal degree of risk to the patient while observing standard precautions. Cerumen removal is indicated when cerumen impaction interferes with visualization of the tympanic membrane (TM); the patient is exhibiting symptoms of pain, pressure, hearing loss, or dizziness; or with the presence of any foreign body in the external ear canal. The procedure is contraindicated when the patient is uncooperative, TM rupture is suspected, or if irrigation will cause the foreign body to expand. The procedure may be contraindicated if the foreign body is lodged against the TM.[1,2]

Equipment

- Ear irrigation water bottle kit (30- to 60-mL syringe)
- Otoscope
- Body temperature water
- Cerumen spoon, loop
- Alligator forceps
- Lidocaine, mineral oil
- Small diameter suction cup (if available)
- Basin
- Towel
- Magnet (for metal object)

Procedure

IRRIGATION
1. Gather appropriate equipment
2. Introduce self to patient

3. Describe procedure
4. Obtain patient consent
5. Wash hands
6. Perform otoscope examination to check for perforation or bleeding
7. Fill ear irrigation medium with tap water at body temperature (attach catheter to syringe if required)
8. Have patient hold irrigation basin to the ear
9. Pull auricle upward, outward, and backward to straighten canal
10. Irrigate with a gentle, continuous stream directed in the open area adjacent to the wax, or if occluded, along the posterior superior canal wall, inspecting frequently for trauma
11. Repeat procedure as needed until clear, or patient says to stop
12. If unsuccessful, remove manually with curettage (see section "Procedure: Curettage")
13. If wax is hard, ceruminolytics or softeners can be tried (few drops of hydrogen peroxide 3%, triethanolamine polypeptide oleate-condensate, carbamide peroxide, or mineral oil)

CURETTAGE

1. Gather appropriate equipment
2. Introduce self to patient
3. Describe procedure
4. Obtain patient consent
5. Wash hands
6. Describe procedure and advise the patient to remain perfectly still
7. Perform otoscope examination to check for perforation or bleeding
8. Pull auricle upward, outward, and backward to straighten canal
9. Place cerumen spoon at one end of impaction in attempt to pull distally
10. Pass instrument beyond cerumen
11. Remove cerumen with instrument
12. If unsuccessful, irrigate and repeat extraction
13. At completion, perform otoscope examination to assess tympanic membrane

FOREIGN BODY REMOVAL

1. Gather appropriate equipment
2. Introduce self to patient
3. Describe procedure
4. Obtain patient consent
5. Wash hands
6. Instrument choice is dependent upon type of foreign body and can include any of the following:
   a. Alligator forceps
   b. Cup-shaped forceps for round objects
   c. Suction
7. Avoid irrigation if foreign body is absorbable or if a battery is lodged in the ear canal
8. Direct the instrument toward the superior edge of the foreign body, slide behind object, and pull forward
9. Inspect canal for any damage

Follow-Up

1. Dry canal with hair dryer on low, if available
2. Report any signs of localized pain, erythema, swelling
3. Consider prescribing a topical antibiotic solution such as ofloxacin/ciprofloxacin, if surface is disrupted from removal wax

Complications of the procedure may include TM perforation, ossicle damage, abrasion of the canal, advancement of the foreign body further into the canal, temporary vertigo, tinnitus, or otitis externa. If TM rupture occurs, schedule eye, nose, and throat (ENT) evaluation within 1 to 2 weeks, treat pain, and reassure patient.

REFERENCES

1. Roberts JR, Custalow CB, Thomsen TW. *Roberts and Hedges' Clinical Procedures in Emergency Medicine and Acute Care / Editor-in-Chief.* 7th ed. Philadelphia, PA: Elsevier; 2019.
2. Kasper D, Fauci A, Hauser S, et al. *Harrison's Principles of Internal Medicine.* 19th ed. New York, NY: McGraw-Hill Professional Publishing; 2018.

INCISION, DRAINAGE, CULTURE, AND PACKING

Indication

The goal of this procedure is to incise and drain a localized collection of pus that is tender and is not resolving spontaneously, with minimal degree of risk to the patient while observing standard precautions. The cardinal signs of infection (pain, fever, redness, swelling, and loss of function) are usually present. Contraindications to this procedure include facial furuncles due to the risk of septic phlebitis with intracranial extension. Abscesses in the rectal or perineal area should be referred to a general or colorectal surgeon for management. Caution should be used with abscesses in the following areas due to close proximity to major vessels: peritonsillar and retropharyngeal regions, anterior triangle of the neck, supraclavicular fossa, deep axilla, antecubital space, groin, and popliteal space.[1-3]

Equipment

- Personal protective equipment (gloves, face shield)
- Skin cleansing agent (chlorhexadine or povidone-iodine solution)
- Needles (large and small, e.g., 25–30 gauge)
- Syringe (3–10 mL)
- Anesthetic agent: 1% lidocaine 4.5 mg/kg, max. vol. 31 mL; 1% lidocaine with epinephrine, 7 mg/kg, max. vol. 49 mL; 0.25% bupivacaine, 3 mg/kg, max. vol. 84 mL
- Culture swab
- Sterile drapes, 4″× 4″ gauze, ¼″ or ½″ packing gauge, and gauze bandage

- Blades: 11 open abscess, 15 debride tissue
- Kelly clamps
- Tissue forceps
- Curved hemostats
- Saline solution, syringes, splash guards, intravenous (IV) catheter needles, sterile container for solution for irrigation
- Tissue, bandage scissors
- Dressings to cover wound

Procedure

1. Gather materials, equipment
2. Introduce self, explain procedure, address all patient questions
3. Obtain patient consent
4. Wash hands
5. Complete the appropriate neurovascular examination
6. Carefully open all materials prior to beginning the procedure
7. Don clean gloves
8. Prepare skin surface with povidone-odine solution or chlorhexadine at least a 1 to 2 inches beyond border surrounding the base of the abscess
9. Prepare anesthetic agent (5–10 mL)
10. Prepare appropriate needle 25–30 g ½ to 1½-inch needle
11. Appropriately drape area to absorb abscess contents and prevent area/equipment contamination by drainage
12. Assess area to assure anesthesia
13. Swap to sterile gloves for incision and drainage
14. Insert needle with the appropriate approach approximately 1 cm away from the erythematous border of the abscess (may perform intradermal injection over the dome of the abscess)
    a. Can be inserted at the junction of the dermis and subcutaneous fat if skin is intact
    b. Can be inserted directly into wound or dome of abscess
    c. Insert the needle into the skin and advance to the hub parallel to the dermis and subcutaneous fat
    d. Aspirate to assure not within vessel; if so, withdraw and redirect
    e. After aspiration, slowly inject anesthetic as needle is withdrawn
    f. Reinsert the needle at the end of the first tract, repeat procedure while testing patient to assure adequate result and the area is sufficiently anesthetized
15. Utilizing a number 11 blade, nick the skin over the abscess, to facilitate drainage
16. Make a simple linear incision conforming to skin creases or natural folds, (Langer's lines). Extend the incision to create an opening large enough to ensure adequate drainage and to prevent recurrent abscess formation; the incision may need to extend the length of the abscess borders
17. If indicated, obtain abscess specimen for culture
18. Apply gentle external pressure to express purulent material

19. Explore the abscess cavity by inserting the curved hemostat (open and close tip to break up loculations or cotton tipped applicator
20. Irrigate the wound, holding edges open with hemostat if required
21. Explore for foreign body with forceps
22. Irrigate again until clear
23. Perform final inspection for foreign body, septa prior to packing
24. Pack the wound with ¼″ gauze, layering lightly, leaving 1 cm out of cavity. This packing may need to be removed every 12 to 24 hours depending upon amount of drainage
25. Apply the outer nonadherent sterile dressing layer and stabilizing (packing, 4″ × 4″ gauze, gauze bandage wrap) dressing
26. Correctly dispose of all used supplies
27. Provide correct documentation of the procedure including date, time, procedure, site, and patient disposition

Follow-Up

- Instruct the patient on follow-up and local wound care
  - Keep wound clean and dry, elevate to reduce edema and pain, minimize mobility (hand and foot) as it may impede the healing process
- The patient should return for reexamination of the wound within 48 to 72 hours to remove initial packing; replace sterile dressings daily (may be required more frequently depending upon discharge)
- Once packing is no longer needed, the patient may begin warm soaks several times per day until healing occurs (typically in 7–10 days)
- Advise the patient to watch for fever or chills, reaccumulation of pus in the area, increased pain or redness, red streaks, and increased swelling
- NSAIDS are recommended for discomfort, with acetaminophen as an alternative for those with aversion

Complications of the procedure may include cellulitis, recollection of purulent material, deep tissue infection, injection pain, local reactions such as bruising, local pain of injection, neuritis, neuropathy, infection, hematoma, local ischemia, and thrombophlebitis. The patient may experience a vasovagal event or anesthesia reaction (most often secondary to inadvertent intravascular injection). Cardiovascular effects may include conduction delays, bradycardia, and hypotension. Central nervous system (CNS) effects may include tinnitus, metallic taste, agitation, dysarthria, and seizures.

REFERENCES

1. Roberts JR, Custalow CB, Thomsen TW. *Roberts and Hedges' Clinical Procedures in Emergency Medicine and Acute Care / Editor-in-Chief.* 7th ed. Philadelphia, PA: Elsevier; 2019.
2. Kasper D, Fauci A, Hauser S, et al. *Harrison's Principles of Internal Medicine.* 19th ed. New York, NY: McGraw-Hill Professional Publishing; 2018.
3. Pfenninger J, Fowler G. *Procedures for Primary Care.* 3rd ed. Philadelphia, PA: Saunders; 2010.

JOINT (KNEE) INJECTIONS

Indications

The goal of a joint injection is to properly aspirate/inject a joint or bursa while observing standard precautions and with minimal degree of risk to the patient. Joint injections are indicated for the administration of medications in acute and chronic inflammatory joint conditions and pain relief in acute hemarthrosis or tense effusion. Joint aspiration is used to perform diagnostic testing in the setting of a septic joint, crystal-induced arthritis, ligamentous or bony injury, anterior cruciate ligament (ACL) rupture, intra-articular fracture, obtaining fluid for analysis (various inflammatory, noninflammatory, hemorrhagic, and infectious sources of joint pain), or determining whether a laceration communicates with the joint space by injecting methylene blue dye. The technical approach for common joint injections is outlined in Table 6.1.

Absolute contraindications to this procedure include cellulitis involving the skin overlying the injection site, significant skin atrophy near the injection site, bacteremia or sepsis, septic arthritis, history of allergy or anaphylaxis to the injectable, acute bleeding, acute fracture, or joint prosthesis. Relative contraindications are coagulopathy, anticoagulant treatment, uncontrolled diabetes, joint instability, adjacent skin lesions or abrasions, and severe osteoporosis.[1,2]

Equipment

- Syringes: 3 mL, 5 mL, 10 mL for injection; 10 mL to 60 mL for aspiration
- Needles: 22, 25, 27, 30 g for injection; 18 to 22 g for aspiration, ½ to 1 ½ length
- Alcohol, povidone-iodine solution, or chlorhexidine gluconate to clean skin
- 4″ × 4″ gauze pads
- Hemostat: Used to help remove syringe from the needle when aspirating a large joint
- Green top test tube, sterile urine cup
- Gloves (sterile or nonsterile)
- Meds: Lidocaine, steroids (methyprednisolone 40 mg/mL or triamcinolone 20 mg/mL), hyaluronan injections

Procedure

INJECTION
1. Gather appropriate equipment
2. Introduce self to patient
3. Describe procedure
4. Obtain patient consent
5. Wash hands
6. Position and drape the patient
7. Put on gloves
8. Palpate bony landmarks to determine the site for needle insertion. Refer to Table 6.1

TABLE 6.1 Technical Approach for Common Joint Injections

Joint	Approach
AC Joint Injection	1. Insert the needle above the AC joint and perpendicular to the clavicle at the point of maximum pain 2. Aiming slightly medial 3. Walk the needle along the lateral clavicle just beyond the distal clavicle and into the joint
Glenohumeral Joint Injection	**Anterior approach:** 1. Insert the needle one thumb width lateral and one thumb width inferior to the coracoid process. 2. Direct the needle perpendicular and slightly lateral to enter the joint. **Posterior approach:** 1. 2 cm inferior and 1 cm medial to the posterolateral acromion 2. Aim needle toward coracoid.
Subacromial	1. Locate the posterior lateral tip of the acromion 2. Insert the needle 1 cm below that landmark. Advance the needle in a perpendicular direction under the acromion, aiming toward the coracoid process. Inject while slowly pulling back on the syringe. 3. Pull back and redirect the needle if resistance is felt
Elbow Joint	**Approach olecranon process:** 1. Extend elbow 2. Palpate the depression between the radial head and the lateral epicondyle of the humerus 3. Flex the elbow to 90 degrees. 4. Pronate the forearm and place the palm flat 5. Insert needle from the lateral aspect just distal to the lateral epicondyle and direct medially **Approach lateral epicondyle:** 1. Flex elbow 90 degrees. 2. Insert the needle perpendicular to the epicondyle, over the site of maximum tenderness at the origin common extensor. 3. Insert the needle deeply into the subcutaneous tissue, advancing to the tender area. 4. Slowly inject while pulling the needle back and then advancing in a fan pattern.
Trochanteric Bursitis	1. Perform with patient lying on the unaffected side. 2. Direct the needle perpendicular to the skin at the site of maximal tenderness and advance just down to the greater trochanter. 3. Pull back slightly while injecting in a fanlike pattern in the area of tenderness.
Knee Joint	1. With the patient seated and the knee flexed to 90 degrees, insert the needle 45 degrees just medial or lateral to the patella tendon at the "divot" of the knee joint 2. Advance toward the intercondylar notch of the tibia. 3. Alternative approach: mid-patella medial or lateral with knee in extension

AC, acromioclavicular.

9. Mark the injection site by indenting the skin with a needle cap
10. Clean the injection site with betadine, alcohol, or chloroprep
11. Do not touch the injection site once it has been cleaned
12. Insert the needle perpendicular to the skin with bevel side up at the designated spot, aspirate to check for blood, then slowly inject med
13. Remove needle and dispose in sharps container
14. Apply bandage
15. Massage the injected area and move the joint through a full range of motion to help distribute the medication

ASPIRATION TECHNIQUE
Follow the Injection Procedure steps, as well as these steps:

1. Consider anesthetizing more difficult to aspirate joints with lidocaine or freeze spray prior to aspiration. A 25- to 30-g needle can be used to numb the skin and soft tissue
2. Use a 18-g needle with a 10- to 60-mL syringe, depending on the amount of aspirate anticipated
3. Insert the needle into the designated site, aspirate for blood, and then aspirate fluid. If syringe becomes full, leave needle in, remove syringe, and replace with an empty one
4. Aspirated fluid should be sent for analysis when indicated. If the aspirate is bloody, hold it up to the light to look for fat globules floating in the blood, indicating an associated fracture
5. Apply bandage and ace wrap
6. Provide patient education

Follow-Up

1. Avoid general use of the joint for 48 hours (minimum)
2. Avoid pressure on the joint
3. Call the office if the patient develops fever or if the joint becomes warm, swollen, increased erythema, or pain increases in severity

Complications: Infection, pain locally at the site of injection, allergic reactions, crystal-induced synovitis, atrophy or depigmentation of the skin overlying the area injected, potential hyperglycemia in patients with diabetes, menstrual irregularities, worsening a preexisting joint infection, cartilage or joint deterioration, tendon rupture, nerve or blood vessel injury.

REFERENCES

1. Stephens MB. Musculoskeletal injections: a review of the evidence. *Am Fam Physician.* 2008;78(8):971–976.
2. Dehn RW, Asprey DP. *Essential Clinical Procedures.* 3rd ed. Philadelphia, PA: Saunders; 2013.

LOCAL ANESTHESIA

Indication

The goal of performing local anesthesia is to provide localized, short-term anesthesia to an area prior to performing a broad range of medical and minor surgical procedures. There are no absolute contraindications to local anesthesia. Relative contraindications include prior allergic reaction, large target areas requiring large doses of anesthetic, underlying liver disease (amides), pseudocholinesterase deficiency (esters), and seizure disorders.[1]

Equipment

- Personal protective equipment (gloves, face shield)
- Skin cleansing agent (chlorhexidine or povidone-iodine solution)
- Needles (large and small, e.g., 27–30 gauge)
- Syringe (e.g., 10 mL)
- Anesthetic agent: 1% lidocaine; 4.5 mg/kg, max. vol. 31 mL; 1% lidocaine with epinephrine 7 mg/kg, max. vol. 49 mL; 0.25% bupivacaine, 3 mg/kg, max. vol. 84 mL

Procedure

1. Gather appropriate equipment
2. Introduce self to patient
3. Describe procedure
4. Obtain patient consent
5. Wash hands
6. Complete the appropriate neurovascular examination
7. Don nonsterile gloves
8. Prepare anesthetic agent (5–10 mL)
9. Replace needle 27–30 g 1½-inch needle
10. Appropriately drape site
11. Prepare skin surface
12. Insertion approach at shallow angle:
    a. Can be inserted at the junction of the dermis and subcutaneous fat if skin is intact
    b. Can be inserted directly into wound as well as dome of abscess
    c. Insert the needle into the skin and advance to the hypodermis and subcutaneous fat
    d. Slowly inject small volumes of anesthetic. During anesthetic infiltration, either slowly advance the needle or initially insert needle to the hub and infiltrate as the needle is withdrawn. Aspiration is not necessary prior to each infiltration unless the area undergoing local anesthesia is close to major blood vessels
    e. Reinsert the needle at the end of the first tract, repeat procedure
    f. Periodic testing to assure adequate result and that the area is sufficiently anesthetized

13. Perform indicated procedure
14. Dress site
15. Correctly dispose of all equipment
16. Give patient instructions for wound/dressing care, analgesia, elevation
17. Provide correct documentation regarding equipment used, patient disposition, dressing changes, follow-up instructions

Complications of the procedure may include local reactions (bruising), local pain, neuritis, neuropathy, infection, hematoma, local ischemia, thrombophlebitis, vasovagal syncope, anesthesia reaction (most often secondary to inadvertent intravascular injection), conduction delays, bradycardia, hypotension, tinnitus, metallic taste, agitation, dysarthria, seizures.

Reference

1. Pfenninger J, Fowler G. *Procedures for Primary Care*. 3rd ed. Philadelphia, PA: Saunders; 2010.

Punch Biopsy

Indication

The goal of this procedure is to definitively diagnose a suspicious-appearing lesion or a rash in which the diagnosis is unclear. Although simple to perform and with minimal risk to the patient, punch biopsy may not provide a sufficient sample for definitive diagnosis and staging. Contraindications include adjacent infection, coagulopathy, or if there is concern the patient will be noncompliant with wound care and follow-up. Specialist referral may be required for lesions around the eyelids, nose, palms, or soles.[1]

Equipment

- Skin cleansing agent (chlorhexadine or povidone-iodine solution)
- Needles (large and small, e.g., 25–30 gauge)
- Syringe (3–10 mL)
- Anesthetic agent: 1% lidocaine, 4.5 mg/kg, max. vol. 31 mL; 1% lidocaine with epinephrine, 7 mg/kg, max. vol. 49 mL; 0.25% bupivacaine, 3 mg/kg, max. vol. 84 mL
- Ferric subsulfate 20% solution, white petrolatum
- Skin punches (2, 3, 4, 6, and 8 mm)
- Forceps
- Scissors
- Needle driver (punch)
- Gauze pads
- Nonabsorbable sutures or adhesive
- Nonsterile gloves
- Small adhesive bandages (circular or square)
- Enough 10% formalin containers

Procedure

1. Gather appropriate equipment
2. Introduce self to patient
3. Describe procedure.
4. Obtain patient consent
5. Wash hands
6. Determine skin line orientation using Langer lines, producing an oval area that can be easily approximated
7. Prep area with cleansing solution, drape
8. Inject site with 1% lidocaine solution
9. Hold punch biopsy instrument perpendicular to the surface of the lesion
10. Obtain punch biopsy to create plug for excision by placing punch over lesion after pulling perpendicular to Langer lines; firmly, gently rotate through skin until a decrease in tension on the tissue is felt
11. With Adson's forceps, gently (to avoid crushing) lift plug and sever base with iris scissors
12. Cauterize open punch with Ferric subsulfate 20% solution using cotton wick or swab
13. If larger than 4 mm, punch wound may require suture closure
14. Apply sterile dressings, with petroleum gel to cover wound

Follow-Up

Provide instructions on local wound care and advise the patient to keep dressing in place for 24 hours. After dressing removal, keep the area clean with soap and water and keep it dry. Advise the patient to look for signs of bleeding and local infection. Instruct the patient to call the office in 5 to 7 days for results, if not contacted sooner.

Complications: The most common complications include bleeding and infection.

Reference

1. Pickett H. Shave and punch biopsy for skin lesions. *Am Fam Physician.* 2011;84(9):995–1002.

7

Common Abbreviations in Family Medicine

AAA: Abdominal aortic aneurysm
A&O: Alert and oriented
AAO: Awake, alert, oriented. AAOx3 indicates the patient is AAO to person, place, and time
ABG: Arterial blood gas. Used to differentiate and evaluate for metabolic acidosis, metabolic alkalosis, respiratory acidosis, and respiratory alkalosis (see Table 7.1)

TABLE 7.1 Arterial Blood Gas Used to Evaluate for Respiratory Acidosis, Respiratory Alkalosis, Metabolic Acidosis, and Metabolic Alkalosis

ABG	pH	PaCO$_2$	HCO$_3$
Respiratory acidosis	↓	↑	normal
Respiratory alkalosis	↑	↓	normal
Metabolic acidosis	↓	normal	↓
Metabolic alkalosis	↑	normal	↑

AC: Acromioclavicular
ac: Before meals
ACL: Anterior cruciate ligament
AD: Right ear
ad lib: As often as desired
ADLs: Activities of daily living
AKA: Above-the-knee amputation
ALT: Alanine transaminase (also known as SGPT)
AMA: Against medical advice
ANA: Antinuclear antibody
AROM: Active range of motion
AS: Aortic stenosis
AS: Left ear
ASA: Aspirin (acetylsalicylic acid)
ASAP: As soon as possible

ASD: Atrial septal defect
ASO: Antistreptolysin O
AST: Aspartate transaminase (also known as SGOT)
AU: Both ears
AVR: Aortic valve replacement or aortic valve regurgitation
BKA: Below-the-knee amputation
BMI: Body mass index (see Table 7.2)

TABLE 7.2 Body Mass Index Classifications

Classification	BMI (kg/m^2)
Underweight	<18.5
Normal weight	18.5–24.9
Overweight	25–29.9
Obesity class I	30–34.9
Obesity class II	35–39.9
Obesity class III	≥40

BP: Blood pressure
BPH: Benign prostatic hypertrophy
BPM: Beats per minute
Bx: Biopsy
C&S: Culture and sensitivity
CABG: Coronary artery bypass graft
CAD: Coronary artery disease
CEA: Carcinoembryonic antigen
CHF: Congestive heart failure
CHO: Carbohydrate
CIS: Carcinoma in situ
CMV: Cytomegalovirus
CN: Cranial nerves (see Table 7.3)

TABLE 7.3 Names of Cranial Nerves

Nerve	Name
I	Olfactory
II	Optic
III	Oculomotor
IV	Trochlear
V	Trigeminal
VI	Abducens
VII	Facial
VIII	Vestibulocochlear

(continued)

TABLE 7.3 Names of Cranial Nerves (*continued*)

Nerve	Name
IX	Glossopharyngeal
X	Vagus
XI	Accessory
XII	Hypoglossal

CTA: Clear to auscultation
CXR: Chest x-ray
D/C: Discontinue
D&C: Dilation and curettage
D&E: Dilation and evacuation
DBP: Diastolic blood pressure
DJD: Degenerative joint disease
DOE: Dyspnea on exertion
DTR: Deep tendon reflexes (see Table 7.4)

TABLE 7.4 Reflexes and Their Associated Main Spinal Roots

Reflex	Main Spinal Root
Ankle	S1
Knee	L4
Brachioradialis	C6
Biceps	C5/6
Triceps	C7

DX: Diagnosis
EBV: Epstein–Barr virus
ECT: Electroconvulsive therapy
EOM: Extraocular movements (see Table 7.5)

TABLE 7.5 Extraocular Movements and Associated Cranial Nerves and Muscles

Cranial Nerve	Muscle	Function
Oculomotor nerve (III)	Medial rectus	Adduction
Oculomotor nerve (III)	Inferior rectus	Downward gaze
Oculomotor nerve (III)	Superior rectus	Upward gaze
Trochlear nerve (IV)	Superior oblique	Downward gaze
Abducens nerve (VI)	Lateral rectus	Abduction

EOMI: Extraocular movements intact
ERCP: Endoscopic retrograde cholangiopancreatography

ETOH: Ethanol

FB: Foreign body

FEV$_1$: Forced expiratory volume in 1 second. This is the volume of air exhaled in the first second which is evaluated by spirometry

FUO: Fever of unknown origin

FVC: Forced vital capacity. This is the total volume of air exhaled upon spirometry testing

Fx: Fracture

GC: Gonorrhea (gonococcus)

GFR: Glomerular filtration rate

GH: Growth hormone

H&H: Hemoglobin and hematocrit

HA: Headache

HMO: Health maintenance organization

HNP: Herniated nucleus pulposus

HOB: Head of bed

HR: Heart rate

HTN: Hypertension

I&D: Incision and drainage

IBS: Irritable bowel syndrome

ICS: Intercostal space

IM: Intramuscular, given intramuscularly

IUD: Intrauterine device

IUP: Intrauterine pregnancy

JVD: Jugular venous distension

KUB: Kidney, ureter, bladder. A type of x-ray

LAD: Left anterior descending artery

LBBB: Left bundle branch block

LLD: Left lateral decubitus position

LLL: Left lower lobe of lung

LMP: Last menstrual period

LOC: Loss of consciousness

LP: Lumbar puncture

LUL: Left upper lobe of lung

MCL: Medial collateral ligament

MCL: Mid-clavicular line

MCP: Metacarpophalangeal

mEq: Milliequivalents

MI: Myocardial infarction

MMM: Moist mucous membranes

MRSA: Methicillin-resistant *Staphylococcus aureus*

MS: Mitral stenosis

MS: Multiple sclerosis

MVA: Motor vehicle accident

MVC: Motor vehicle crash or collision

MVP: Mitral valve prolapse

NAD: No acute distress

NSR: Normal sinus rhythm

NTG: Nitroglycerin

N/V/D: Nausea/vomiting/diarrhea
O&P: Ova and parasites
OD: Right eye
OM: Otitis media
ORIF: Open reduction internal fixation
OS: Left eye
OS: Opening snap
OU: Both eyes
P: Pulse
PCL: Posterior cruciate ligament
PCP: Primary care provider
PDA: Patent ductus arteriosus
PERRLA: Pupils equal, round, reactive to light and accommodation
PIP: Proximal interphalangeal
PKU: Phenylketonuria
PMI: Point of maximal impulse
PND: Paroxysmal nocturnal dyspnea
PND: Postnasal drip
PRN: As needed
PROM: Passive range of motion
PROM: Premature rupture of membranes (in pregnancy)
Pt: Patient
PT: Physical therapy
PT: Prothrombin time
PTA: Prior to admission/arrival
Q: Every (as a measure of frequency)
RA: Rheumatoid arthritis
RBBB: Right bundle branch block
RML: Right middle lobe of lung
R/O: Rule out
ROM: Range of motion
ROS: Review of systems
RPR: Rapid plasma reagin
RR: Respiratory rate
RRR: Regular rate and rhythm
RSV: Respiratory syncytial virus
RTC: Return to clinic
RUL: Right upper lobe of lung
SBP: Systolic blood pressure
SGGT: Serum gamma-glutamyl transpeptidase
SGOT: Serum glutamic-oxaloacetic transaminase (also known as AST)
SGPT: Serum glutamic-pyruvic transaminase (also known as ALT)
SL: Sublingual. Commonly used as an instruction for medication administration
SOAP: Mnemonic of Subjective, Objective, Assessment, and Plan
SOB: Shortness of breath, or dyspnea
S/P: Status post
Sub-Q, SQ: Subcutaneous tissue
T&A: Tonsillectomy and adenoidectomy

TAH: Total abdominal hysterectomy
TB: Tuberculosis
TIA: Transient ischemic attack
TM: Tympanic membrane
TMJ: Temporomandibular joint
tPA: Tissue plasminogen activator
Tx: Treatment
U/A or UA: Urinalysis
U/S or US: Ultrasound/sonogram
V/Q scan: Ventilation–perfusion scan
VDRL: Venereal Disease Research Laboratory tests
VSD: Ventricular septal defect
VSS: Vital signs stable
WD: Well-developed
WDWN: Well-developed, well-nourished
WN: Well-nourished
x: Times; by (size)
y/o: years old

Appendix A

SELECTED RESOURCES FOR THE FAMILY MEDICINE PHYSICIAN ASSISTANT STUDENT

1. A depository of tools and resources for preventative care: U.S. Preventive Services Task Force (USPSTF).
   https://www.uspreventiveservicestaskforce.org/Page/Name/browse-tools-and-resources
2. Cultural Competence Self-Assessments
   a. https://nccc.georgetown.edu/assessments
   b. https://implicit.harvard.edu/implicit/takeatest.html
3. Health Maintenance
   a. Obesity Guidelines and Calculation
      https://www.cdc.gov/obesity/adult/defining.html
      https://www.cdc.gov/obesity/childhood/defining.html
   b. Dietary Guidelines
      https://health.gov/dietaryguidelines/2015/guidelines
      https://www.choosemyplate.gov
   c. Physical Activity Guidelines
      https://health.gov/paguidelines/guidelines
4. Endocrinology
   a. Diabetes: American Diabetes Association 2018 Standards of Care
      https://diabetesed.net/wp-content/uploads/2017/12/2018-ADA-Standards-of-Care.pdf
5. Respiratory
   a. Asthma Action (or management) Plan
      i. Children: https://www.aap.org/en-us/Documents/Asthma_Action_Plan.pdf
      ii. Adults: https://portal.ct.gov/-/media/Departments-and-Agencies/DPH/dph/hems/asthma/pdf/AAP12yrsolderfinalengspanpdf.pdf?la=en
   b. Pneumonia
      Guidelines and CURB-65—A tool for evaluating outpatient versus hospital treatment of pneumonia
      https://evidencebasedpractice.osumc.edu/Documents/Guidelines/pneumonia.pdf

    c. Obstructive Sleep Apnea
        i. Guidelines for evaluation, management, and care
           https://www.ncbi.nlm.nih.gov/pmc/articles/PMC2699173
        ii. Epworth Sleepiness Scale
           https://web.stanford.edu/~dement/epworth.html
        iii. Stanford Sleepiness Scale
           https://web.stanford.edu/~dement/sss.html
        iv. STOP-BANG
           http://www.stopbang.ca/osa/screening.php
    d. COPD Global Initiative for Obstructive Lung Disease (GOLD) Guidelines
        https://goldcopd.org/wp-content/uploads/2017/11/GOLD-2018 -v6.0-FINAL-revised-20-Nov_WMS.pdf

6. Cardiovascular
    a. Framingham Risk Score: Calculates risk of having an MI in the next 10 years
        http://tools.acc.org/ASCVD-Risk-Estimator-Plus/#!/calculate/estimate
    b. Dietary Approaches to Stop Hypertension (DASH)
        https://www.nhlbi.nih.gov/files/docs/public/heart/dash_brief.pdf
    c. 2017 Guidelines for the Management of Heart Failure
        https://www.ahajournals.org/doi/pdf/10.1161/CIR.0000000000000509
    d. 2017 Guidelines for the Prevention, Detection, Evaluation and Management of High Blood Pressure in Adults
        https://www.acc.org/education-and-meetings/image-and-slide -gallery/media-detail?id=CF4EBD8CC6F343B98989AB1793ADCF19

7. Psychiatry/Behavioral Health
    a. PHQ-2 (Patient Health Questionnaire): Simplified assessment of depression in adolescents and adults. If positive, administer PHQ-9
        http://www.cqaimh.org/pdf/tool_phq2.pdf
    b. PHQ-9 (Patient Health Questionnaire): Used to support diagnosis of depression and monitor progress
        http://www.cqaimh.org/pdf/tool_phq9.pdf
    c. MDQ (Mood Disorder Questionnaire)
        http://www.cqaimh.org/pdf/tool_mdq.pdf
    d. EPDS (Edinburgh Postnatal Depression Scale)
        https://psychology-tools.com/epds
    e. SRQ-R (Suicide Risk Questionnaire-Revised)
        http://www.cqaimh.org/pdf/tool_sbq-r.pdf
    f. Substance Abuse Screening Tools
        https://www.drugabuse.gov/nidamed-medical-health-professionals/ tool-resources-your-practice/screening-assessment-drug-testing -resources/chart-evidence-based-screening-tools
    g. Alcohol Use Disorders Identification Test (AUDIT)
        https://www.drugabuse.gov/sites/default/files/files/AUDIT.pdf
    h. Alcohol, Smoking and Substance Involvement Screening Test (ASSIST)
        https://www.ct.gov/dmhas/lib/dmhas/publications/SBIRT -ASSIST.pdf

8. Urology
   a. American Urology Association BPH Symptoms Score
      http://www.bostonscientific.com/content/dam/bostonscientific
      -anz/patients/downloads/Enlarged_Prostate_Symptom_Score_
      Questionnaire.pdf
   b. National Institute of Health Prostatitis Symptom Index (NIH-CPSI)
      http://www.upointmd.com/NIHCPSIEnglish.pdf
9. Gynecology
   a. Due date calculator
      http://www.yourduedate.com
   b. FDA Birth Control Guide
      https://www.fda.gov/downloads/forconsumers/byaudience/forwomen/
      freepublications/ucm517406.pdf
   c. Algorithms for managing women with cytological abnormalities
      http://www.asccp.org/asccp-guidelines
10. Neurology
   a. AHA ACLS Adult Suspected Stroke Algorithm
      https://acls-algorithms.com/wp-content/uploads/2016/03/Website
      -Adult-Suspected-Stroke-Algorithm.pdf
11. Pediatrics
   a. Immunization schedules
      https://www.cdc.gov/vaccines/schedules/index.html
   b. Bright Futures Guidelines and Pocket Guide
      https://brightfutures.aap.org/materials-and-tools/guidelines-and
      -pocket-guide/Pages/default.aspx
   c. Modified Checklist for Autism in Toddlers (M-CHAT)
      https://m-chat.org/en-us/page/take-m-chat-test/online
12. Geriatric
   a. Beers criteria for potentially inappropriate medication use in older
      adults
      http://bcbpsd.ca/docs/part-1/PrintableBeersPocketCard.pdf
   b. Lawton Instrumental Activities of Daily Living (IADL) Scale
      https://consultgeri.org/try-this/general-assessment/issue-23.pdf
   c. Mini-Mental State Exam
      https://www.ncbi.nlm.nih.gov/projects/gap/cgi-bin/GetPdf.cgi?id
      =phd001525.1

Appendix B

Insulin Use in Primary Care

Using insulin to treat diabetes mellitus[1]

I. Type 1 Diabetes
- In type 1 diabetes, autoimmune destruction of pancreatic beta cells necessitates treatment with exogenous insulin, usually 0.5 to 1.0 units per kilogram of body weight per day.
- The hallmark of treatment is to mimic the pancreas, which produces a basal insulin, which peaks with meals.

II. Type 2 Diabetes
- There are variable combinations of treatment using oral, noninsulin, and insulin injectables.
- For most patients, lifestyle therapy and oral agents are the first line of treatment.
- Insulin therapy may be used together with oral and noninsulin injectables to reach glycemic target.
- Patients with HgA1c >7.5 while on oral and/or noninjectable agents can be considered for insulin therapy.
- Treatment naïve patients with initial HgA1c of ≥9% with symptoms of hyperglycemia may be started on insulin with or without other agents.

Starting insulin therapy

a. Long-acting insulin is usually the first insulin agent to be added.
   i. If A1c <8%: Long-acting insulin at 0.1 to 0.2 units per kilogram once daily
   ii. If A1c >8%: Long-acting insulin at 0.2 to 0.3 units per kilogram once daily
   iii. In general, titrate insulin by 2 units every 2 to 3 days to reach glycemic target
   iv. Other adjustment regimens based on daily fasting blood glucose can also be used

b. If using a long-acting insulin does not achieve glycemic target, either add another noninsulin agent, add meal-time insulin, or change to an insulin mix.

> **CLINICAL PEARL:**
> - Diet and exercise, including medically assisted weight loss, should accompany all treatment plans.
> - Adjustment of therapy is determined by HgA1c progression and patient symptoms.
> - Prior to starting an insulin regimen, ensure that the patient is capable and willing to use injectables, and is not at risk for hypoglycemia.

There are more than 20 types of insulin in the United States. Those presented in Table 1 are the most commonly used. This table summarizes their activity profiles.

TABLE 1 Commonly Used Types of Insulin

	Brand Name	Generic Name	Onset	Peak	Duration
Long Acting	Levermir	Insulin detemir	1.6 hours	No peak	Up to 24 hours
	Lantus	Insulin glargine	1.5 hours	No peak	24 hours
	Insulin glargine*	Toujeo	6 hours	No peak	24–36 hours
	Insulin degludec*	Tresiba	1 hour	No peak	Up to 42 hours
Intermediate Acting	Humulin N	NPH	1–2 hours	2–8 hours	14–24 hours
	Novolin N	NPH	1.5 hours	4–12 hours	24 hours
Short Acting	Humulin R	Regular	30–60 minutes	2–4 hours	5–8 hours
	Novolin R	Regular	30 minutes	1.5–3.5 hours	8 hours
Rapid Acting	Humalog	Insulin lispro	15–30 minutes	0.5–3 hours	5 hours or less
	Novolog	Insulin aspart	10–20 minutes	1–3 hours	3–5 hours
	Apidra	Insulin glulisine	15–30 minutes	0.5–2.5 hours	5 hours or less
	Afrezza*	Insulin human (inhalation powder)	Immediate	12–15 minutes	3 hours

(continued)

TABLE 1 Commonly Used Types of Insulin (*continued*)

	Brand Name	Generic Name	Onset	Peak	Duration
Insulin Mix: Intermediate/ Rapid Acting	50% lispro protamine suspension, 50% insulin lispro	Humalog Mix 50/50	15–30 minutes	0.5–3 hours	14–24 hours
	75% lispro protamine suspension, 25% lispro injection	Humalog Mix 75/25	15–20 minutes	0.5–2.5 hours	14–24 hours
	70% aspart protamine suspension, 30% insulin aspart	Novolog Mix 70/30	10–20 minutes	2.4 hours	Up to 24 hours
Insulin Mix: Intermediate/ Short Acting	70% NPH/30% regular	Humulin Mix 70/30	30–90 minutes	1.5–6.5 hours	18–24 hours
	70% NPH/30% regular	Novolin Mix 70/30	30 minutes	2–12 hours	24 hours

* Less commonly used.

NPH, neutral protamine Hagedorn.

Source: Donner T. Insulin – pharmacology, therapeutic regimens and principles of intensive insulin therapy. [Updated 2015 Oct 12]. In: Feingold KR, Anawalt B, Boyce A, et al, eds. *Endotext* [Internet]. South Dartmouth, MA: MDText.com, Inc.; 2000.[2]

REFERENCES

1. American Diabetes Association. 9. Pharmacologic approaches to glycemic treatment: standards of medical care in diabetes 2019. *Diabetes Care.* 2019; 42(suppl 1): S90–S102.
2. Donner T. Insulin – pharmacology, therapeutic regimens and principles of intensive insulin therapy. [Updated 2015 Oct 12]. In: Feingold KR, Anawalt B, Boyce A, et al, eds. *Endotext* [Internet]. South Dartmouth, MA: MDText.com, Inc.; 2000.

Appendix C

ASTHMA AND CHRONIC OBSTRUCTIVE PULMONARY DISEASE INHALATION FORMULATIONS

Asthma and Chronic Obstructive Pulmonary Disease (COPD) Inhalation Formulations[1]

Rescue Therapy

Brand Name	Generic Name	Formulation
SABA		
Albuterol	Generic	MDI and nebulizer
Levalbuterol	Generic	MDI and nebulizer
Proair HFA	Albuterol	MDI
Proair RespiClick	Albuterol	DPI
Proventil HFA	Albuterol	MDI
Ventolin HFA	Albuterol	MDI
Xopenex	Levalbuterol	Nebulizer
Xopenex HFA	Levalbuterol	MDI
SAMA (Anticholinergics)		
Atrovent	Ipratropium bromide	MDI
Ipratropium bromide	Generic	Nebulizer
Combination SABA + SAMA		
Combivent Respimat	Albuterol + ipratropium	MDI
Duoneb	Albuterol + ipratropium	Nebulizer
Albuterol + Ipratropium	Generic	Nebulizer

DPI, dry powder inhaler; MDI, metered dose inhaler, SABA, short-acting beta2-agonist; SAMA, short-acting muscarinic antagonist.

Maintenance/Control Therapy

Brand Name	Generic Name	Formulation
	CS	
Alvesco	Ciclesonide	MDI
ArmonAir RespiClick	Fluticasone propionate	DPI
Arnuity Ellipa	Fluticasone furoate	DPI
Asmanex	Mometasone	MDI and DPI
Budesonide Inhaled	Generic	Nebulizer
Flovent	Fluticasone propionate	MDI and DPI
Pulmicort	Budesonide	DPI and nebulizer
QVAR RediHaler	Beclomethasone	MDI
	LABA	
Arcapta Neohaler	Indacaterol	DPI
Brovana	Arformeterol	Nebulizer
Perforomist	Formoterol	Nebulizer
Serevent Diskus	Salmetrol	DPI
Striverdi Respimat	Olodaterol	MDI
	LAMA (Anticholinergics)	
Incruse Ellipta	Umeclidinium	DPI
Lonhala Magnair	Glycopyrrolate	Nebulizer
Seebri Neohaler	Glycopyrrolate	DPI
Spiriva	Tiotropium	MDI and DPI
Tudorza Pressair	Aclidinium bromide	DPI

MDI, metered dose inhaler; DPI, dry powder inhaler; ICS, inhaled corticosteroids; LABA, long-acting beta2-agonist; LAMA, long-acting muscarinic antagonist; SABA, short-acting beta2-agonist; SAMA, short-acting muscarinic antagonist.
Source: Sin, D. D., Man, J., Sharpe, H., et al. (2004). Pharmacological management to reduce exacerbations in adults with asthma: a systematic review and meta-analysis. JAMA, 292(3):367–376.

Combination Therapies

Brand Name	Generic Name	Formulation
	ICS + LABA	
Advair	Fluticasone propionate + salmetrol	MDI and DPI
AirDuo RespiClick	Fluticasone propionate + salmetrol	DPI
Breo Ellipta	Fluticasone furoate + vilanterol	DPI
Dulera	Mometasone + formoterol	MDI
Fluticasone propionate + salmetrol	Generic	DPI
Symbicort	Budesonide + formoterol	MDI
	LAMA + LABA	
Anoro Ellipta	Umeclidinium + vilaterol	DPI
Bevespi	Glycopyrrolate + formoterol	MDI

(*continued*)

Combination Therapies (*continued*)

Brand Name	Generic Name	Formulation
Stiolto	Tiotropium + olodaterol	MDI
Utibron	Glycopyrrolate/indacaterol	DPI
	ICS + LABA + LAMA	
Trelegy Ellipta	Fluticasone Furoate/umeclidinium/vilanterol	DPI
TBD	Budesonide/formoterol fumarate/glycopyrronium*	MDI

MDI, metered dose inhaler; DPI, dry powder inhaler; ICS, inhaled corticosteroids; LABA, long-acting beta2-agonist; LAMA, long-acting muscarinic antagonist; SABA, short-acting beta2-agonist; SAMA, short-acting muscarinic antagonist; TBD, to be determined.

* in development.

Source: Barnes, P. J. (2002). Scientific rationale for inhaled combination therapy with long-acting β2-agonists and corticosteroids. European Respiratory Journal, 9(1):182–191.

REFERENCE

1. http://www.epocrates.com. Updated continuously. Accessed January 28, 2019. Source: www.epocrates.com.

Index

NOTES

NOTES

NOTES

NOTES

9 780826 195227